# CHRONICLES OF DRUG DISCOVERY

CHRONICLES OF DRUG DISCOVERY

# CHRONICLES OF DRUG DISCOVERY

## Volume 2

Edited by

**JASJIT S. BINDRA**
*Pfizer Inc.*
*Groton, Connecticut*

**DANIEL LEDNICER**
*Adria Laboratories Inc.*
*Columbus, Ohio*

*A Wiley-Interscience Publication*
**John Wiley & Sons**

*New York* • *Chichester* • *Brisbane* • *Toronto* • *Singapore*

*Library of Congress Cataloging in Publication Data*
Main entry under title:

Chronicles of drug discovery.

"A Wiley-Interscience publication."

Includes bibliographical references and index.
1. Pharmaceutical research—History—Addresses,
essays, lectures.   2. Drugs—History—Addresses,
essays, lectures.   3. Drugs—Personal narratives.
4. Research—Personal narratives.   5. Technology,
Pharmaceutical—Personal narratives.   I. Bindra,
Jasjit S.   II. Lednicer, Daniel, 1929-    . [DNLM:
QV 11.1 C553 1982]

RS122.C48                    615'.1'09047                81-11471
ISBN 0-471-06516-1 (v. 1)
ISBN 0-471-89135-5 (v. 2)

Printed in the United States of America

10 9 8 7 6 5 4 3 2 1

# Preface

When we set in motion the project which resulted in "Chronicles of Drug Discovery", the scope of the undertaking was not at all clear. We had no idea, for example, whether discoverers of drugs would even be willing to take the trouble to write about their experience. We were thus surprised and gratified to find that such a high proportion of individuals who were approached agreed to contribute to the volume. The acceptance rate was, in fact, so high that the contributions could not be contained in a single book. At about the same time too, some additional new drugs came to our attention which demanded inclusion. It thus became clear that we might well be faced with at least an additional book and perhaps a series rather than a single volume.

The book in hand is thus the second of what we hope will be a continuing series of volumes describing new drugs. Since the process of drug development is somewhat sporadic in nature, timing of subsequent additions to this series is expected to also be uneven. Books will be organized and published each time a sufficient volume of new material becomes available.

The first volume discussed drugs belonging to a rather broad selection of therapeutic areas; many different approaches to the discovery process were represented. The present volume mirrors both the breadth in content and in philosophy. The reader will thus meet an antihypertensive agent, a CNS drug, five antibiotics, and one drug each for the treatment of helminthiasis and fungal infections. We have, for the first time, included cancer chemotherapy agents; two are included in this book.

Approaches to the discovery process cover a similarly broad range. To name a few, several chapters describe the development of a new drug based on very directed synthesis. At the other end of the spectrum several sections describe drugs which were the results of serendipitous discovery. It is of note that these very different approaches and philosophies are apparently equally fruitful in producing new drugs.

*Jasjit S. Bindra*
*Daniel Lednicer*

*Groton, Connecticut*
*Columbus, Ohio*
*October 1983*

# Contents

# Contributors
# to Volume 2

**Frederico Arcamone,** Farmitalia Carlo Erba S.p.A., Milano, Italy

**K. H. Büchel,** Mitglied des Vorstandes du Bayer AG, Bayerwerk, West Germany

**R. R. Chauvette,** The Lilly Research Laboratories, Indianapolis, Indiana

**David W. Cushman,** Squibb Institute for Medical Research, Princeton, New Jersey

**B. Ekström,** Astra Lakemedel AB, Södertälje, Sweden

**W. O. Godtfredsen,** Leo Pharmaceutical Products, Ballerup, Denmark

**M. Gorman,** The Lilly Research Laboratories, Indianapolis, Indiana; Present address: Bristol-Myers Co., Syracuse, New York

**P. A. J. Janssen,** Department of Theoretical Medicinal Chemistry, Janssen Pharmaceutica, Beerse, Belgium

**Hiroshi Kawaguchi,** Bristol-Banyu Research Institute, Ltd., Tokyo, Japan

**S. Kukolja,** The Lilly Research Laboratories, Indianapolis, Indiana

**Frantz J. Lund,** Leo Pharmaceutical Products, Ballerup, Denmark

**James W. McFarland,** Pfizer Central Research Laboratories, Groton, Connecticut

**John A. Montgomery,** Organic Chemistry Research, Southern Research Institute, Birmingham, Alabama

**Takayuki Naito,** Bristol-Banya Research Institute, Ltd., Tokyo, Japan

**Miguel A. Ondetti,** Squibb Institute for Medical Research, Princeton, New Jersey

**M. Plempel,** Mitglied des Vorstandes du Bayer AG, Bayerwerk, West Germany; Present address: Bayer AG, Leverkusen, West Germany

**Bernard Rubin,** Squibb Institute for Medical Research, Princeton, New Jersey

**B. Sjöberg,** Astra Lakemedel AB, Södertälje, Sweden; Present address: Vitrum AB, Stockholm, Sweden

**J. P. Tollenaere,** Department of Theoretical Medicinal Chemistry, Janssen Pharmaceutica, Beerse, Belgium

# CHRONICLES OF DRUG DISCOVERY

CHRONICLES OF DRUG DISCOVERY

# Captopril

1

Miguel A. Ondetti, David W. Cushman and
Bernard Rubin

## 1. INTRODUCTION

The observations of Tigerstedt and Bergman in 1898 on the extraction of a
hypertensive principle from the kidney[1] and the development of an experimental model of renal hypertension by Goldblatt and collaborators in 1934[2] are the
most significant milestones in the research trail that led to an understanding of
the role of the kidney in hypertension. The independent and convergent work
of Braun-Menendez and coworkers[3] and of Page and Helmer[4] during the late
thirties and early forties established on solid foundations the nature of the
humoral mechanism that supports this important role of the kidneys in
hypertension, and that is now known as the renin-angiotensin system. The
chemical characterization of the final steps of this sequence (Figure 1) had to
await the isolation studies of Bumpus et al.,[5] Peart,[6] and Skeggs et al.,[7] the
identification of the two forms of angiotensin and the isolation of the
angiotensin-converting enzyme by Skeggs et al.,[8] and finally the synthetic
studies that confirmed the structure proposed for angiotensin II.[9,10]

Angiotensin II was thus established as one of the most potent vasoconstrictor
agents known, but its significance as a mediator of elevated blood pressure in
clinical or experimental renovascular hypertension was still unclear. In 1960
and 1961 several independent groups of investigators[11-15] provided conclusive
proof that angiotensin was involved in the release of the sodium-retaining hor-
mone aldosterone by the adrenal gland, thus establishing that the renin-
angiotensin system could affect blood pressure by a dual mechanism of
vasoconstriction and sodium retention.

1

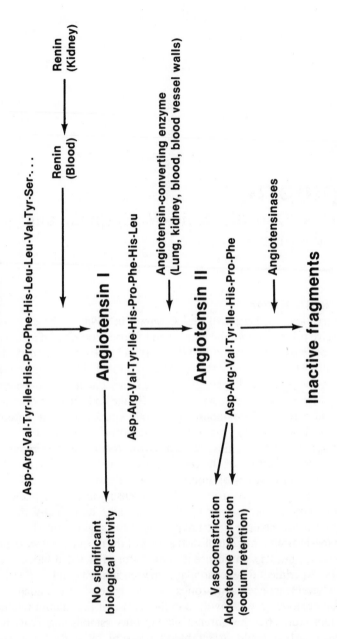

**Figure 1.** The renin-angiotensin system.

2

In spite of these brilliant contributions, the role of the renin-angiotensin system in relation to the elevated blood pressure in experimental and human hypertension remained doubtful, particularly when the blood levels of renin and/or angiotensin were elevated only slightly or not at all. To quote W. S. Peart[16]: "it seems unlikely that the system usually operates as a direct pressor system, but the various ways in which the pressor effects can be modified by electrolyte changes, by aldosterone, and by interaction with the nervous system would allow widely varying quantitative relations in different physiological and pathological states."

## 2. THE SEARCH FOR ANGIOTENSIN-CONVERTING ENZYME INHIBITORS

Against this background of potential biological significance and inconclusive therapeutic relevance, we initiated our studies directed at blocking the renin-angiotensin system through inhibition of angiotensin-converting enzyme. In retrospect, we can say that these studies exemplify three different approaches to drug discovery: (a) identification of a naturally occurring biologically active lead, followed by total synthesis of the original structure and analogues; (b) random screening of a wide variety of chemical structures to obtain a new biologically active lead suitable to further chemical modification; and (c) *ab initio* drug design based on a molecular model of the receptor site. No explanations are necessary for the first two approaches, but it is important to point out that the expression "drug design" has been normally applied to the optimization of a biologically active lead obtained from approach *a* or *b* by a careful study of the physicochemical parameters implicated in the drug action.[17] In the development of the orally active angiotensin-converting enzyme inhibitors, the process of design was critically applied in *generating the leads,* before any optimization process could take place. Thus the expression *"ab initio* drug design" has been coined to distinguish this approach from that usually implied with the use of the "drug design" terminology.

### 2.1 The Natural Product Approach

One of us (D.W.C.) had already begun in 1968 to study the properties of angiotensin-converting enzyme, at that time a rather novel and poorly characterized peptidase. However, the great impetus for beginning a search for inhibitors was provided by the observation of Ng and Vane[18] and Bakhle[19] that crude extracts of the venom of *Bothrops jararaca* inhibited the conversion of angiotensin I to II. Ferreira had shown in 1965 that these extracts potentiated the biological activities of the nonapeptide bradykinin,[20] particularly its hypotensive effect. In collaboration with L. J. Greene, he undertook the fractionation of the crude venom extract, with the aim of isolating "bradykinin potentiating peptides."[21-23]

## Table 1
### Angiotensin-Converting Enzyme Inhibitors
### (Bradykinin Potentiators) Isolated from *Bothrops jararaca*

| Designation | | Structure[a] | ACE I$_{50}$[b] | | BkP[c] | References |
| --- | --- | --- | --- | --- | --- | --- |
| | | | Cheung et al.[27] | Bakhle et al.[26,28] | | |
| SQ 20,475 | BBP$_{5a}$ | <Glu-Lys-Trp-Ala-Pro | 0.06 | 0.9 | 100 | 26, 27, 29 |
| SQ 20,661 | | <Glu-Trp-Pro-Arg-Pro-Thr-Pro-Gln-Ile-Pro-Pro | 5.0 | | 34 | 27, 29 |
| SQ 20,881 | BBP$_{9a}$ | <Glu-Trp-Pro-Arg-Pro-Gln-Ile-Pro-Pro | 0.56 | 0.02 | 410 | 26, 27, 29 |
| SQ 20,858 | | <Glu-Asn-Trp-Pro-His-Pro-Gln-Ile-Pro-Pro | 5.8 | 0.02 | 47 | 26, 27, 29 |
| SQ 20,859 | BPP$_{10a}$ | <Glu-Ser-Trp-Pro-Gly-Pro-Asn-Ile-Pro-Pro | 34.0 | 3.2 | 80 | 26, 27, 29, 47 |
| SQ 20,861 | | <Glu-Asn-Trp-Pro-Arg-Pro-Gln-Ile-Pro-Pro | 2.5 | | 100 | 27, 29 |
| SQ 20,718 | BPP$_{13a}$ | <Glu-Gly-Gly-Trp-Pro-Arg-Pro-Gly-Pro-Glu-Ile-Pro-Pro | 14 | 0.2 | 200 | 27, 29, 47 |
| | V-3-B | <Glu-Ser-Trp-Pro-Gly-Pro[d] | | >5.0 | 9 | 28, 29 |
| | V-1-A | <Glu-Glx-Trp-Ala-Trp-Pro-Arg-Pro-Gln-Ile-Pro-Pro[d] | | | 380 | 28, 29, 47 |
| | BPP$_{13b}$ | <Glu-Gly-Gly-Leu-Pro-Arg-Pro-Gly-Pro-Glu-Ile-Pro-Pro[d] | | 0.4 | 90 | 28, 29, 47 |

[a] The standard three-letter abbreviations for amino acids have been used. All amino acids are of the L-configuration.

[b] Micromolar concentration required to inhibit 50% of the activity of angiotensin-converting enzyme.

[c] Relative specific activity, on a molar basis, for the potentiation of the action of bradykinin on guinea-pig ileum. The activity of BPP$_{5a}$ is arbitrarily taken as 100.

[d] The sequence of these peptides was not determined, but was deduced from physical properties and comparison with related peptides.[29]

Since it was not quite clear to us that bradykinin potentiation would be a desirable property for an antihypertensive agent, in view of the putative pro-inflammatory actions of bradykinin, we began our studies on the fractionation of the *Bothrops jararaca* venom, following not the bradykinin potentiating activity but the angiotensin-converting enzyme inhibitory activity.[24,25] As it turned out, both activities were found to reside in the same peptides, and the amino acid compositions of peptides that we isolated were identical to those of the peptides isolated by Greene and Ferreira (Table 1).[26-29] A synthetic sample of one of the most active peptides we isolated (the nonapeptide SQ 20,881) was found to be identical with the nonapeptide BPP$_{9a}$ (bradykinin potentiating peptide 9a), the most active bradykinin potentiator isolated by Greene, Ferreira, and collaborators.[28] In addition to the peptide inhibitors that were isolated from the venom, all their synthetic analogues showed both activities in a guinea pig ileum test; that is, all inhibited the contractile response of angiotensin I and potentiated the contractile activity of bradykinin without affecting the action of any other smooth muscle agonist, (*e.g.*, angiotensin II and acetylcholine). Finally, the studies of Erdös, Sofer, and other investigators utilizing homogeneous angiotensin-converting enzyme showed that both peptides, angiotensin I and bradykinin, are substrates for this enzyme and that the bradykinin-hydrolyzing enzyme previously designated as kininase II is indeed angiotensin-converting enzyme.[30,104]

The structure-activity relationships elaborated on the basis of inhibitory activity versus isolated angiotensin-converting enzyme correlate extremely well with those obtained using the bradykinin potentiating activity in guinea pig ileum,[98] supporting the contention that the effects of these inhibitors on the agonistic activities of angiotensin I and bradykinin in this smooth muscle preparation are due to their interaction with the converting enzyme present in this tissue. Thus the isolated smooth muscle test became a very useful tool in discriminating between specific angiotensin-converting enzyme inhibitors and compounds that nonspecifically antagonize a variety of other agonists in addition to angiotensin I.

Extensive *in vivo* studies were carried out with SQ 20,881 (teprotide) in our own laboratories, and those of other investigators.[31-33] Both inhibition of hypertension induced by exogenous angiotensin I and potentiation of hypotension induced by bradykinin were observed in several animal species. The duration of action after parenteral administration was considerable, keeping in mind that SQ 20,881 is a peptide and that peptides are often known to have rather fleeting activity.

When tested in animal models of hypertension, SQ 20,881 produced the most significant lowering of blood pressure in those that had been suspected to be dependent on the renin-angiotensin system for the maintenance of elevated blood pressure, such as the two-kidney one-clip classical Goldblatt model.[34,35] In the one-kidney one-clip dog model, the antihypertensive effect was only manifested for a brief period after renal artery constriction.[36] The first studies in the spontaneously hypertensive rat (SHR), using the same doses that were effective in the renal hypertensive rat, showed no hypotensive effect.[32] However, it was later shown that larger doses do indeed produce a modest but significant lowering of blood pressure.[37] These results correlated fairly well with the then prevailing understanding of the functioning of the renin-angiotensin system. Based on circulating levels of renin, the only animal model of hypertension in which the renin-angiotensin system was thought to be important for the maintenance of blood pressure was the two-kidney one-clip renal hypertensive rat, the classical Goldblatt model. In the one-kidney one-clip model or in the SHR, the levels of renin were normal or returned to normal very soon after renal artery constriction and nephrectomy.[36,38]

More or less concurrently with our studies on angiotensin-converting enzyme inhibitors, researchers in other laboratories had finally developed angiotensin II receptor antagonists, thereby opening a new avenue for the blockade of the renin-angiotensin system.[39-41] From the point of view of potency and duration of action, the most effective of these antagonists was saralasin, the 1-sarcosine-5-valine-8-alanine angiotensin II.[41] This agent was also shown to lower blood pressure in the two-kidney one-clip rats, but not in the one-kidney one-clip or the SHR.[41-43] These results, being in good agreement with those obtained with angiotensin-converting enzyme inhibitors, confirmed the unique but restricted importance of the renin-angiotensin system in hypertension. Since the duration of the antihypertensive activity of these angiotensin II antagonists was shorter than that of SQ 20,881, and since they still retained a small amount of agonistic activity, we felt that converting enzyme inhibition was still the preferable approach to renin-angiotensin system blockade, in spite of the ambiguity introduced by the potentiation of the kinin system.

Studies in human volunteers confirmed that potent and fairly long lasting inhibition of the pressor activity of exogenous angiotensin I could be obtained with reasonable intravenous doses of SQ 20,881,[44] and the first clinical report on the use of this converting enzyme inhibitor showed that lowering of blood pressure could be obtained in those patients with elevated blood renin levels.[45,46] These observations demonstrated a point of the utmost importance, namely, that any compound capable of inhibiting isolated angiotensin-converting enzyme and specifically antagonizing angiotensin I contractile activity in smooth muscle preparations had potential for use as an antihypertensive agent. However, two very basic problems were still unresolved: (1) SQ 20,881 and any of its peptide analogues could only be used parenterally, and any serious attempt at the development of an antihypertensive agent for

# Table 2

## Peptidic Angiotensin-Converting Enzyme Inhibitors with Modified Peptide Bonds[48]

| No. | Structure[a] | Rabbit lung ACE $I_{50}$[b] |
|---|---|---|
| 1 | $NH_2$ / $(CH_2)_4$ ... CO—NHCHCO—NHCHCO—N—$CO_2H$ (with $CH_3$ and benzyl substituents; succinyl ring with HN, O=) | 0.1 |
| 2 | $NH_2$ / $(CH_2)_4$ ... CO—NHCHCO—NHCHCH$_2$—OCH$_2$CO—N—$CO_2H$ (benzyl substituent; succinyl ring with HN, O=) | 44 |
| 3 | $NH_2$ / $(CH_2)_4$ ... CO—NHCHCO—NHCHCH$_2$—OCHCO—N—$CO_2H$ (with $CH_3$ and benzyl substituents; succinyl ring with HN, O=) | 34 |
| 4 | $NH_2$ / $(CH_2)_4$ ... CO—NHCHCH$_2$CO—NHCHCO—N—$CO_2H$ (with $CH_3$ and benzyl substituents; succinyl ring with HN, O=) | 0.4 |

[a] All amino acids are of the L-configuration.

[b] Concentration ($\mu M$) required to inhibit 50% of rabbit lung angiotensin-converting enzyme (ACE) activity.

7

chronic use required oral administration; and (2) if blockade of the renin-angiotensin system was only effective in reducing blood pressure in those patients with elevated plasma renin levels, this approach was going to be of limited utility, since hypertensive patients with high plasma renin constitute only 10-20% of the total hypertensive population. Further clinical studies by Laragh and collaborators were to provide some very important clues to resolve the second problem, but it was the first that constituted the major challenge for the medicinal chemist.

Our first attempts at increasing the stability of peptidic inhibitors, with the aim of achieving oral activity, were directed at modifying the peptidic backbone of one of the most active and the smallest of the venom inhibitors, the pentapeptide $BPP_{5a}$. We had observed that this peptide and its 3-phenylalanine analogue were more inhibitory than SQ 20,881 in the isolated enzyme assay,[27] but since they were substrates for the converting enzyme, and possibly also for trypsin-like endopeptidases, they showed a rather poor activity in the guinea pig ileum and *in vivo*.[23,32,47] However, the synthetic analogues of $BPP_{5a}$ in which the peptide bond susceptible to cleavage by converting enzyme was replaced by an ether or $\beta$-homopeptide bond did not lead to useful inhibitors.[48] (1-4, Table 2). The ether linkage decreased substantially the affinity of the inhibitor for the enzyme, and the $\beta$-homopeptide derivative (4), even though fairly active and stable to angiotensin-converting enzyme, did not show an improved duration of action *in vivo*.

## 2.2 The Screening Approach
During 1973 and 1974 the clinical studies with SQ 20,881 (teprotide) began to show that an antihypertensive effect with SQ 20,881 could also be observed in essential hypertensive patients with normal renin levels, indicating that converting enzyme inhibitors might have wider applicability than originally thought.[26,49] Studies with chronically hypertensive one- and two-kidney rats with renal artery constriction showed that sodium depletion made these models responsive to angiotensin II antagonists, indicating that the renin dependence of these hypertensive models had been "covered up" by a volume-dependent hypertension.[50,51] It was then reasoned that a similar situation might be operative in human hypertension with normal renin levels.

These observations rekindled our interest in orally active and longer lasting angiotensin-converting enzyme inhibitors and prompted us to expand the previously initiated screening of a large variety of nonpeptidic chemical structures, utilizing an *in vitro* assay with isolated rabbit lung enzyme. The results of this screening were rather disappointing, since out of approximately 2000 compounds only a few showed any significant inhibitory activity, and practically all of them were not specific when tested in the guinea pig ileum smooth muscle assay, that is, besides inhibiting the contractile activity of angiotensin I, they also inhibited that of bradykinin and usually that of other agonists such as acetylcholine and angiotensin II. Only one compound, 2,3-quinoxalinedithiol (5),[52] showed the typical specificity of an angiotensin-converting enzyme inhibitor in the smooth muscle test. The metal-chelating ability of this compound

**5**

explains its inhibitory activity on angiotensin-converting enzyme, a metalloprotease. However, the significant toxicity of the compound precluded any further development of this lead.

It is interesting to speculate why the approach of random screening did not produce any significant lead. Our later studies on the design of active-site-directed specific inhibitors of this enzyme have shown that considerable attention must be paid to the detailed molecular architecture and functionality to obtain potent inhibitors. The presence of at least one acidic group is essential to obtain significant interaction with the enzyme and specificity in the smooth muscle assay. Compounds of this type of functionality were very poorly represented among the different types of chemicals available for random screening. Besides, the two main groups of compounds that we later found to provide efficient and specific inhibitors, namely, carboxyalkanoyl and mercaptoalkanoyl amino acids, had been the subject of very few literature reports before we started our studies, and therefore, it would have been very unlikely for us to come across representative samples of these classes during the random screening process.

### 2.3  The Design of Active-Site-Directed Inhibitors

**2.3.1  Preliminary Studies**  In March of 1974, shortly after Byers and Wolfenden published their studies on benzylsuccinic acid as a biproduct analogue inhibitor of carboxypeptidase A,[53] we initiated a program aimed at the design of active-site-directed inhibitors of angiotensin-converting enzyme, utilizing the rationale expounded by those investigators.

According to Byers and Wolfenden, benzylsuccinic acid is a potent inhibitor of carboxypeptidase A because it combines in one molecule the modes of binding of the two products of the enzymatic reaction: the original C-terminal

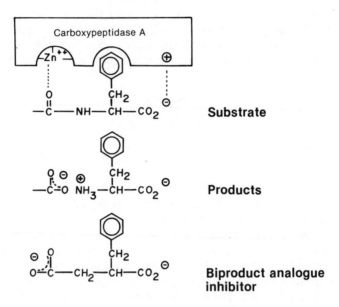

**Figure 2.**   Modes of binding of substrate, products, and inhibitor to the active site of carboxypeptidase A.

amino acid and the peptide chain with its new C-terminal amino acid (Figure 2). Enzyme interactions that contribute to the binding of the amino acid product include: (a) the interaction of its benzyl ring with the hydrophobic pocket of the enzyme and (b) the electrostatic attraction between its carboxyl group and arginine residue 145 on the enzyme surface. Both of these interactions are reproduced by benzylsuccinic acid, with the electrostatic attraction to the arginine residue of the enzyme being even stronger than that in the amino acid product because of the absence of a positively charged ammonium group.[99] Of all the potential enzyme interaction sites of the other product, the peptide chain minus one amino acid, the biproduct analogue benzylsuccinic acid retains only one, the carboxyl group. However, this is probably the strongest interaction in the case of carboxypeptidase A, because it provides an anionically charged ligand for the positively charged zinc ion.

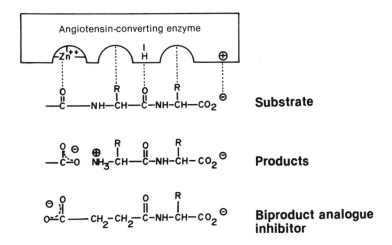

**Figure 3.** Modes of binding of substrate, products, and inhibitor to the hypothetical active site of angiotensin-converting enzyme.

To extend these considerations to the design of biproduct analogue inhibitors of angiotensin-converting enzyme, we had to keep in mind that this exopeptidase cleaves a dipeptide from the C-terminal end of peptide chains. Therefore, the enzyme residues involved in cleavage of the scissile amide bond are separated from the carboxyl binding site by a somewhat longer distance than in carboxypeptidase A. Thus the compound that we thought would combine the main enzyme binding interactions of the two products of angiotensin-converting enzyme activity was a succinyl amino acid (Figure 3). The first compound synthesized to test this hypothesis was succinyl-L-proline (7, Table 3), which turned out to be a weak but specific inhibitor of angiotensin-converting enzyme; that is, in the smooth muscle test it inhibited the contractile activity of angiotensin I and potentiated the contractile activity of bradykinin without affecting the action of other agonists (Table 3).[54] In view of the disappointing results obtained in the random screening that preceded these studies, the results obtained with succinyl-L-proline had to be considered remarkable in spite of its borderline value and emphasized the utility of a hypothetical model of the active site in the selection of structures to be synthesized and tested for enzyme inhibitory activity.

## Table 3
### Carboxyalkanoyl Amino Acid Inhibitors of Angiotensin-Converting Enzyme[54,57]

| No. | Structure[a] | Rabbit lung ACE $I_{50}$[b] | Guinea pig ileum Angiotensin I $IC_{50}$[c] | Guinea pig ileum Bradykinin $AC_{50}$[d] |
|---|---|---|---|---|
| 6 | <Glu-Trp-Pro-Arg-Pro-Gln-Ile-Pro-Pro (SQ 20,881) | 0.9 | 0.06 | 0.001 |
| 7 | $HO_2C-CH_2-CH_2-CO-N$ (pyrrolidine) $-CO_2H$ | 330 | 440 | 37 |
| 8 | $HO_2C-CO-N$ (pyrrolidine) $-CO_2H$ | 4800 | >500 | >500 |
| 9 | $HO_2C-CH_2-CO-N$ (pyrrolidine) $-CO_2H$ | 2600 | 273 | 12 |
| 10 | $HO_2C-CH_2-CH_2-CH_2-CO-N$ (pyrrolidine) $-CO_2H$ | 70 | 29 | 4 |
| 11 | $HO_2C-CH_2-CH_2-CH_2-CH_2-CO-N$ (pyrrolidine) $-CO_2H$ | >4000 | >400 | 86 |

12

| | | | | |
|---|---|---|---|---|
| 12 | HO$_2$C—CH$_2$—CH—CO—N⟨ ⟩—CO$_2$H (SQ 13,297) (with CH$_3$ wedge) | 22 | 20 | 0.7 |
| 13 | HO$_2$C—CH$_2$—CH—CO—N⟨ ⟩—CO$_2$H (with CH$_3$) | 1480 | >400 | 65 |
| 14 | HO$_2$C—CH—CH$_2$—CO—N⟨ ⟩—CO$_2$H (with CH$_3$) | 610 | >400 | 57 |

[a]The standard three-letter abbreviations for amino acids have been used. All amino acids are of the L-configuration.
[b]Concentration ($\mu M$) required to inhibit 50% of rabbit lung angiotensin-converting enzyme (ACE) activity.
[c]Concentration ($\mu M$) required to inhibit 50% of the contractile effect of angiotensin I in excised guinea pig ileum.
[d]Concentration ($\mu M$) required to augment 50% of the contractile effect of bradykinin in excised guinea pig ileum.

13

## Table 4
### Angiotensin-Converting Enzyme Inhibitory Activity of Acyl Amino Acid Derivatives[55]

| No. | Structure[a] | Rabbit lung ACE $I_{50}$[b] | Guinea pig ileum Angiotensin I $IC_{50}$[c] | Guinea pig ileum Bradykinin $AC_{50}$[d] |
|---|---|---|---|---|
| 15 | $HO_2C-CH_2-CH_2-CO-Phe$ | 550 | >300 | 130 |
| 16 | $CH_3-CO-CH_2-CH_2-CO-Phe$ | 1990 | >300 | 240 |
| 17 | $CH_3-\overset{OH}{\underset{S}{CH}}-CH_2-CH_2-CO-Phe$ | >3000 | >300 | >300 |
| 18 | $HONHCO-CH_2-CH_2-CO-Phe$ ($CH_3$) | 58 | 172 | 33 |
| 19 | $HONHCO-CH_2-CH-CO-Pro$ ($CH_3$) | 0.6 | 2 | 0.9 |
| 20 | $HONH-CO-CH_2-CH_2-CH-CO-Pro$ ($NH_2$) | 7.7 | 13 | 6.5 |
| 21 | $HO_2C-CH-CH_2-CH_2-CO-Pro$ | 4100 | 1300 | 140 |

| | | | |
|---|---|---|---|
| **22** | NH$_2$—CH$_2$—CH$_2$—CO—Pro | 910 | >500 | 215 |
| **23** | ![pyridine] CH$_2$—NH—CH$_2$—CH$_2$—CO—Pro | 2900 | >300 | >300 |
| **24** | HS—[pyridine]—CO—Pro | 830 | 190 | 47 |
| **25** | HS—CH$_2$—CH$_2$—CO—Pro (SQ 13,863) <br> CH$_3$ | 0.2 | 0.3 | 0.02 |
| **26** | HS—CH$_2$—CH—CO—Pro (SQ 14,225, captopril) | 0.02 | 0.02 | 0.002 |

[a]The standard three-letter abbreviations for amino acids have been used. All amino acids are of the L-configuration.
[b]Concentration ($\mu M$) required to inhibit 50% of rabbit lung angiotensin-converting enzyme (ACE) activity.
[c]Concentration ($\mu M$) required to inhibit 50% of the contractile effect of angiotensin I in excised guinea pig ileum.
[d]Concentration ($\mu M$) required to augment 50% of the contractile effect of bradykinin in excised guinea pig ileum.

15

As is pointed out above, in this approach to biproduct inhibition most of the binding interactions of the biproduct inhibitor correspond to those of the C-terminal dipeptide of the substrate. Structure-activity studies with analogues of succinyl-*L*-proline confirmed these predictions, since the highest inhibitory activity was obtained with derivatives that mimicked the structure of those dipeptides serving as *C*-terminal residues of the most efficient substrates. There are, however, some unexplained exceptions. The model of the active site and the concept of a biproduct analogue require that succinyl-*L*-proline (**7**) be more active than glutarylproline (**10**), and the opposite is the case (Table 3).

Substituents on the succinyl or glutaryl moieties increased inhibitory activity when introduced in the position alpha to the amide bond and with the stereochemistry required for making the resulting derivatives isosteric with *L,L*-dipeptides. One of the most active of these derivatives, *D*-2-methylsuccinyl-*L*-proline (**12**, SQ 13,297), was subjected to extensive tests *in vivo*. Inhibition of the pressor activity of angiotensin I in normotensive rats was achieved with intravenous doses of 3-10 mg/kg. Clear antihypertensive effects were observed with 100 mg/kg i.v. in two-kidney one-clip hypertensive rats. Similar results, although not as pronounced, were obtained in spontaneously hypertensive rats. However, the most encouraging aspect of these *in vivo* studies was the observation that this derivative was capable of inhibiting the pressor response to angiotensin I when given orally, albeit at considerably high doses.

**2.3.2   The Development of Captopril**    A comparison of the potencies of SQ 20,881 (**6**) and *D*-2-methylsuccinyl-*L*-proline (**12**) as antagonists of angiotensin I action in the guinea pig ileum and in the normotensive rat made it clear that a substantial increase in intrinsic activity was required to convert this new lead into a successful drug.

To obtain this increase in intrinsic activity we had to develop new possibilities for stronger interactions between the inhibitor and the enzyme. Modification of the amino acid and the carboxyalkanoyl moiety did not seem to provide the possibilities for obtaining a dramatic increase in activity, and we decided to concentrate on optimizing the interaction we believed to exist between the carboxyl group of the carboxyalkanoyl moiety and the zinc atom at the active site.

Different types of nitrogen-containing functional groups were tested as potential monodentate ligands since nitrogen was expected to be a better ligand than oxygen (Table 4). However, these substitutions led only to a decrease in the inhibitory activity, and the same results were obtained with bidentate ligands containing only nitrogen (**23**). It is possible that lacking the negative charge of the carboxylate anion these functional groups cannot disperse the charge of the zinc ion and become efficient ligands. Attempts at designing bidentate ligands with nitrogen and oxygen, such as α-aminocarboxylic acids (21), were not more successful.[55] A significant finding was the observation that the hydroxamic acid derivative of succinyl-L-phenylalanine (18) was approximately 50 times as active as the corresponding carboxylic acid precursor. Here, the possibility of bidentate ligand interaction with two oxygens and a negative charge might be the most important factor in increasing the strength of the interaction with zinc. When we later explored in more detail the requirements for optimal activity in this type of derivative, we found that, in contrast to the carboxylic acid-containing analogues, the hydroxamic acid derivative of D-2-methylsuccinyl-L-proline (19) was more potent than the corresponding analogue with the glutaryl side chain (20). Substitution of the oxygen of the hydroxyamino group was more detrimental for inhibitory activity than nitrogen substitution, which is in agreement with the type of binding postulated for these analogues. Nishino and Powers[56] have shown that hydroxamic acid derivatives patterned after the substrate are also potent inhibitors of thermolysin, a zinc-containing endopeptidase.

In spite of the promising activity of the hydroxamic acid derivative of succinylphenylalanine we did not choose to pursue this lead any further at that time. Instead we continued to search for other functional groups that could provide a more efficient ligand interaction with zinc. And thus we came to synthesize 3-mercaptopropanoyl-L-proline (SQ 13,863, 25, Table 4), which showed an activity three orders of magnitude greater than that of succinyl-L-proline, our prototype inhibitor. A further tenfold increase in activity was obtained by introducing a methyl substituent alpha to the amide bond with the S-configuration to make it isosteric with the D-methylsuccinyl derivatives and the L-L dipeptides. With the synthesis of the S-3-mercapto-2-methylpropanoyl-L-proline (26, SQ 14,225, captopril) we obtained an active-site-directed angiotensin-converting enzyme inhibitor that was even more potent than our present goal, SQ 20,881, in the isolated enzyme assay and still retained the characteristic specificity of the nonapeptide inhibitor in the smooth muscle assay.

**2.3.3   Structure-Activity Relationships in Mercaptoalkanoyl Amino Acid Inhibitors**   When one considers the interaction of captopril with the hypothetical active site of angiotensin-converting enzyme, it is clear that the high degree of binding achieved with this compound is the consequence of the cooperative effect of several interactions that could be artificially dissected as indicated in the scheme of Figure 4.

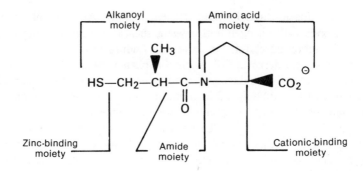

**Figure 4.**    Schematic dissection of functional groups in the captopril structure.

To establish how important each one of these contributions was, we synthesized analogues in which each of the functional groups or moieties in question had been deleted without, whenever possible, affecting the rest of the molecule. The inhibitory activities of these analogues are given in Tables 5, 6, and 7.

It is immediately apparent that the carboxyl function makes a very important contribution to binding, since its elimination or inversion of its stereochemistry leads to a substantial decrease in inhibitory activity. The amino acid moiety in which this carboxyl function is included also has an important role to play in the interaction with the active site.[57,103] Proline and tryptophan stand out as the amino acid moieties that lead to the best inhibitors, even though the reasons for efficient binding might be considerably different in each case. Tryptophan can probably establish a very strong hydrophobic bonding with the active site, while in the case of proline the increased binding is more likely to be provided by the conformational rigidity introduced by the pyrrolidine ring (Table 5).

Study of the contribution to binding of the amide function (Table 6) exemplified how the modification of one functional group might affect other properties of the molecule and complicate interpretation.[58] If in compound **25** we replace the carbonyl of the amide by a methylene (compound **43**), the loss in activity might be due not only to the elimination of the amide function but also to the fact that we now have, instead of a neutral function (amide), a positively charged one (amine). To restore the neutrality, we introduced a carbonyl on the pyrrolidine ring (compound **44**), but this modification did not restore activity. However, this substitution might have introduced some detrimental effect —steric, electronic, or otherwise—that could have vitiated the comparison. To eliminate this possibility, we synthesized compound **45** with the two carbonyls, and, since this compound is as active as captopril, it is safe to conclude that the lack of activity of **43** and **44** is due mostly to elimination of the carbonyl of the amide function. This conclusion is supported by the observation that the ketone analogue **46**, in which only the carbonyl portion of the amide bond is retained, shows significant inhibitory activity.[59] The oxygen atom of this carbonyl group is probably hydrogen bonded to a hydrogen donor group on the enzyme (Figure 3).

Two factors had to be considered in the modification of the alkanoyl moiety: size and degree of substitution.[57] The optimal activity was obtained with a three-carbon alkanoyl moiety bearing substituents alpha to the amide function (Table 7). As pointed out earlier, the S-configuration of this moiety, which is isosteric with an L (or S) amino acid, is the one that affords the highest degree of binding. Finally, it is evident that this alkanoyl side chain with the most suitable amino acid moiety, proline, but without the proper zinc-binding functionality contributes very little to binding (see **51**).

From these comparisons it is obvious that no one of the interactions that captopril can establish with the active site of angiotensin-converting enzyme is capable by itself of producing the necessary binding to give an efficient inhibitor. It is also important to point out that captopril does not function as a zinc chelator, since it can only contribute one ligand to the zinc ion at the active site. Mercaptopropanoyl amino acids, like $\alpha$-mercaptopropanoylglycine, can form stable chelates because they have an ionizable NH bond and the three ligands (S, N, and O) required to form two 5-membered-ring structures of great stability (**52**).[60] These features are not present in captopril, since the sulfhydryl

**52**

group is beta to the amide bond and the amide bond has no ionizable hydrogen.

Captopril and its predecessor, SQ 13,297 (**12**, Table 3), have been shown to be reversible competitive inhibitors of angiotensin-converting enzyme by kinetic and dialysis studies.[57] This, and the structure-activity studies outlined above, confirm that these inhibitors bind at the active site of angiotensin-converting enzyme. The fact that these compounds had been tailored to fit the active site

## Table 5
## Mercaptopropanoyl Amino Acid Inhibitors
## of Angiotensin-Converting Enzyme[57,103]

| No. | Structure[a] | Rabbit lung ACE $I_{50}$[b] | Guinea pig ileum Angiotensin I $IC_{50}$[c] | Bradykinin $AC_{50}$[d] |
|---|---|---|---|---|
| 27 | HS—CH$_2$—CH$_2$—CO—Trp | 0.07 | 0.5 | 0.007 |
| 25 | HS—CH$_2$—CH$_2$—CO—Pro (SQ 13,863) | 0.2 | 0.3 | 0.02 |
| 28 | HS—CH$_2$—CH$_2$—CO—$\Delta^2$—Pro | 0.6 | 1.8 | 0.12 |
| 29 | HS—CH$_2$—CH$_2$—CO—$\Delta^3$—DL—Pro | 0.3 | 0.05 | 0.2 |
| 30 | HS—CH$_2$—CH$_2$—CO—Tca | 0.1 | 1.1 | 0.76 |
| 31 | HS—CH$_2$—CH$_2$—CO—Arg | 0.65 | 3.4 | 0.07 |
| 32 | HS—CH$_2$—CH$_2$—CO—Phe | 0.43 | 2.0 | 0.2 |
| 33 | HS—CH$_2$—CH$_2$—CO—Ala | 0.85 | 1.3 | 1.2 |

20

| No. | Structure | [b] | [c] | [d] |
|---|---|---|---|---|
| 34 | HS—CH$_2$—CH$_2$—CO—Leu | 1.6 | 9.1 | 0.07 |
| 35 | HS—CH$_2$—CH$_2$—CO—Gly | 2.8 | 27 | 0.7 |
| 36 | HS—CH$_2$—CH$_2$—CO—Lys | 2.4 | 4.2 | 1.1 |
| 37 | HS—CH$_2$—CH$_2$—CO—Asp | 68 | 67 | 19 |
| 38 | HS—CH$_2$—CH$_2$—CO—$\beta$—Ala | 490 | >500 | >500 |
| 39 | HS—CH$_2$—CH$_2$—CO—D—Pro | 1800 | >500 | 210 |
| 40 | CH$_3$<br>HS—CH$_2$—CH—CO—N | 250 | 280 | >300 |

[a]The standard three-letter abbreviations for amino acids have been used. All amino acids are of the L-configuration. Tca = 4-thiazolidine car-boxylic acid.

[b]Concentration ($\mu M$) required to inhibit 50% of rabbit lung angiotensin-converting enzyme (ACE) activity.

[c]Concentration ($\mu M$) required to inhibit 50% of the contractile effect of angiotensin I in excised guinea pig ileum.

[d]Concentration ($\mu M$) required to augment 50% of the contractile effect of bradykinin in excised guinea pig ileum.

21

## Table 6

### Amide Bond Modifications in Mercaptoalkanoyl Amino Acid Inhibitors of Angiotensin-Converting Enzyme[48,59]

| No. | Structure[a] | Rabbit lung ACE $I_{50}$[b] | Guinea pig ileum | |
|---|---|---|---|---|
| | | | Angiotensin I $IC_{50}$[c] | Bradykinin $AC_{50}$[d] |
| 41 | $HS-CH_2-CH_2-CO-NH-CH_2-CO_2H$ | 2.7 | 27 | 0.7 |
| 42 | $HS-CH_2-CH_2-CH_2-CH_2-CO_2H$ | 1800 | 540 | 364 |
| 25 | $HS-CH_2-CH_2-CO-N$⟨ring⟩$CO_2H$ (SQ 13,863) | 0.2 | 0.3 | 0.02 |
| 43 | $HS-CH_2-CH_2-CH_2-N$⟨ring⟩$CO_2H$ | 238 | 500 | 211 |
| 44 | $HS-CH_2-CH_2-CH_2-N$⟨ring⟩$CO_2H$ | 640 | 500 | 100 |
| 45 | $HS-CH_2-CH(CH_3)-CO-N$⟨ring⟩$CO_2H$ | 0.009 | 0.011 | 0.002 |
| 46 | $HS-CH_2-CH_2-CO$⟨ring⟩$CO_2H$ | 2.4 | 4.7 | 0.5 |

[a]The standard three-letter abbreviations for amino acids have been used. All amino acids are of the L-configuration.
[b]Concentration ($\mu M$) required to inhibit 50% of rabbit lung angiotensin-converting enzyme (ACE) activity.
[c]Concentration ($\mu M$) required to inhibit 50% of the contractile effect of angiotensin I in excised guinea pig ileum.
[d]Concentration ($\mu M$) required to augment 50% of the contractile effect of bradykinin in excised guinea pig ileum.

**Table 7**

**Alkanoyl Moiety Modifications in Mercaptoalkanoyl Amino Acid Inhibitors of Angiotensin-Converting Enzyme[57]**

| No. | Structure[a] | Rabbit lung ACE $I_{50}$[b] | Guinea pig ileum Angiotensin I $IC_{50}$[c] | Guinea pig ileum Bradykinin $AC_{50}$[d] |
|---|---|---|---|---|
| 25 | 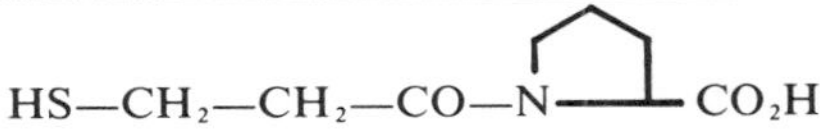 $HS-CH_2-CH_2-CO-N\langle\text{pyrrolidine}\rangle-CO_2H$ (SQ 13,863) | 0.3 | 0.2 | 0.02 |
| 47 | 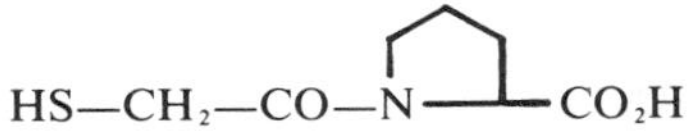 $HS-CH_2-CO-N\langle\text{pyrrolidine}\rangle-CO_2H$ | 1.1 | 0.2 | 0.04 |
| 48 | 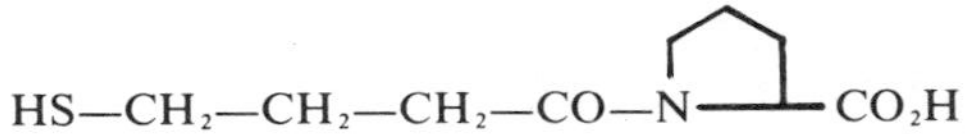 $HS-CH_2-CH_2-CH_2-CO-N\langle\text{pyrrolidine}\rangle-CO_2H$ | 9.7 | 12 | 5.0 |
| 26 | 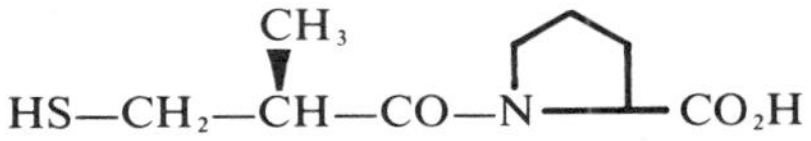 $HS-CH_2-\underset{CH_3}{CH}-CO-N\langle\text{pyrrolidine}\rangle-CO_2H$ (SQ 14,225, captopril) | 0.02 | 0.02 | 0.002 |
| 49 | 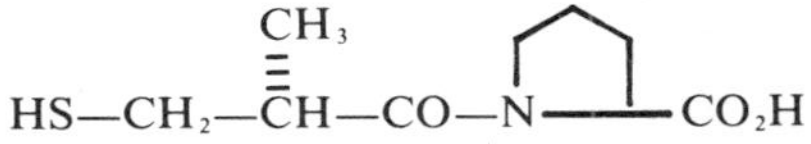 $HS-CH_2-\underset{CH_3}{C}-CO-N\langle\text{pyrrolidine}\rangle-CO_2H$ | 2.4 | 7.8 | 14 |
| 50 | 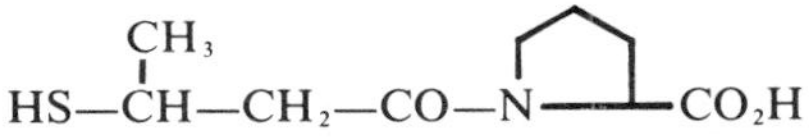 $HS-\underset{CH_3}{CH}-CH_2-CO-N\langle\text{pyrrolidine}\rangle-CO_2H$ | 1.1 | 2.3 | 0.2 |
| 51 | 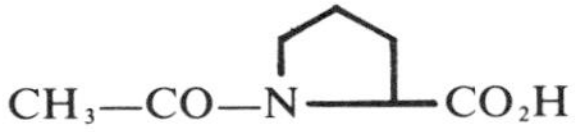 $CH_3-CO-N\langle\text{pyrrolidine}\rangle-CO_2H$ | 550 | — | — |

[a]The standard three-letter abbreviations for amino acids have been used. All amino acids are of the L-configuration.

[b]Concentration ($\mu M$) required to inhibit 50% of rabbit lung angiotensin-converting enzyme (ACE) activity.

[c]Concentration ($\mu M$) required to inhibit 50% of the contractile effect of angiotensin I in excised guinea pig ileum.

[d]Concentration ($\mu M$) required to augment 50% of the contractile effect of bradykinin in excised guinea pig ileum.

23

of this rather peculiar peptidase was the basis of our expectations that they would be specific as well as potent. Our expectations were fully justified, since captopril is not an inhibitor of other common peptidases, even of those containing zinc at their active site, such as carboxypeptidases A and B,[100] carbonic anhydrase, and liver alcohol dehydrogenases.[98] Leucine aminopeptidase is moderately inhibited by captopril.[57]

## 3. BIOLOGICAL STUDIES WITH CAPTOPRIL
### 3.1 Pharmacology

The very high and specific inhibitory activity that captopril had shown in the isolated enzyme in guinea pig ileum assays indicated that, in view of our previous experience with SQ 20,881, we then had at our disposal a potent, specific, and orally active blocker of the renin-angiotensin system for *in vivo* studies.

The first and most conclusive evidence that this expectation was justified was the profound inhibition of the pressor effect of angiotensin I observed in normotensive conscious rats when captopril was administered in doses as low as 0.1-1 mg/kg intravenously or orally.[54,61] As expected, a pronounced potentiation of the hypotensive effect of bradykinin was also observed. Similar results were then obtained in several other animal species[62] and eventually in humans,[63] where total inhibition of the angiotensin I response for at least 2 hours was obtained with oral doses of about 0.3 mg/kg.

A marked hypotensive effect was observed when captopril was administered to two-kidney one-clip renal hypertensive rats in doses of 3-30 mg/kg orally.[64,65] This hypotensive effect was maintained after one year of continuous daily dosage and was potentiated by the simultaneous administration of a diuretic.[66]

A significant finding of these early pharmacological studies was that captopril can lower blood pressure in an animal model of chronic hypertension in which the renin-angiotensin system is apparently not involved: the spontaneously hypertensive rat (SHR).[64,67] The oral doses needed to obtain a substantial reduction in blood pressure were higher in this model than in the case of the renal hypertensive rat, 30-100 mg/kg, but after 6 months of daily dosage the blood pressure of the spontaneously hypertensive rat had been normalized.[68] It was later shown that administration of captopril to weanling spontaneously hypertensive rats prevented the development of hypertension.[69]

Another hypertensive model with normal circulating levels of renin, and in which captopril lowers blood pressure, is the one-kidney one-clip renal hypertensive rat.[65,70] In this model, the blood-pressure-lowering effect of captopril is progressive and not as pronounced as in the two-kidney one-clip model.[65]

Various hypotheses have been advanced to explain the hypotensive effect of captopril in those animal models in which the renin-angiotensin system is apparently not involved, at least when judged by the normal circulating levels of renin. In the one-kidney one-clip model the progressive lowering of the blood pressure was attributed to the small, but persistent, diuresis and natriuresis observed.[65] This might be due to a direct intrarenal inhibition of the renin-angiotensin system or potentiation of the kallikrein-kinin system. Potentiation of the hypotensive effect of bradykinin has also been incriminated in the hypotensive effect of captopril in these models, but most of the evidence produced to support this involvement is indirect and inconclusive.

The possibility has been considered[71,72] that the angiotensin generated locally by the renin and converting enzyme present in the arterial wall might be more important during the chronic stages of hypertension than the angiotensin generated by renal renin and lung-converting enzyme. If that were the case, circulating enzyme inhibitors would still be effective antihypertensive agents, provided they could reach the sites of angiotensin generation within the arterial wall.

Captopril also has been useful in studying the involvement of the renin-angiotensin system in other pathological processes besides hypertension. In animal models of hemorrhagic shock, angiotensin-converting enzyme inhibitors increase survival rates by increasing blood perfusion of critical organs after fluid replacement therapy has been initiated.[73] The involvement of the renin-angiotensin system has also been demonstrated in animal models of cardiac failure utilizing angiotensin-converting enzyme inhibitors such as SQ 20,881[74] and captopril.[75,76] These agents increase sodium excretion, lower plasma aldosterone levels, and prevent formation of edema. The above studies support the expectation that captopril could be of significant value in the treatment of hemorrhagic shock and cardiac failure.

### 3.2   Pharmacokinetics and Toxicology

Captopril is rapidly and efficiently absorbed after oral administration. In normal subjects an average of 68% of an oral dose of 100 mg was recovered from the urine in 5 days with 66% recovered in the first 24 hours.[77,78] The major component of the metabolic profile is unchanged captopril, but a significant amount of the administered dose is present in the blood and urine as disulfides, either symmetrical disulfide or mixed disulfides formed between captopril and other thiols such as cysteine and glutathione.

Captopril can interact with and bind to plasma proteins through covalent disulfide bridges.[79] This binding can be reversed by incubation with other thiols such as cysteine, glutathione, and dithiothreitol.

Captopril has a very low degree of acute or subacute toxicity. The intravenous $LD_{50}$ in mice is about 1000 mg/kg and the oral $LD_{50}$ in mice and rats is approximately 6000 mg/kg. No overt effects were observed in mice, rats, dogs, and monkeys after oral administration of captopril in doses of 2800, 4000, 200, and 375 mg/kg, respectively. Only minor effects were observed in monkeys after daily oral administration of 450 mg/kg for three months.[80]

## 4. CLINICAL STUDIES WITH CAPTOPRIL

In view of the promising results obtained in the short term clinical studies that had been undertaken with SQ 20,881, captopril was quickly moved from the clinical pharmacological studies briefly described above[63,78] to the full-scale treatment of hypertensive patients. Significant lowering of the blood pressure was observed in the large majority of patients[81-90] even though many of those involved in the initial studies had been refractory to other forms of antihypertensive therapy.[81,82]

Correlation between the pretreatment blood levels of renin and the magnitude of the blood pressure decrease was not always found.[84-86,89,91] However, it can be stated that the largest decreases in blood pressure upon captopril administration were obtained in those patients with high renin levels. Further demonstration of this positive correlation was found in the dramatic efficacy of captopril in the treatment of malignant hypertension.[101,102] These observations support the contention that the antihypertensive effect of captopril is due, to a major extent, to the blockade of the renin-angiotensin system.

In a significant number of patients, the addition of a diuretic or a low sodium diet was required to normalize the blood pressure.[84,89,91] This was not surprising in view of the results obtained with renal hypertensive rats (see above). On the other hand, the addition of a converting enzyme inhibitor to the diuretic therapy could be very useful in preventing the secondary hyperaldosteronism and the resultant hypokalaemia that follows diuretic administration[91] and weakens the effectiveness of the diuretic.[92]

The most common side effects of captopril therapy are rash[83-85,89,91] and taste alterations.[87,93] In many cases the side effects disappear when therapy is continued with a lower dosage.[84,89,91] More recent studies[94] have shown that good efficacy combined with a low level of side effects can be achieved in the treatment of mild to moderate hypertension.

No evidence of tachyphylaxis has been observed during therapy with captopril. On the contrary, the hypotensive effect becomes more pronounced after a few weeks,[83,88] probably because of the progressive effect on reduction of aldosterone levels.[88]

The clinical experience with the widespread antihypertensive effect of captopril had, as expected, raised questions concerning the mechanism or mechanisms by which it reduces blood pressure in hypertensive patients. The weak correlation between pretreatment plasma renin activity and captopril antihypertensive effects leads many investigators to postulate a mechanism of action for captopril other than blockade of the renin-angiotensin system. However, it could be argued that this apparent lack of correlation is only an indication that plasma renin activity may not necessarily be a good barometer for measuring activation of the renin-angiotensin system.

Potentiation of the kinin system by inhibiting degradation of bradykinin has been proposed as an additional mechanism for captopril antihypertensive action. However, no significant changes in levels of circulating kinins have been observed[91] and patients do not show symptoms of raised bradykinin concentration.[84,87] The possibility that angiotensin-converting enzyme inhibitors might influence the kinin system intrarenally and thereby affect the electrolyte-water balance remains to be demonstrated. It is likely that the most important influence of captopril in relation to electrolyte balance is through the reduction of aldosterone levels, a logical consequence of the blockade of the renin-angiotensin system.[88]

The evidence accumulated through the years that the renin-angiotensin system is implicated in the pathology of cardiac failure in animal models[75,76] has prompted the evaluation of captopril in a similar clinical situation. All the studies so far reported have confirmed the expected beneficial effect of this agent in those cases in which conventional therapy with digitalis and diuretics failed.[95-97] These observations could be considered a confirmation of the involvement of the renin-angiotensin system in congestive heart failure and indicate that a new therapeutic tool is now available for treatment of this serious disease.

## 5.   CONCLUSIONS

The studies that led to the development of captopril exemplify a new approach in the search for novel therapeutic agents, the *"ab initio* drug design."* In this approach assumptions concerning the chemical structure of the receptor, in this case the active site of an enzyme of key biological importance, guide the design of potent and specific inhibitors. This *ab initio* approach to drug design can, of course, only be applied to receptors for which molecular structural features are known or can be hypothesized on the basis of the knowledge accumulated for similar biological structures. At the present time, the only type of receptors for which such knowledge is available, and here only on a limited basis, are enzyme active sites. However, since many important biological processes are controlled by key enzymatic steps, this truly basic approach to drug design holds a great potential for the development of completely novel molecules as "tailor-made" therapeutic agents.

## REFERENCES

1. R. Tigerstedt and P. G. Bergman, *Scand. Arch Physicol.,* **8**, 223 (1898).
2. H. Goldblatt, J. Lynch, R. F. Hanzal, and W. W. Summerville, *J. Exp. Med.,* **59**, 347 (1934).
3. E. Braun-Menendez, J. C. Fasciolo, L. F. Leloir, and J. M. Munoz, *Rev. Soc. Argent. Biol.,* **15**, 420 (1939).
4. I. H. Page and O. M. Helmer, *J. Exp. Med.,* **71**, 29 (1940).
5. F. M.Bumpus, A. A. Green, and I. H. Page, *J. Biol. Chem.,* **210**, 287 (1954).
6. W. S. Peart, *Biochem. J.,* **62**, 520 (1956).
7. L. T. Skeggs, W. H. Marsh, J. R. Kahn, and N. P. Shumway, *J. Exp. Med.,* **100**, 363 (1954).
8. L. T. Skeggs, W. H. Marsh, J. R. Kahn, and N. P. Shumway, *J. Exp. Med.,* **103**, 295 (1956).
9. F. M. Bumpus, H. Schwarz, and I. H. Page, *Science,* **125**, 3253 (1957).
10. W. Rittel, B. Iselin, H. Kappeler, B. Riniker, and R. Schwyzer, *Helv. Chim. Acta,* **40**, 614 (1957).
11. F. Gross, *Klin. Wochenschr.,* **36**, 693 (1958).
12. J. H. Laragh, M. Angers, W. G. Kelly, and S. Lieberman, *J. Am. Med. Assoc.,* **174**, 234 (1960).
13. J. E. Genest, E. Koiw, W. Nowaczynski, and T. Sandor, Abstracts, 1st International Congress of Endocrinology, Copenhagen, 1960, p. 173; see also *J. Clin. Invest.,* **40**, 338 (1961).
14. J. O. Davis, C. C. J. Carpenter, C. R. Ayers, J. E. Holman, and R. C. Bahn, *J. Clin. Invest.,* **40**, 684 (1961).
15. W. F. Ganong and P. J. Mulrow, *Nature,* **190**, 1115 (1961).
16. W. S. Peart, *Pharmacol. Rev.,* **17**, 143 (1965).
17. Y. C. Martin, *Quantitative Drug Design,* Dekker, New York, p. 6.
18. K. K. F. Ng and J. R. Vane, *Nature,* **218**, 144 (1968).
19. Y. S. Bakhle, *Nature,* **220**, 919 (1968).
20. S. H. Ferreira, *Br. J. Pharmacol.,* **24**, 163 (1965).
21. L. J. Greene, J. M. Stewart, and S. H. Ferreira, *Pharmacol. Res. Commun.,* **1**, 159 (1969).
22. S. H. Ferreira, D. C. Bartlet, and L. J. Greene, *Biochemistry,* **9**, 2583 (1970).
23. J. M. Stewart, S. H. Ferreira, and L. J. Greene, *Biochem. Pharmacol.,* **20**, 1557 (1971).
24. M. A. Ondetti, N. J. Williams, E. F. Sabo, J. Pluscec, E. R. Weaver and O. Kocy, in *Progress in Peptide Research,* S. Lande, Ed., Proceedings of the 2nd American Peptide Symposium, August 1970, Gordon and Breach, New York, 1972, p. 251.
25. M. A. Ondetti, N. J. Williams, E. F. Sabo, J. Pluscec, E. R. Weaver, and O. Kocy, *Biochemistry,* **10**, 4033 (1971).
26. Y. S. Bakhle, in *Hypertension, '72,* J. Genest and E. Koiw, Eds., Springer-Verlag, New York, 1972, p. 541.
27. H. S. Cheung and D. W. Cushman, *Biochem. Biophys. Acta.,* **293**, 451 (1973).
28. S. H. Ferreira, L. J. Greene, V. A. Alabaster, Y. S. Bakhle, and J. R. Vane, *Nature,* **225**, 379 (1970).
29. J. M. Stewart, in *Chemistry and Biology of the Kallikrein-Kinin System in Health and Disease,* J. J. Pisano and K. F. Austen, Eds., U. S. Government Printing Office, Washington, D. C., 1977, p. 299.

30. See E. G. Erdös, *Circ. Res.,* **36,** 247 (1975) for a review.
31. S. L. Engel, T. R. Schaeffer, B. I. Gold, and B. Rubin, *Proc. Soc. Exp. Biol. Med.,* **140,** 240 (1972).
32. A. Bianchi, D. B. Evans, M. Cobb, M. E. Peschka, T. R. Schaeffer, and R. J. Laffan, *Eur. J. Pharmacol.,* **23,** 90 (1973).
33. L. J. Greene, A. C. M. Camargo, E. M. Krieger, J. M. Stewart, and S. H. Ferreira, *Circ. Res.,* **30,** II-62 (1972).
34. S. L. Engel, T. R. Schaeffer, M. H. Waugh, and B. Rubin, *Proc. Soc. Exp. Biol. Med.,* **143,** 483 (1973).
35. T. G. Coleman and A. C. Guyton, *Clin. Sci. Mol. Med.,* **48,** 45S (1975).
36. E. D. Miller, A. I. Samuels, E. Haber, and A. C. Barger, *Am. J. Physiol.,* **228,** 448 (1975).
37. R. J. Laffan, M. E. Goldberg, J. P. High, T. R. Schaeffer, M. H. Waugh, and B. Rubin, *J. Pharmacol. Exp. Ther.,* **204,** 281 (1978).
38. S. Koletsky, P. Shook, and J. Rivera-Velez, in *Hypertension, Its Pathogenesis and Complications,* K. Okamota, Ed., Springer-Verlag, New York, 1972, p. 199.
39. P. A. Khairallah, A. Toth, and F. M. Bumpus, *J. Med. Chem.,* **13,** 181 (1970).
40. G. R. Marshall, W. Vine, and P. Needleman, *Proc. Natl. Acad. Sci.,* **67,** 1624 (1970).
41. D. T. Pals, F. D. Masucci, G. S. Dening, Jr., F. Sipos, and D. C. Fessler, *Circ. Res.,* **29,** 673 (1971).
42. H. Gavras, H. R. Brunner, H. Thurston, and J. H. Laragh, *Science,* **188,** 1316 (1975).
43. C. M. Ferrario, F. M. Bumpus, Z. Masaki, M. C. Khosla, and J. W. McCubbin, *Prog. Biochem. Pharmacol.,* **12,** 86 (1976).
44. J. G. Collier, B. F. Robinson, and J. R. Vane, *Lancet,* **1,** 72 (1973).
45. H. Gavras, H. R. Brunner, J. H. Laragh, J. E. Sealey, I. Gavras, and R. A. Vukovich, *N. Engl. J. Med.,* **291,** 817 (1974).
46. J. G. Johnson, W. D. Black, R. A. Vukovich, F. E. Hatch, Jr., B. I. Friedman, C. F. Blackwell, A. N. Shenouda, L. Share, R. E. Shade, S. R. Acchiardo, and E. E. Muirhead, *Clin. Sci. Mol. Med.,* **48,** 53S (1975).
47. L. J. Greene, A. C. M. Camargo, E. M. Krieger, J. M. Stewart, and S. H. Ferreira, *Circ. Res.,* **30,** II-62 (1972).
48. M. A. Ondetti, J. Pluscec, E. R. Weaver, N. Williams, E. F. Sabo, and O. Kocy, in *Chemistry and Biology of Peptides,* J. Meienhofer, Ed., Ann Arbor Science Publishers, Ann Arbor, Michigan, 1972, p. 525.
49. D. B. Case, J. M. Wallace, H. J. Keim, M. A. Weber, J. I. M. Brayer, R. P. White, J. E. Sealey, and J. H. Laragh, *Am. J. Med.,* **61,** 790 (1976).
50. H. Gavras, H. R. Brunner, E. D. Vaughan, Jr., and J. H. Laragh, *Science,* **180,** 1369 (1973).
51. H. Gavras, H. R. Brunner, H. Thurston, and J. H. Laragh, *Science,* **188,** 1316 (1975).
52. B. Rubin, E. H. O'Keefe, D. G. Kotler, D. A. DeMaio, and D. W. Cushman, *Fed. Proc.,* **34,** 770 (1975).
53. L. D. Byers and R. Wolfenden, *Biochemistry,* **12,** 2070 (1973).
54. M. A. Ondetti, B. Rubin, and D. W. Cushman, *Science,* **196,** 441 (1977).
55. M. A. Ondetti, E. F. Sabo, K. Losee, H. S. Cheung, D. W. Cushman, and B. Rubin, in *Peptides, Proceedings of the 5th American Peptide Symposium,* M. Goodman and J. Meienhofer, Eds., Wiley, New York, 1977, p. 576.
56. N. Nishino and J. C. Powers, *Biochemistry,* **18,** 4340 (1979).
57. D. W. Cushman, H. S. Cheung, E. F. Sabo, and M. A. Ondetti, *Biochemistry,* **16,** 5484 (1977).

58. M. A. Ondetti, E. W. Petrillo, Jr., M. E. Condon, D. W. Cushman, M. Puar, J. E. Heikes, E. F. Sabo, and J. Reid, *Fed. Proc.,* **37,** 1386 (1978).
59. M. E. Condon, J. A. Reid, K. A. Losee, D. W. Cushman, and M. A. Ondetti, Abstracts, 177th Meeting of the American Chemical Society, April 1979, MEDI-64.
60. Y. Sugiura, Y. Hirayama, H. Tanaka, and K. Ishizu, *J. Am. Chem. Soc.,* **97,** 5577 (1975).
61. B. Rubin, R. J. Laffan, D. G. Kotler, E. H. O'Keefe, D. A. DeMaio, and M. E. Goldberg, *J. Pharm. Exp. Ther.,* **204,** 271 (1978).
62. B. Rubin, M. J. Antonaccio, and Z. P. Horovitz, *Prog. Cardiovasc. Res. Dis.,* **21,** 183 (1978).
63. R. K. Ferguson, H. R. Brunner, G. A. Turini, H. Gavras, and D. N. McKinstry, *Lancet,* **1,** 775 (1977).
64. R. J. Laffan, M. E. Goldberg, J. P. High, T. R. Schaeffer, M. H. Waugh, and B. Rubin, *J. Pharm. Exp. Ther.,* **204,** 281 (1978).
65. R. G. Bengis, T. G. Coleman, D. B. Young, and R. E. McCaa, *Circ. Res.,* **43,** I-45 (1978).
66. M. J. Antonaccio, B. Rubin, Z. P. Horovitz, G. B. Mackaness, and R. Panasevich, *Clin. Exp. Hypertension,* **1,** 505 (1979).
67. E. E. Muirhead, R. J. Prewitt, Jr., B. Brooks, and W. L. Brosius, Jr., *Circ. Res.,* **43,** I-53 (1978).
68. M. J. Antonaccio, B. Rubin, Z. P. Horovitz, R. J. Laffan, M. E. Goldberg, D. N. Harris, and I. Zaidi, *Jpn. J. Pharmacol.,* **29,** 275 (1979).
69. R. A. Ferrone and M. J. Antonaccio, *Eur. J. Pharmacol.,* **60,** 131 (1979).
70. S. Sen, R. R. Smeby, F. M. Bumpus, and J. G. Turcotte, *Hypertension,* **1,** 427 (1979).
71. H. Thurston, J. D. Swales, R. F. Bind, B. C. Hurst, and E. S. Marks, *Hypertension,* **1,** 643 (1979).
72. M. Asaad and M. J. Antonaccio, *Pharmacologist,* **21,** 212 (1979).
73. G. Trachte and A. M. Lefer, *Proc. Soc. Exp. Biol. Med.,* **162,** 54 (1979).
74. L. Watkins, Jr., J. A. Burton, E. Haber, J. R. Cant, F. W. Smith, A. C. Barger, S. E. McNeill, and S. M. Sherrill, *J. Clin. Invest.,* **57,** 1606 (1976).
75. G. M. Williams, J. O. Davis, R. H. Freeman, J. M. DeForrest, A. A. Seymour, and B. P. Rowe, *Am. J. Physiol.,* **236,** F-541 (1979).
76. R. H. Freeman, J. O. Davis, G. M. Williams, J. M. DeForrest, A. A. Seymour, and B. P. Rowe, *Circ. Res.,* **45,** 540 (1979).
77. S. M. Shinghvi, K. J. Kripalani, D. N. McKinstry, J. M. Shaw, D. A. Willard, and B. H. Migdalof, *Pharmacologist,* **20,** 214 (1978).
78. D. N. McKinstry, S. M. Singhvi, K. J. Kripalani, J. Dreyfuss, D. A. Willard, and R. A. Vukovich, *Clin. Pharmacol. Ther.,* **23,** 121 (1978).
79. K. K. Wong, S. Lan, and B. Migdalof, *Pharmacologist,* **21,** 173 (1979).
80. P. L. Sibley, G. R. Keim, C. H. Keysser, J. S. Kulesza, M. M. Miller, and I. H. Zaidi, *Toxicol. Appl. Pharmacol.,* **45,** 315 (1978).
81. E. L. Bravo and R. C. Tarazi, *Hypertension,* **1,** 39 (1979).
82. D. N. McKinstry, D. A. Willard, and R. A. Vukovich, *Clin. Pharmacol.,* **25,** 237 (1979).
83. B. D. Case, S. A. Atlas, J. H. Laragh, J. E. Sealey, P. A. Sullivan, and D. N. McKinstry, *Prog. Cardiovasc. Dis.,* **21,** 195 (1978).
84. H. R. Brunner, H. Gavras, B. Waeber, G. A. Turini, D. N. McKinstry, R. A. Vukovich, and I. Gavras, *Br. J. Clin. Pharmacol.,* **7,** Suppl. 2, 2055 (1979).
85. H. Gavras, H. R. Brunner, G. A. Turini, G. R. Kershaw, C. P. Tifft, S. Cuttelod, I. Gavras, R. A. Vukovich, and D. N. McKinstry, *N. Engl. J. Med.,* **298,** 991 (1978).
86. J. M. Sullivan, B. A. Ginsburg, T. E. Ratts, J. G. Johnson, B. R. Barton, D. H. Kraus, D. N. McKinstry, and E. R. Muirhead, *Hypertension,* **1,** 397 (1979).

87. G. A. MacGregor, N. D. Markandu, J. E. Roulston, and J. C. Jones, *Br. Med. J.*, **2**, 1106 (1979).
88. S. A. Atlas, D. B. Case, J. E. Sealey, J. H. Laragh, and D. N. McKinstry, *Hypertension*, **1**, 274 (1979).
89. E. L. Bravo and R. C. Tarazi, *Hypertension*, **1**, 39, (1979).
90. H. R. Brunner, H. Gavras, B. Waeber, G. R. Kershaw, G. A. Turini, R. A. Vukovich, D. N. McKinstry, and I. Gavras, *Ann. Int. Med.*, **90**, 19 (1979).
91. C. I. Johnston, J. A. Miller, B. P. McGrath, and P. G. Matthews, *Lancet*, **2**, 493 (1979).
92. H. Ibsen, A. Leth, H. Hollnagel, A. M. Kappelgaard, M. D. Nielsen, N. J. Christensen, and J. Giese, *Acta Med. Scand.*, **205**, 547 (1979).
93. R. H. Vlasses and R. K. Ferguson, *Lancet*, **2**, 526 (1979).
94. Veterans Administration Cooperative Study Group on Antihypertensive Agents, *Clin. Sci.*, **63**, 443s (1982).
95. G. A. Turini, M. Gribic, H. R. Brunner, B. Waeber, and H. Gavras, *Lancet*, **1**, 1213 (1979).
96. R. Davis, H. S. Ribner, E. Keung, E. H. Sonnenblick, and T. H. LeJemmtel, *N. Engl. J. Med.*, **301**, 117 (1979).
97. R. C. Tarazi, F. M. Fouad, J. K. Ceimo, and E. L. Bravo, *Am. J. Cardiol.*, **44**, 1013 (1979).
98. M. A. Ondetti and D. W. Cushman, in *The Biochemical Regulation of Blood Pressure*, R. L. Soffer, Ed., Wiley, Interscience, New York, 1981, p. 165.
99. S. Nakagawa and H. Umeyana, *J. Am. Chem. Soc.*, **100**, 7716 (1978).
100. M. A. Ondetti, M. E. Condon, J. Reid, E. F. Sabo, H. S. Cheung, and D. W. Cushman, *Biochemistry*, **18**, 1427 (1979).
101. S. E. Oberfield, D. B. Case, L. S. Levine, R. Rapaport, W. Rauh, and M. I. New, *J. Pediat.*, **95**, 641 (1979).
102. A. B. Atkinson, J. J. Brown, D. L. Davies, R. Fraser, R. Leckie, A. F. Lever, J. J. Morton, and J. I. S. Robertson, *Lancet*, **2**, 606 (1979).
103. S. Natarajan, M. E. Condon, M. S. Cohen, J. Reid, D. W. Cushman, B. Rubin, and M. A. Ondetti, in *Proceedings Sixth American Peptide Symposium*, E. Gross, Ed., Pierce Chemical Company, Rockford, Ill., 1980, p. 463.
104. R. L. Soffer in *The Biochemical Regulation of Blood Pressure*, R. L. Soffer, Ed., Wiley, Interscience, New York, 1981, p. 123.

# Pimozide 2

## P.A.J. Janssen and J.P. Tollenaere

*The man who doesn't make up his mind to cultivate the habit of thinking misses the greatest pleasures in life.*

*Thomas Alva Edison*

## 1. INTRODUCTION

Looking back over the decade or so prior to our discovery of pimozide, it occurs to us that pimozide was to a large extent a logical outcome within the framework of our thinking and our activities at that time. In this sense pimozide was not all that much the result of serendipity but rather the offspring of stubborn work along the track that we knew from past experience had led us to success.

Reconstructing the past to describe a scientific process that occurred 18 years ago is quite a challenge to the mind of today because of the knowledge acquired since that time and the all too comfortable vantage point offered by hindsight. A plain account of the daily business, as strictly as possible in terms of our knowledge of that time, may lead to a historically faithful but utterly dull diary which, unless generously spiced with aspects of the human endeavor behind it, nobody would care to read. The addition of present-day knowledge could give rise to a much more readable but historically less accurate account. Striking a balance between these two alternatives appears to be a worthwhile strategy for our present task and might be helpful for drawing lessons from the past in order to more efficiently exploit the research effort we are conducting today.

## 2. TOWARDS HALOPERIDOL

Writing the story of the discovery of pimozide in our laboratory and its subsequent establishment as a useful, potent, and long-acting neuroleptic is essentially writing the story of our laboratory from its early beginnings. Before the

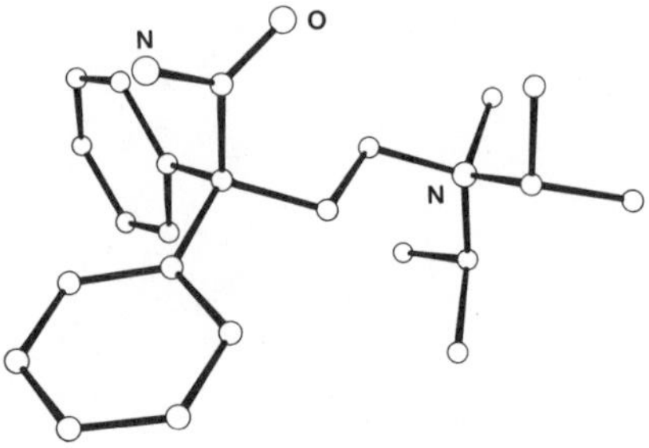

**Figure 1.**  Isopropamide iodide.

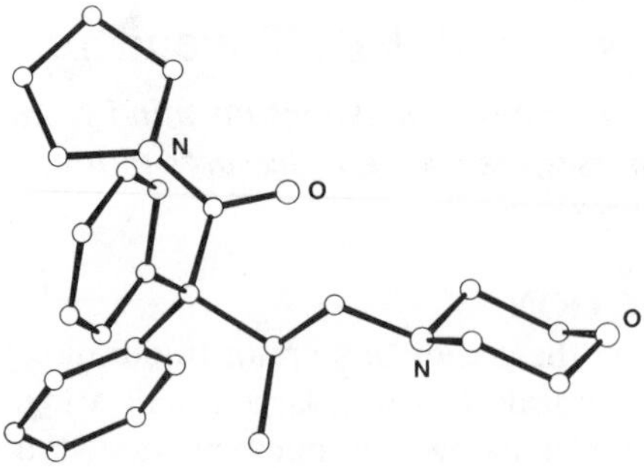

**Figure 2.**  Dextromoramide.

discovery of the butyrophenone derivatives we were acutely aware of the necessity and the importance of trying to better understand the relationship between pharmacological effects and chemical and physicochemical properties of compounds. Analyzing this relationship in the field of diphenylpropylamines, with methods markedly different from those employed today, led us to the discovery in 1954 of R 79 or isopropamide iodide, a long-acting anticholinergic, and in 1956 to the potent analgesic dextromoramide with the research or serial number R 875.

Knowledge of the detailed conformation of these compounds, such as that shown in Figures 1 and 2, was of course totally nonexistent in the mid-1950s. In fact, the only detailed stereochemical pictures available to the medicinal chemist at that time were those of morphine[1] and codeine.[2] The systematic investigation of the crystal structure conformation of drugs did not begin in earnest until the late 1960s. More specifically, more than 20 years elapsed between the original syntheses of isopropamide iodide and dextromoramide and their crystal structure determinations by X-ray crystallography.[3,4]

As early as 1954 we were investigating the 4-phenylpiperidine derivatives with the objective of increasing the analgesic potency of meperidine or pethidine. Contrary to the belief of that time that a small group on the tertiary nitrogen atom was optimal for analgesic activity,[5] the propiophenone derivative (R 951) of normeperidine was synthesized in 1956 and turned out to be about a hundred times more potent as an analgesic than meperidine.[6,7,8]

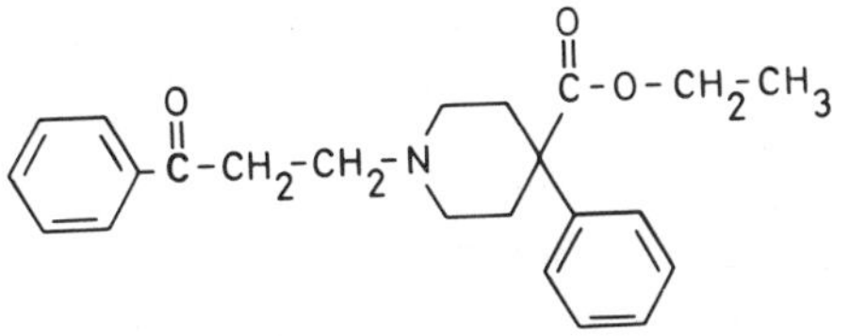

**Figure 3.** R 951.

Our interest in and work with the diphenylpropylamines in the meantime[9] led to the specific antidiarrheal, diphenoxylate, R 1132.[10] Further structural modification of R 951 produced the compound R 1187.

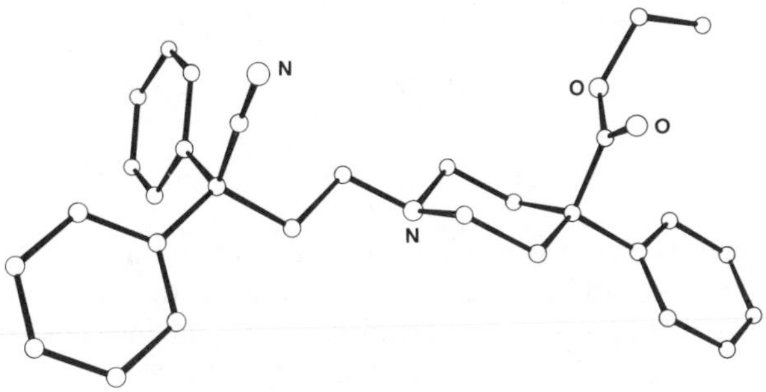

**Figure 4.** Diphenoxylate.

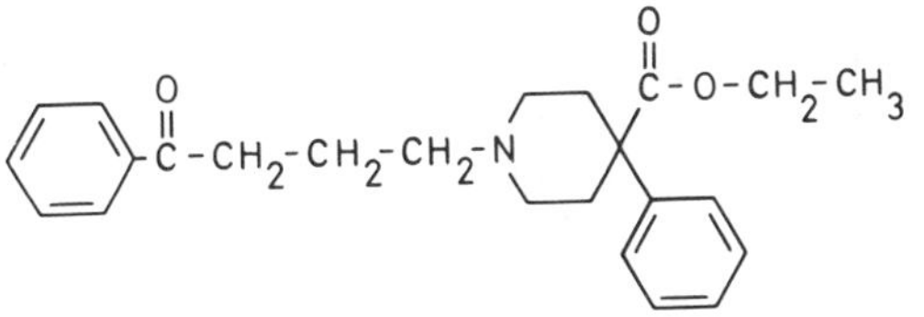

**Figure 5.** R 1187.

As it was common laboratory practice[11] to determine the ratio of the median effective dose levels for hot plate activity ($AD_{50}$) and mydriatic activity ($MD_{50}$) (analgetic to anticholinergic ratio), R 1187 revealed the unusual property of having its ratio $AD_{50}/MD_{50}$ significantly lower than unity.[12] What really interested us was that R 1187 shared the property $AD_{50}/MD_{50} \ll 1$ with chlorpromazine-like neuroleptics and reserpine despite the absence of any structural resemblance with the latter compounds. In fact, what we saw with R 1187, immediately after injection in mice at $AD_{50}$ dose levels, was a morphine-like excitement, mydriasis, and reduced nociception, followed by sedation and mild catatonia. However, owing to its mixed morphine like and chlorpromazine-like properties, the R 1187 synthesized in early 1957 did not lead to a drug but proved to be an important and memorable milestone in our odyssey towards a useful neuroleptic. Some nine months later we learned that replacement of meperidine's carbethoxy ester by a tertiary alcohol group led to an enhancement of the chlorpromazine-like activity with a concomitant decrease of the morphine-like activity. A typical compound was R 1472.

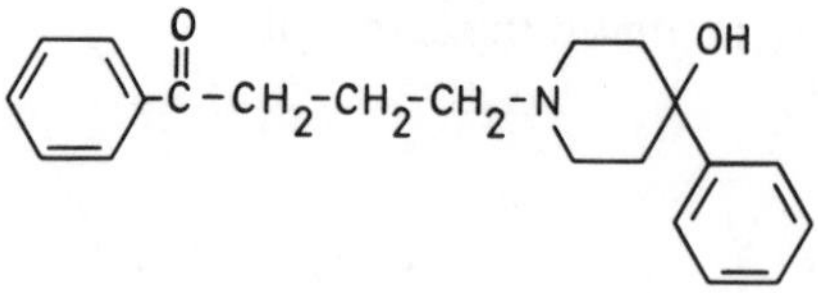

**Figure 6.**  R 1472.

Convinced that we had a valuable lead compound in our hands, we started investigating the effect of substitution on both aromatic rings. Within a few months we knew that appropriate substitution could enhance both the potency and the duration of R 1472's neuroleptic activity.[13] In fact, of the many hundreds of related ketones synthesized and tested, R 1625, now known as haloperidol, was a far more potent and longer acting neuroleptic than chlorpromazine.[13-17] An account of the discovery of haloperidol and its congeners may be found elsewhere.[18]

The advent of haloperidol and its related analogues heralded an era of frantic activity in the field of antipsychotics. Our own research continued and within a relatively short time other neuroleptics of the butyrophenone type, such as meperone (R 1658), azaperone (R 1919), fluanisone (R 2028), trifluperidol (R 2498), and pipamperone (R 3345) were tested pharmacologically and clinically, and are currently used as drugs in human and veterinary medicine.[16,19-23]

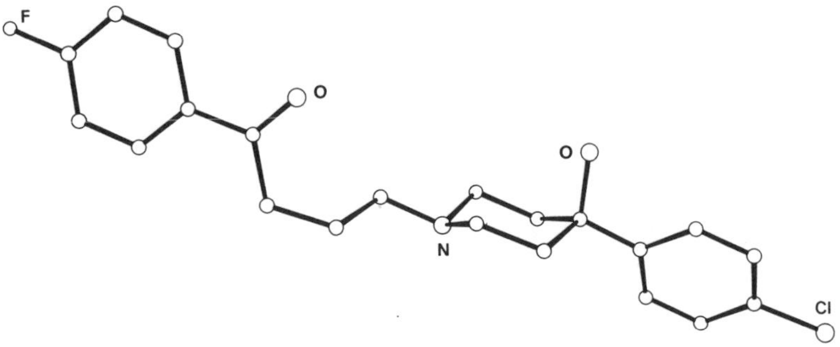

**Figure 7.** Haloperidol.

Concomitant with our search for novel chemical structures, reliable and efficient screening methods were investigated for the evaluation of neuroleptic drugs. Within a few years the tests presented in Table 1 were considered adequate for our objectives.

This series of pharmacological tests not only enabled us to accurately predict[19-22] the gross clinical behavior of neuroleptics but also permitted a fine-tuned evaluation of the compounds that were being continually created in our organic synthesis department. In short, our activities in the late 1950s and early 1960s consolidated the expertise of our laboratory in the field of drugs acting on the central nervous system (CNS) and equipped us for the things to come.

## 3. MODIFICATION OF THE AMINE MOIETY

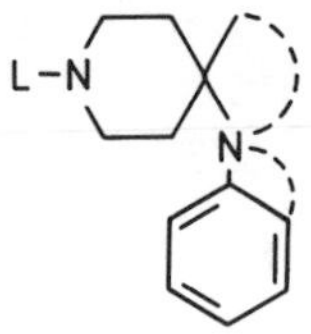

**1**

A first indication of what lay ahead was our interest in compounds containing moiety **1**, where $L$ could be, for example, diphenylpropyl, benzyl, phenethyl, or butyrophenone. In fact, at the end of 1960, fentanyl (R 4263) was synthesized and proved to be an extremely potent analgesic.[34]

Fentanyl, its congeners, and the synthesis of compounds containing moiety **1** afforded us a rich harvest of many interesting CNS agents, such as benperidol (R 4584), droperidol (R 4749), bezitramide (R 4845), and spiperone (R 5147).

**Table 1**

*In Vivo* **Tests for the Evaluation of Neuroleptic Drugs**

| Test | Observed effect | References |
|---|---|---|
| Hot plate (mice) | Typical licking reflex | 9, 11, 16 |
| Catalepsy ptosis (rats) | Cataleptic immobility; palpebral ptosis | 16, 24, 25 |
| Jumping box (rats; dogs) | Loss of avoidance of punishment | 16, 25, 26, 27, 28, 29 |
| Antiamphetamine (rats) | Blockade of compulsory gnawing movements | 16, 25, 26 |
| Antiapomorphine (rats) | Blockade of compulsory gnawing movements | 16, 25, 26, 30 |
| Weight increase, ΔW (rats) | Depression of weight increase and food consumption | 16, 25, 26 |
| Open field (rats) | Inhibition of exploratory ambulation, rearing, preening, and emotional defecation | 16, 25, 26, 31 |
| Antiepinephrine and antinorepinephrine (rats) | Protection against lethal effects of both catecholamines | 16, 25, 26 |
| Antitryptamine (rats) | Protection against clonic seizures of forepaws | 16, 25, 26 |
| Noble and Collip drumming (rats) | Protection against shock-induced mortality | 16, 25, 26 |
| Antiapomorphine (dogs) | Protection against emesis | 16, 25, 26, 32, 33 |

38

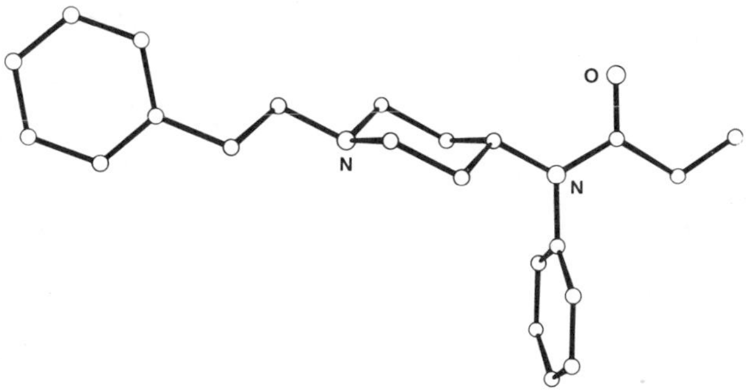

**Figure 8.**   Fentanyl.

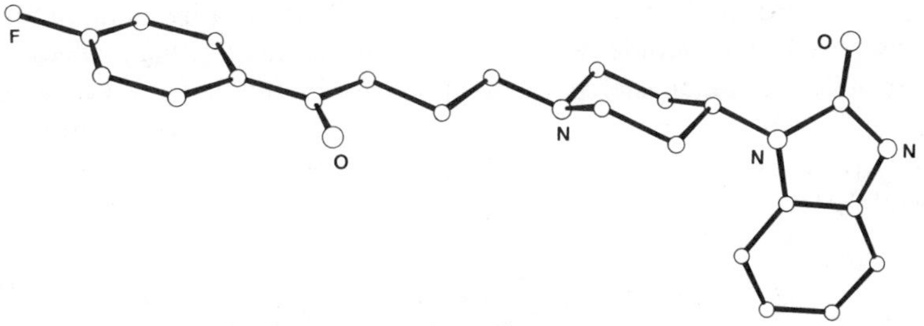

**Figure 9.**   Benperidol.

Benperidol was synthesized in mid-1961 and was subsequently identified and characterized as a neuroleptic many times more potent than haloperidol; it was, in fact, the most potent neuroleptic known at that time.[35,26]

The reaction scheme[37] and our interest in structural variations involving the piperidine ring led us to use moiety **2** in the synthetic efforts that resulted in droperidol.[38]

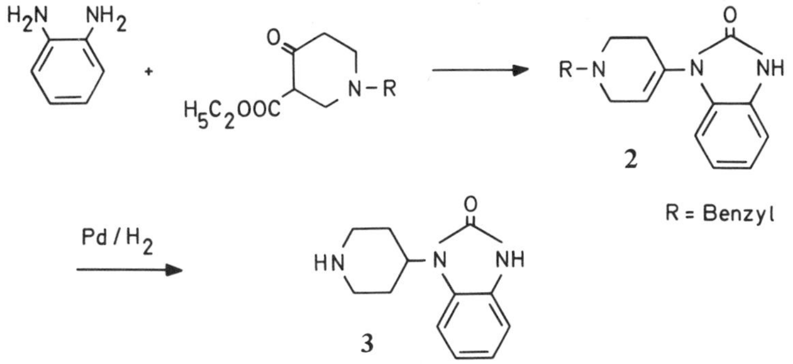

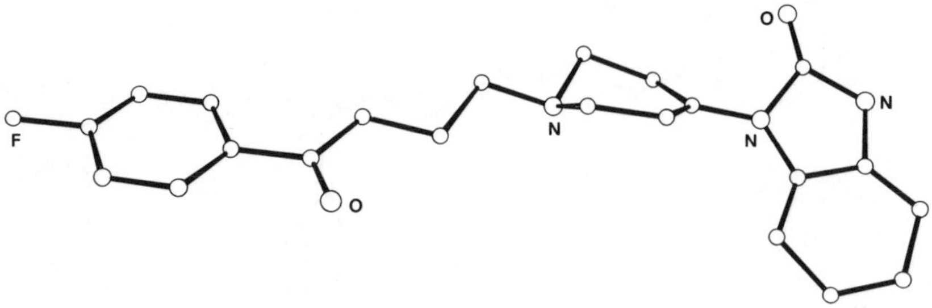

**Figure 10.**    Droperidol.

As experience had taught us that lengthening, shortening, and branching the *L* of **1** was a profitable way to obtain biologically interesting compounds, we soon discovered bezitramide (R 4845), a potent and long-acting analgesic.[39]

Meanwhile, as we mastered the synthetic skills involving 1,3-diazaspiro-decane and related compounds,[40,41] we succeeded in synthesizing spiperone (R 5147), which turned out to be an even more potent neuroleptic than benperidol.[19]

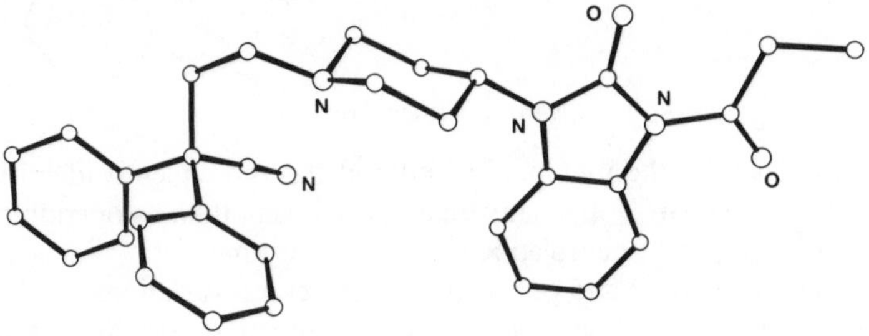

**Figure 11.**    Bezitramide.

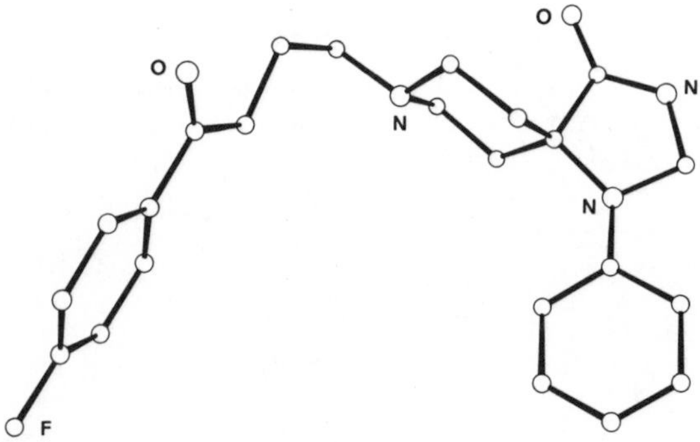

**Figure 12.**    Spiperone.

## 4. MODIFICATION OF THE BUTYROPHENONE CHAIN

At this stage, one of our synthetic programs was already built around the general structure 4 where R represented, among many other things, the corresponding fragments of haloperidol, benperidol, and spiperone. It is obvious that 4 represents thousands of compounds, but our limited manpower

prevented us from synthesizing most of them. One of the proposed modifications, substituting the benzoyl terminus with a benzhydryl moiety, was not one of the urgent priorities of our synthetic program. Based on earlier experience we believed that such an introduction of a diphenyl grouping into the molecule would lead to morphine-like compounds. Moreover, having successfully broken away in the past from chlorpromazine-like structures we were hesitant to return to structures with even a formal resemblance such as that conferred by the diphenyl moiety.

In other words, the wisdom of robbing our cherished butyrophenone chain of its keto function and replacing it by a $p$-$F$-phenylmethine moiety ($5 \rightarrow 6$) was not readily evident to us. Despite our vastly increased knowledge regarding the conformational aspects of the butyrophenone, diphenylbutyl, and tricyclic types of neuroleptics[42] we feel even today, let alone some 18 years ago, that the move from 5 to 6 was a bold one. This foray into the unknown rewarded us

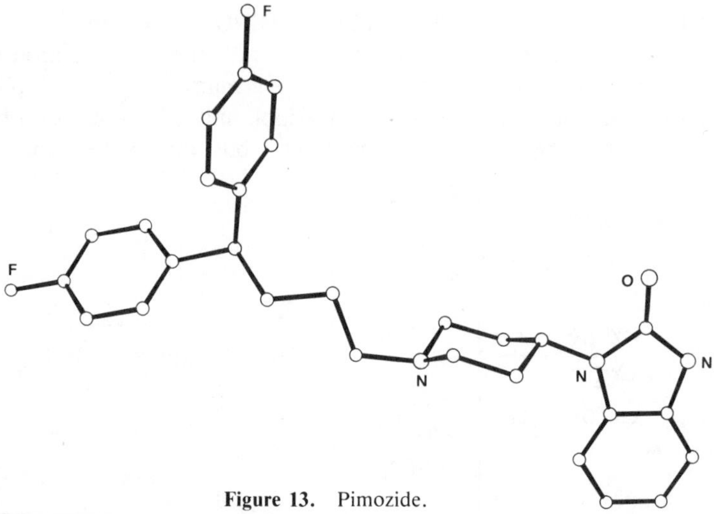

**Figure 13.** Pimozide.

with R 6238, or pimozide, which was synthesized in January 1963. A patent application was filed in June 1963 and the U.S. patent was granted in 1965.[43]

Pimozide, 1-{1--[4,4-bis(4-fluorophenyl)butyl]-4-piperidinyl}-1,3-dihydro-2H-benzimidazol-2-one, is a weak organic base (p$K$ = 8.63), almost insoluble in water, and one of the most lipophilic (log P = 6.23) neuroleptics known.[44] The dipole moment of pimozide measured in benzene at 20 °C is $\mu$ = 2.68D.[45]

The report mentioning pimozide for the first time in the open literature introduced it as "a prototype of a new chemical series of long-acting neuroleptic drugs."[22] In a series of papers[46-48] pimozide was described, in spite of its novel chemical structure, as a typical neuroleptic with a pharmacological profile resembling the profile of haloperidol rather than that of chlorpromazine.[46] From the animal data presented, it was predicted that pimozide would be particularly well suited as a neuroleptic for long-term oral treatment of psychotic patients at a single daily dose of 2.4 mg.[46] In the meantime, clinical trials with pimozide were already well under way. The first reports were published in 1968[49-52] by essentially the same team of psychiatrists who had clinically evaluated haloperidol, the compound that was exactly ten years earlier at the origin of our adventuring into the fascinating world of neuroleptics. In the following decade, pimozide continued to live up to our expectations and unabatedly drew attention, as can be gathered from the fact that up to the middle of 1979 almost a thousand publications were devoted to pimozide, including 503 papers on its pharmacology, 24 on pharmacokinetics, 12 on toxicology and teratology, and 410 on its clinical aspects.[53] For the interested reader, an excellent review article covering the most important literature on pimozide up to 1976 is available.[54]

In 1970, seven years after the original synthesis, pimozide, or Orap, was introduced on the Belgian market; since that time it has been gradually made available in more than 70 countries of the world. As was predicted many years earlier,[46] Orap proves to be an effective long-acting neuroleptic indicated for the long-term oral treatment of psychiatric patients susceptible to the specific effect of neuroleptics.

From the historical point of view it is interesting that the experience gained with a long-acting neuroleptic such as pimozide happened to be once again a stepping stone for the synthesis and development over the past decade of three other long-acting diphenylbutyl-type neuroleptics, fluspirilene or Imap,[55] penfluridol or Semap,[56] and clopimozide or Clorap.[57]

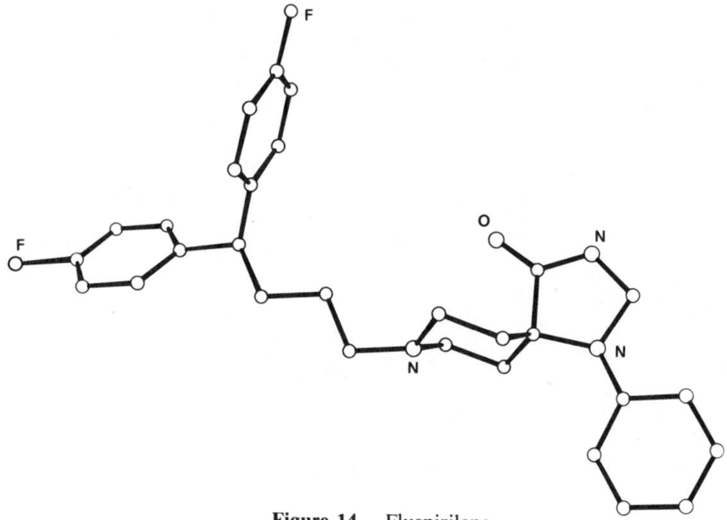

Figure 14.   Fluspirilene.

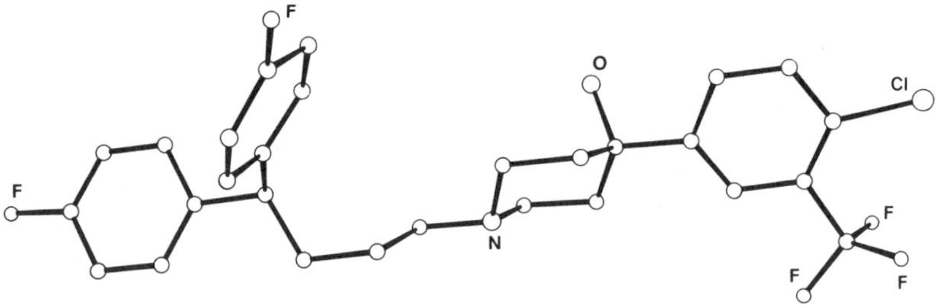

Figure 15.   Penfluridol.

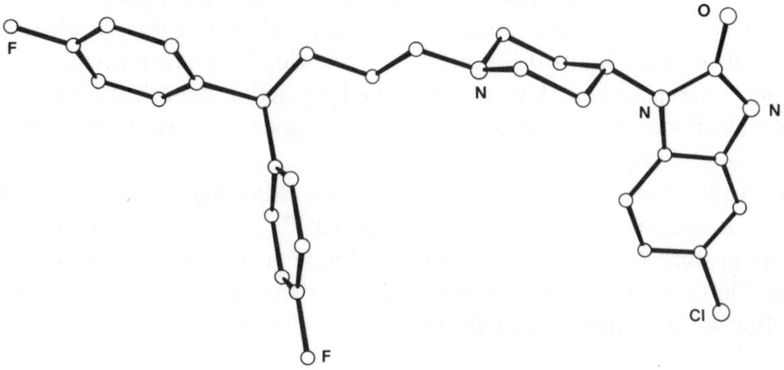

**Figure 16.** Clopimozide.

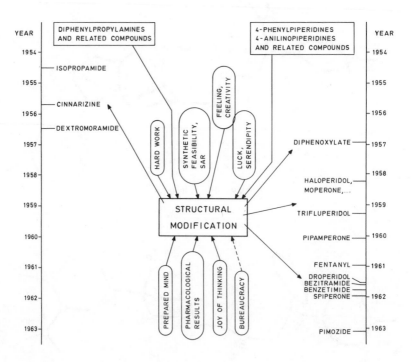

**Figure 17.** Schematic representation of the operational approach to drug design.

## 5.   CONCLUSION

A decade of research, starting in 1953, introduced us to the fields of anticholinergics, analgesics, and neuroleptics. When the diphenylpropylamines were subjected to systematic and thorough structural modification, our primary goal of producing new powerful analgesics was reached with the discovery of dextromoramide. When we tackled pethidine in the belief that thorough structural modification should lead to more potent morphinomimetics, we were soon successful. At this point we temporarily dropped the pursuit of analgesic activity of our leads and moved on to develop their CNS-depressing property, which eventually culminated in a structurally novel neuroleptic compound. The discovery of haloperidol set the scene for further discoveries in the field of analgesics and neuroleptics. Structural modification of haloperidol resulted in a number of valuable analogs and in a series of long-acting neuroleptics of which pimozide was the prototype. There is no clear-cut answer to the question how pimozide came about. Figure 17, nevertheless, is an attempt to answer this question. It summarizes in some ways what we did to foster a scientific atmosphere that created the opportunity for pimozide to be synthesized.

## REFERENCES

1.  M. Mackay and D. C. Hodgkin, *J. Chem. Soc.,* 3261 (1955).
2.  J. M. Lindsey and W. H. Barnes, *Acta Crystallogr.,* **8,** 227 (1955).
3.  N. Datta, P. Green, and P. Pauling, *J. Chem. Soc.,* Perkin Trans., **2,** 781 (1977).
4.  E. Bye, *Acta Chem. Scand. Ser. B.,* **30,** 95 (1976).
5.  O. J. Braenden, N. B. Eddy, and H. Halbach, *Bull. W. H. O.,* **13,** 937 (1955).
6.  P. A. J. Janssen, A. H. Jageneau, E. G. Van Proosdy-Hartzema, and D. K. De Jongh, *Acta Physiol. Pharmacol. Neerl.,* **7,** 373 (1958).
7.  P. A. J. Janssen, A. H. M. Jageneau, P. J. A. Demoen, C. Van de Westeringh, A. H. M. Raeymaekers, M. S. J. Wouters, S. Sanczuk, B. K. F. Hermans, and J. L. M. Loomans, *J. Med. Pharm. Med.,* **1,** 105 (1959).
8.  P. A. J. Janssen, A. H. M. Jageneau, P. J. A. Demoen, C. Van de Westeringh, J. H. M. De Cannière, A. H. M. Raeymaekers, M. S. J. Wouters, S. Sanczuk, and B. K. F. Hermans, *J. Med. Pharm. Med.,* **1,** 309 (1959).
9.  P. A. J. Janssen, in D. H. R. Barton and W. Doering, Eds., *Synthetic Analgesics, Part I: Diphenylpropylamines,* Vol. 3, International Series of Monographs on Organic Chemistry, Macmillan (Pergamon), New York, 1954.
10.  P. A. J. Janssen, A. H. M. Jageneau, and J. Huygens, *J. Med. Pharm. Med.,* **1,** 299 (1959).
11.  A. H. M. Jageneau and P. A. J. Janssen, *Arch. Int. Pharmacodyn. Ther.,* **106,** 199 (1956).
12.  P. A. J. Janssen, A. H. M. Jageneau, P. J. A. Demoen, C. Van de Westeringh, J. H. M. Cannière, A. H. M. Raeymaekers, M. S. J. Wouters, S. Sanczuk, and B. K. F. Hermans, *J. Med. Pharm. Chem.,* **2,** 271 (1960).
13.  P. A. J. Janssen, C. Van de Westeringh, A. H. M. Jageneau, P. J. A. Demoen, B. K. F. Hermans, C. H. P. Van Daele, K. H. L. Schellekens, C. A. M. Van der Eycken, and C. J. E. Niemegeers, *J. Med. Pharm. Med.,* **1,** 281 (1959).
14.  P. Divry, J. Bobon, and J. Collard, *Acta Neurol. Psychiatr. Belg.,* **58,** 878 (1958).
15.  P. Divry, J. Bobon, J. Collard, A. Pinchard, and E. Nols, *Acta Neurol. Psychiatr. Belg.,* **59,** 337 (1959).

16.  P. A. J. Janssen, *Arzneim.-Forsch.*, **11**, 819, 932 (1961).
17.  P. A. J. Janssen, *Int. Rev. Neurobiol.*, **8**, 221 (1965).
18.  P. A. J. Janssen in F. J. Ayd, Jr., and B. Blackwell, Eds., *Discoveries in Biological Psychiatry*, J. B. Lippincott, Philadelphia, 1970, p. 165.
19.  P. A. J. Janssen, C. J. E. Niemegeers, and K. H. L. Schellekens, *Arzneim.-Forsch.*, **15**, 104 (1965).
20.  P. A. J. Janssen, C. J. E. Niemegeers, and K. H. L. Schellekens, *Arzneim.-Forsch.*, **15**, 1196 (1965).
21.  P. A. J. Janssen, C. J. E. Niemegeers, and K. H. L. Schellekens, *Arzneim.-Forsch.*, **16**, 339 (1966).
22.  P. A. J. Janssen, C. J. E. Niemegeers, K. H. L. Schellekens, and F. M. Lenaerts, *Arzneim.-Forsch.*, **17**, 841 (1967).
23.  P. A. J. Janssen, in M. Gordon, Ed., *Psychopharmacological Agents*, Vol. 2, Academic Press, New York, 1967, p. 199.
24.  P. A. J. Janssen, *Psychopharmacologia*, **2**, 141 (1961).
25.  P. A. J. Janssen, C. J. E. Niemegeers, K. H. L. Schellekens, F. J. Verbruggen, and J. M. Van Nuten, *Arzneim.-Forsch.*, **13**, 205 (1963).
26.  P. A. J. Janssen, *Encéphale*, **51**, 582 (1962).
27.  P. A. J. Janssen, C. J. E. Niemegeers, and, J. G. H. Dony, *Arzneim.-Forsch.*, **13**, 401 (1963).
28.  C. J. E. Niemegeers and P. A. J. Janssen, *J. Pharm. Pharmacol.*, **12**, 744 (1960).
29.  P. A. J. Janssen and C. J. E. Niemegeers, *Arzneim.-Forsch.*, **11**, 1037 (1961).
30.  P. A. J. Janssen, C. J. E. Niemegeers, and A. H. M. Jageneau, *Arzneim.-Forsch.*, **10**, 1003 (1960).
31.  P. A. J. Janssen, A. H. M. Jageneau, and K. H. L. Schellekens, *Psychopharmacologia*, **1**, 389 (1960).
32.  P. A. J. Janssen and C. J. E. Niemegeers, *Nature*, **190**, 911 (1961).
33.  P. A. J. Janssen, C. J. E. Niemegeers, and K. H. L. Schellekens, *Arzneim.-Forsch.*, **10**, 955 (1960).
34.  P. A. J. Janssen, C. J. E. Niemegeers, and J. G. H. Dony, *Arzneim.-Forsch.*, **13**, 502 (1963).
35.  J. Bobon, J. Collard, and A. Pinchard, *Acta Neurol. Psychiatr. Belg.*, **62**, 566 (1962).
36.  J. Bobon, J. Collard, and R. Lecoq, *Acta Neurol. Psychiatr. Belg.*, **63**, 839 (1963).
37.  A. Rossi, A. Hunger, J. Kebrle, and K. Hoffman, *Helv. Chim. Acta*, **43**, 1298 (1960).
38.  P. A. J. Janssen, C. J. E. Niemegeers, K. H. L. Schellekens, F. J. Verbruggen, and J. M. Van Nueten, *Arzneim.-Forsch.*, **13**, 205 (1963).
39.  P. A. J. Janssen, C. J. E. Niemegeers, R. H. M. Marsboom, V. V. Hérin, W. K. P. Amery, P. V. Admiraal, J. T. Bosker, J. F. Crul, C. Pearce, and C. Zegveld, *Arzneim.-Forsch.*, **21**, 862 (1971).
40.  E. Schipper, *Chem. Ind.*, 464 (1960).
41.  E. Schipper and E. Chinery, *J. Org. Chem.*, **26**, 3597 (1961).
42.  J. P. Tollenaere, H. Moereels, and L. A. Raymaekers, *Atlas of the Three-Dimensional Structure of Drugs*, Elsevier North-Holland Biomedical Press, Amsterdam, New York, Oxford, 1979, p. 100.
43.  P. A. J. Janssen, U.S. Patent No. 3,196,157 (1965); Belg. Patent 633,495 (1963); Fr. Patent 1,360,532 (1964); Brit. Patent 1,039,923 (1966).
44.  Janssen Pharmaceutica, Specification Report No. 561 (740930) — R 6238.
45.  J. Peeters, unpublished results.
46.  P. A. J. Janssen, C. J. E. Niemegeers, K. H. L. Schellekens, A. Dresse, F. M. Lenaerts, A. Pinchard, W. K. A. Schaper, J. M. Van Nueten and F. J. Verbruggen, *Arzneim.-Forsch.*, **18**, 261 (1968).

47. P. A. J. Janssen and F. T. N. Allewijn, *Arzniem.-Forsch.*, **18**, 279 (1968).
48. P. A. J. Janssen, W. Soudijn, I. Van Wijngaarden, and A. Dresse, *Arzneim.-Forsch.*, **18**, 282 (1968).
49. J. Bobon, J. Collard, A. Pinchard, L. Goffioul, D. P. Bobon, and A. Devroye, *Acta Neurol. Belg.*, **68**, 137 (1968).
50. J. Brugmans, *Acta Neurol. Belg.*, **68**, 875 (1968).
51. D. P. Bobon, A. Devroye, L. Goffioul, and A. Pinchard, *Acta Neurol. Belg.*, **68**, 888 (1968).
52. P. Sterkmans, J. Brugmans, and F. Gevers, *Clin. Trials*, **5**, 1107 (1968).
53. J. Van Gestel, Medical Documentation Department, Janssen Pharmaceutica, private communication.
54. R. M. Pinder, R. N. Brogden, P. R. Sawyer, T. M. Speight, R. Spencer, and G. S. Avery, *Drugs*, **12**, 1 (1976).
55. P. A. J. Janssen, C. J. E. Niemegeers, K. H. L. Schellekens, F. M. Lenaerts, F. J. Verbruggen, J. M. Van Nueten, R. H. M. Marsboom, V. V. Hérin, and W. K. A. Schaper, *Arzneim.-Forsch.*, **20**, 1689 (1970).
56. P. A. J. Janssen, C. J. E. Niemegeers, K. H. L. Schellekens, F. M. Lenaerts, F. J. Verbruggen, J. M. Van Nueten, and W. K. A. Schaper, *Eur. J. Pharmacol.*, **11**, 139 (1970).
57. P. A. J. Janssen, C. J. E. Niemegeers, K. H. L. Schellekens, F. M. Lenaerts, and A. Wauquier, *Arzneim.-Forsch.*, **25**, 1287 (1975).

# Cefaclor 3

M. Gorman, R.R. Chauvette,
and S. Kukolja

## 1. INTRODUCTION

In September of 1979, a new, orally absorbed cephalosporin antibiotic, cefaclor, was introduced into the armamentarium against infectious disease. In the United States, cefaclor (CECLOR, Lilly) became the eleventh cephalosporin-derived antibiotic to be available in clinical medicine. Ten other closely related antibiotics are now on clinical trial or available elsewhere around the world. In this chapter we discuss the chemical and biological properties of these compounds and indicate their origins. It is of interest to note the unique chemical structure of cefaclor (**1**). Of the 15 structures shown in Table 1, only cefaclor has no carbon-carbon bond at C-3. In cefaclor, this linkage is replaced by the more electronegative carbon-chlorine bond. The consequence of this alteration upon antibacterial effectiveness is discussed below. Common to all the antibiotics in Table 1 is their genesis from cephalosporin C.

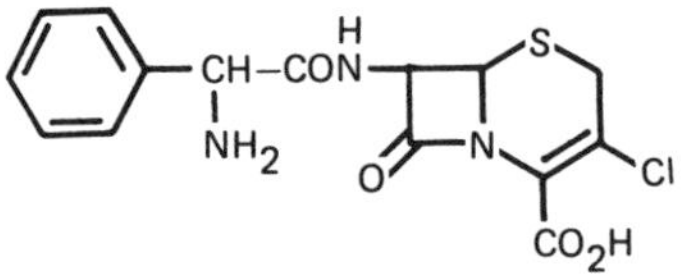

**1**
Cefaclor

## Table 1
## Cephalosporin Antibiotics Clinically Available in 1979

| Antibiotic | $R_1$ | $R_2$ |
|---|---|---|
| *Inside U.S.* | | |
| *Parenterals* | | |
| Cephalothin | (2-thienyl)$-CH_2-$ | $-CH_2OAc$ |
| Cephaloridine | (2-thienyl)$-CH_2-$ | $-CH_2-N^+$(pyridinium) |
| Cephapirin | (4-pyridyl)$-S-CH_2-$ | $-CH_2OAc$ |
| Cefazolin | (tetrazol-1-yl)$-CH_2-$ | $-CH_2S$(1,3,4-thiadiazol-2-yl)$-CH_3$ |
| Cefoxitin (7-methoxy) | (2-thienyl)$-CH_2-$ | $-CH_2OCONH_2$ |
| Cefamandole | D (phenyl)$-\underset{OH}{CH}-$ | $-CH_2S$(1-methyltetrazol-5-yl) $CH_3$ |

**Table 1 (continued)**

| Antibiotic | $R_1$ | $R_2$ |
|---|---|---|
| *Inside U.S.* | | |
| *Orals* | | |
| Cephaloglycin | D—C₆H₄—CH(NH₂)— | $-CH_2OAc$ |
| Cephalexin | D—C₆H₄—CH(NH₂)— | $-CH_3$ |
| Cephradine | D—(cyclohexadienyl)—CH(NH₂)— | $-CH_3$ |
| Cefadroxil | D  HO—C₆H₄—CH(NH₂)— | $-CH_3$ |
| Cefaclor | D—C₆H₄—CH(NH₂)— | $-Cl$ |
| *Outside U.S.* | | |
| *Parenterals* | | |
| Cefuroxime | (furanyl)—C(=N—OCH₃)— | $-CH_2OCONH_2$ |

**Table 1 (continued)**

| Antibiotic | R₁ | R₂ |
|---|---|---|
| Ceftezole | [tetrazole ring]–$CH_2$– | –$CH_2S$–[thiadiazole ring]–H |
| Cefotaxime | 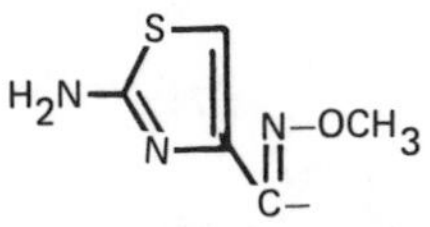 [aminothiazole ring] $C(=N-OCH_3)$– ($H_2N$– substituent) | –$CH_2OAc$ |
| Cefacetrile | $N\equiv C–CH_2$– | –$CH_2OAc$ |
| *Oral* Cefatrizine | D HO–[phenyl]–$CH(NH_2)$– | –$CH_2S$–[tetrazole ring]–H |

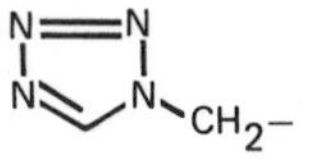

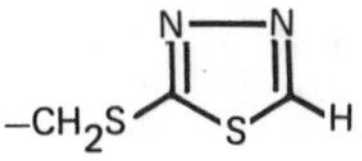

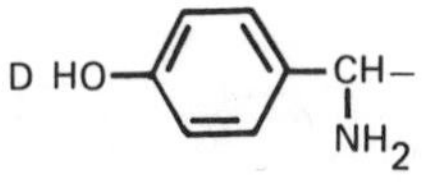

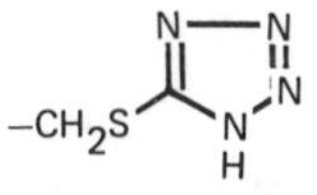

## 2.  HISTORICAL BACKGROUND

The discovery of cephalosporin C dates back to 1945, shortly after the recognition of the medical miracle penicillin. The Italian professor Guiseppe Brotzu,[1] while studying microbial flora off the coast of Sardinia, isolated an antibiotic-producing mold identified as a strain of *Cephalosporium.* He noted that crude extracts from the culture broth, when injected into patients, had a therapeutic effect. In 1948, the culture was sent to Oxford University for further study, and eventually detailed investigations were undertaken by Professors E.P. Abraham and G.G.F. Newton.[2] In addition to a solvent extractable acidic steroid, cephalosporin P, they discovered a water-soluble antibiotic, penicillin N (Figure 1), which was originally designated cephalosporin N. This penicillin was rapidly decomposed by acid, and during a study carried out at low pH it was observed that residual antibiotic activity remained in the solution.

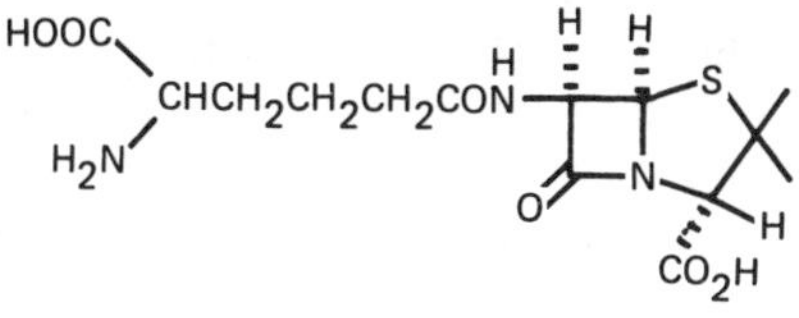

(a)

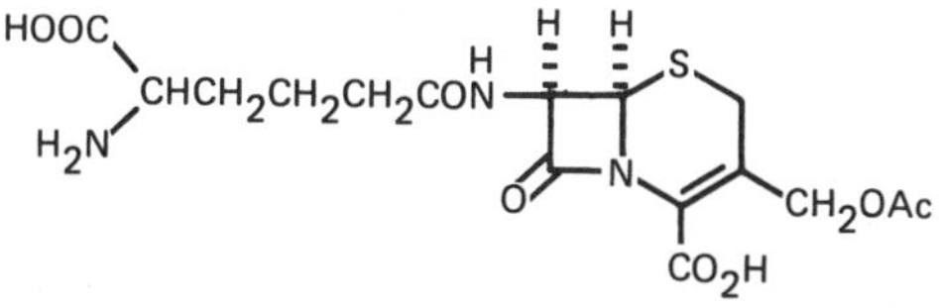

(b)

**Figure 1.** (a) Penicillin N, (b) Cephalosporin C.

A new substance responsible for the antibiotic activity of *Cephalosporium* was eventually isolated and named cephalosporin C. It was purified and found to resemble penicillin N in some ways (Figure 1). While it had only about one-tenth the intrinsic biological activity of penicillin N against penicillin-sensitive strains of bacteria, it nonetheless possessed very impressive biological properties. Notably, it had minimum toxicity and it was stable to the action of penicillinase (the $\beta$-lactamase enzyme produced by gram-positive bacteria which destroys penicillin by opening the $\beta$-lactam ring), consequently rendering a much broader spectrum of antibacterial action to the new antibiotic. The increasing incidence of penicillinase related *Staphylococcus* infection in hospitals spurred the rapid development of this new $\beta$-lactam antibiotic.

It was known at that time that many beneficial changes in activity could be derived from the acylation of the penicillin nucleus (6-APA) with a variety of acids. The acylation reaction could be accomplished either chemically by manipulations or microbiologically by adding the appropriate acid or its derivative to the fermentation. Thus the addition of phenoxyacetic acid to a penicillin fermentation led to the isolation of penicillin V. Alternatively, chemical acylation of 6-APA, the penicillin nucleus, led to many new antibiotics; for example, with 2,6-dimethoxybenzoic acetic acid, methicillin was obtained. It was quickly concluded in the scientific community that while the specific activity of cephalosporin C was too low for it to be considered as a clinical antibiotic, analogous manipulations might lead to more potent antibacterial substances.

In 1960, the National Research Development Corporation in Great Britain made available to a number of pharmaceutical companies the results of research on cephalosporin C. Since then the quantity of research on this subject has escalated rapidly and continues to accelerate, as indicated by the number of new antibiotics listed in Table 1.

Today there are few pharmaceutical companies that are not engaged in some form of research with the cephalosporin molecule. The rapid expansion of this area is due to the tremendous clinical success of many of the early $\beta$-lactam antibiotics. In part, the increase is generated by the realization by various researchers that the tools exist for modifying the cephalosporin molecule, either through chemical manipulation or through total systhesis, to afford novel chemical structures that mimic the parent natural substances. In addition to chemical methods, techniques of microbiology, biochemistry, pharmacology are now available that will rapidly tell interested scientists whether their new compounds hold medicinal promise. Despite this "ideal" medicinal chemistry situation, it has not been possible at this writing to synthesize the perfect antibiotic, one that will inhibit every infecting strain of microorganism with no untoward liability to the patient. We have come closer with each new generation of $\beta$-lactam antibiotic, but just how close, the reader must ascertain.

## 3. PARENTERAL CEPHALOSPORINS
### 3.1  The Early Chemistry of Cephalosporins at C-7
Many scientists involved in the initial research with cephalosporin C believed that the techniques developed for penicillin modifications would apply directly to the preparation of new analogues. Workers in many pharmaceutical laboratories devoted major research efforts to adding precursors to the cephalosporin fermentation or, alternatively, to finding an acylase enzyme capable of cleaving the $D$-$\alpha$-aminoadipic acid from cephalosporin C. After some 20 years of searching, no such biological method has as yet been found. It must be assumed that the side-chain amide bond containing $D$-$\alpha$-aminoadipic acid is inert to enzymatic cleavage. In the Lilly Research Laboratories, the project of functionalization of cephalosporin C was assigned to organic chemists rather than fermentation experts. While significant efforts were directed toward learning to produce large quantities of cephalosporin C, efforts were directed to its modification from a primarily chemical point of view.

Direct acid cleavage explored earlier by Loder et al.[3] had produced 7-ACA, 7-aminocephalosporanic acid, the cephalosporin nucleus, in yields of less than 1% because of a multitude of secondary reactions. In analogy with some selective cleavage methods being applied at that time by Witkop[4] to peptides containing glutamic acid amides, cephalosporin C was treated with aqueous nitrous acid, whereupon 2 moles of nitrogen were evolved. Because the parent molecule has only one diazotizable amine function (Figure 1), the second mole must have arisen from a newly generated amine. It was hypothesized that the second mole of nitrogen was derived from 7-ACA formed *in situ* from cleavage of the C-7 amide bond. It remained to find a suitable reagent that would allow the isolation of the free 7-ACA. Such a reagent was found by Morin *et al.*[5] to be nitrosyl chloride (NOCl). Indeed, for some years, the NOCl cleavage was the only process available for the commercial preparation of 7-ACA. Eventually an improved method was discovered by Fechtig and coworkers,[6] involving the use of phosphorus pentachloride/pyridine followed by an alcohol treatment that converts the C-7 amide first to an imino halide and then to an iminoether. Subsequent hydrolysis led to 7-ACA in very high yields. Figure 2 summarizes the three cleavage procedures just discussed.

The successful cleavage of cephalosporin C and the availability of 7-ACA in larger quantities enabled Chauvette and coworkers[7] to prepare many semi-synthetic cephalosporins. From among them, cephalothin (Keflin, Lilly) was selected for clinical testing. This antibiotic, 7-(thienyl-2-acetamido)-cephalo-sporanic acid, measured up to the early expectation for modification of cephalosporin C. It was resistant to destruction by penicillinase and shared, with the penicillins, a low incidence of side effects in humans. The new anti-biotic was also acid stable and it exhibited a wider antibacterial spectrum than the corresponding penicillin. But cephalothin, was not absorbed when given

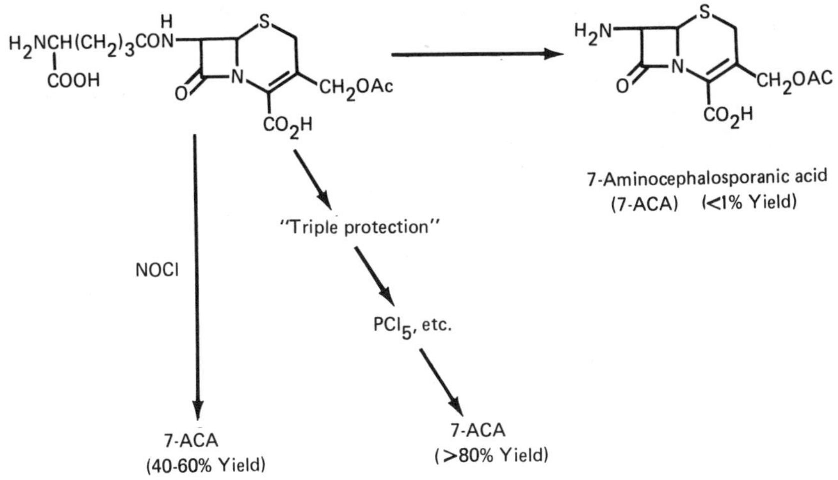

**Figure 2.** Preparation of 7-ACA from cephalosporin C.

**Table 2**

**Microbiological Activity of Some β-Lactam Antibiotics**

| Structure No. | $R_1$ | $R_2$ | S. aureus[a] | E. coli | K. pneumoniae |
|---|---|---|---|---|---|
| 1 | | A | 0.4 | 6.4 | 0.8 |
| | | B | 2.0 | 50 | 16 |
| | | C | 0.8 | 3.3 | 3.3 |
| | | E | 20 | 44 | 110 |
| 2 | $C_6H_5CH_2$— | A | 0.7 | 27 | 1.0 |
| | | B | 5.0 | 50 | 27 |
| | | C | 1.2 | 9.0 | 7.0 |
| | | E | 150 | 52 | 110 |
| 3 | $C_6H_5OCH_2$— | A | 0.2 | 140 | 6.2 |
| | | B | 2.8 | 50 | 50 |
| | | C | 0.2 | 38 | 14 |
| | | E | 140 | 200 | 150 |
| 4 | $C_6H_5CH(NH_3)$— | A | 2.0 | 3.5 | 1.0 |
| | | B | 3.8 | 9.7 | 6.6 |
| | | C | 170 | 6.3 | 110 |
| 5 | $C_6H_5CH(CO_2H)$— | A | 9.3 | 88 | 28 |
| | | E | 14 | 8.8 | 200 |
| 6 | | A | 20 | 200 | 52 |
| | | E | 8.7 | 200 | 110 |

## Table 2 (continued)

| Structure No. | $R_1$ | $R_2$ | S. aureus[a] | E. coli | K. pneumoniae |
|---|---|---|---|---|---|
| 7 | C₆H₅ isoxazole with CH₃ | A | 4.9 | 110 | 3.9 |
|   |   | E | 0.5 | 180 | 29 |
| 8 | NCCH₂— | A | 0.8 | 12 | 10 |
| 9 | pyridyl—SCH₂— | A | 0.5 | 17 | 3.1 |
| 10 | tetrazole NCH₂— | D | 0.5 | 1.0 | 1.0 |

[a]Penicillin resistant strain.

orally and caused pain upon intramuscular injection. These shortcomings limited its use to intravenous administration and prompted further research in the hope of finding compounds more convenient to administer. Table 2 compares a variety of common substituents on different β-lactam nuclei, for example, 1A represents cephalothin (the 7-ACA derivative) and 1E represents the analogous penicillin. Note the 50-fold improvement in activity for the cephalosporin against the penicillinase-producing gram-positive pathogen *Staphylococcus aureus*. The *Klebsiella pneumoniae* activity is of interest since this organism also produces a penicillinase that makes it resistant to most penicillins. This common property is also seen in a comparison of 2 and 3, A and E structures. In Table 2, structures 6 and 7 represent side chains that confer penicillinase resistance to the corresponding penicillins, that is, 6E and 7E. When these functionalities are attached to 7-ACA (6A and 7A), only mediocre biological activity results. This is an example of a common finding: What is optimal for one β-lactam antibiotic nucleus is not necessarily optimal for another.

## Table 3
### Gradient Plate Assay of Minimum Inhibitory Concentrations (μg/ml)

| | S. aureus[a] | Shigella sp. | E. coli | K. pneumoniae | Enterob. aerogenes | Sal. heidelberg | Ps. aeruginosa | Ser. marcescens |
|---|---|---|---|---|---|---|---|---|
| **Parenteral Products** | | | | | | | | |
| Cephalothin | 0.5 | 17.6 | 15.8 | 0.9 | 4.0 | 3.6 | 200 | 200 |
| Cephaloridine | 2.0 | 5.0 | 5.3 | 5.8 | 4.2 | 5.5 | 200 | 124 |
| Cephapirin | 0.7 | 18.2 | 11.3 | 0.8 | 1.0 | 0.8 | 200 | 200 |
| Cephacetrile | 3.1 | 7.6 | 7.7 | 7.3 | 7.0 | 5.6 | 200 | 110 |
| Cephazolin | 0.9 | 2.1 | 1.2 | 1.0 | 0.9 | 0.8 | 200 | 200 |
| Ceftezole | 0.6 | 3.0 | 3.0 | 1.0 | 1.0 | 0.7 | >200 | 180 |
| Cefoxitin | 2.0 | 8.0 | 8.0 | 4.0 | 6.0 | 5.0 | 200 | 6.0 |
| Cefamandole | 0.8 | 0.6 | 0.9 | 0.6 | 0.5 | 0.7 | 200 | 10.7 |
| Cefotaxime | 2.0 | 0.06 | 0.3 | <0.1 | 0.1 | 0.07 | 20.0 | 1.0 |
| Cefuroxime | 0.7 | 3.5 | 8.0 | <0.1 | 6.8 | 5.0 | >200 | >200 |
| **Oral Products** | | | | | | | | |
| Cephaloglycin | 3.4 | 3.9 | 2.3 | 0.9 | 0.8 | 0.8 | 200 | 44.5 |
| Cephalexin | 9.6 | 13.4 | 15.6 | 7.6 | 7.0 | 6.8 | 200 | 126 |
| Cefadroxil | 5.5 | 13.5 | 14.7 | 16 | 16 | 8.0 | >200 | 120 |
| Cephradine | 8.2 | 20.4 | 15.4 | 11.7 | 11.6 | 10.6 | 200 | 122 |
| Cefaclor | 2.9 | 0.7 | 0.8 | 0.6 | 0.6 | 0.5 | >200 | 21.5 |
| Cefatrizine | 3.0 | 2.0 | 3.0 | 1.0 | 2.0 | 0.6 | 200 | 35 |

[a] Penicillin-resistant strain.

## 3.2 The Early Chemistry at the C-3 Position in Cephalosporin C

Since the general theme of this chapter is to present an outline of events leading to the discovery of cefaclor, it is necessary to turn our attention at this time to the 3-position of cephalosporin C (Figure 1). Abraham and Newton[8] had noted that cephalosporin C reacted with pyridine in aqueous solution by replacement of the acetoxyl function on the C-3 methylene with the pyridinium moiety. The new compounds (Table 2, **1, 2**, and **3**, **A** and **C**) were also potent antibiotics and were especially effective against problem gram-positive bacteria such as penicillin-resistant *staphylococci*. When the reaction with pyridine was applied to cephalothin, the product, called cephaloridine (Table 2 **1C**), was deemed to have properties superior to cephalothin and was readily administered by intra-muscular injection. This became the second marketed cephalosporin.

Further research reported by Kariyone and associates[9] paved the way to preparation of the newer antibiotics in Table 1 by showing that heterocyclic thiols such as alkyl-substituted thiadiazole thiol and tetrazole thiol readily displaced the acetoxyl function to yield compounds of much increased potency. The first marketed compound among these new 3-heterocyclic thiomethyl-cephalosporins was cefazolin (Table 2, **10D**). Finland and associates[10] reported that cefazolin, when used parenterally (Table 3), is more potent than cephalothin.

Strominger[11] suggested that $\beta$-lactam antibiotics act as acylating agents on a transpeptidase enzyme that normally cleaves a *d*-alanyl-*d*-alanine peptide bond to form the bacterial cell wall. Consequently, the better the acylating ability, the more potent the antibiotic. Penicillin $\beta$-lactams owe this acylating activity to the chemical strain of the 4,5 bicyclic-ring system (Figure 1). In the 4,6 ring system of the cephalosporin (Figure 1), the acylating ability is enhanced by the electronic effects due to the double bond and the "leavability" of the acetoxyl group.

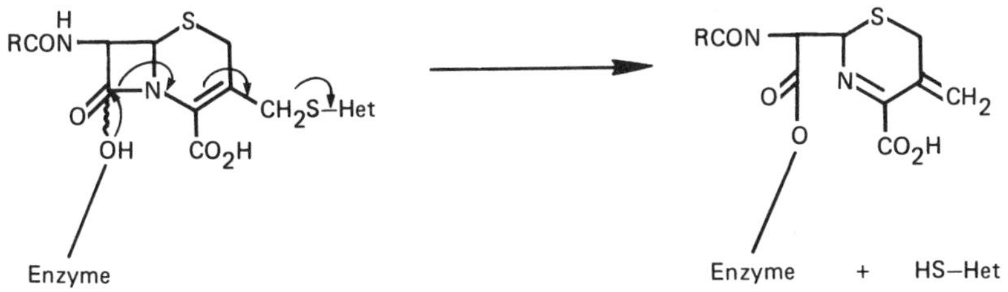

**Figure 3.** Cephalosporin acylation reaction.

The improved potency of heterocyclic thiomethyl cephalosporins is thus believed to be due to the superior leavability of the thioheterocycle over the acetoxyl group. This concept is illustrated in Figure 3. It seems that antibacterial potency is greatly enhanced when the 1-methyltetrazolethio functionality is incorporated at the 3-methylene position of the cephalosporin nucleus (cefamandole, Table 1). The thiol is very acidic, and according to Boyd and Lunn[12] the thioether possesses the best leaving ability of a number of thiols studied.*

## 4. THE DEVELOPMENT OF ORALLY EFFECTIVE CEPHALOSPORINS

The absence of oral efficacy in early cephalosporins was a disappointment to the scientists involved in this project. Simple penicillins such as penicillin G and penicillin V are quite well absorbed upon oral administration if one takes into account their decomposition by stomach acid. The analogous cephalosporins, inherently acid stable, are not absorbed from the gastrointestinal tract to any significant extent.[2]**

### 4.1 Cephaloglycin Development

Ampicillin was prepared by Doyle and coworkers[13] through the acylation of penicillin nucleus (6-APA) with D-phenylglycine. This new penicillin was acid stable and more active against gram negative bacteria than other penicillins known at that time. Although the oral absorption of this new antibiotic was not significantly greater than that of other penicillins, according to Bergan,[14] it led to the preparation of the analogous 7-ACA derivative. Spencer et al.[15] prepared this analogue, cephaloglycin (Kafocin, Lilly), by acylation of 7-ACA with

---

*Among parenteral cephalosporins, cefamandole, cefuroxime, and cefoxitin represent so-called second generation β-lactam antibiotics. This term results from the properties these three compounds possess that cause them to inhibit not only the so-called cephalosporin-sensitive gram-negative bacteria but also certain strains from genera such as *Enterobacter, Proteus,* and *Serratia* normally resistant to earlier cephalosporins. It is beyond the scope of this chapter to describe these newer clinical entitites in depth. Cefoxitin contains a 7-methoxyl function in its structure which imparts almost total β-lactamase resistance to the molecule. It is the subject of another chapter in this volume. The other two antibiotics appear to owe their wider spectrum of activity, compared with the earlier compounds, to a combination of enhanced β-lactamase stability and better crypticity (the ability to pass "unnoticed" through the bacterial cell wall to the site of action).

**It is of interest that the $ED_{50}$'s of the cephaloridine and cephalexin tested in mice orally against *S. pyogenes* compare favorably (1.0 and 1.2 mg/kg x 2, respectively) (Table 4). The reason for these excellent therapeutic effects is a low minimum inhibitory concentration (MIC 0.008 $\mu$g/ml) in the case of cephaloridine and effective oral absorption in the case of cephalexin as seen from peak serum levels of 0.5 and 18.0 $\mu$g/ml, respectively, for the two antibiotics. It is important not to draw pharmacokinetic conclusions from mouse therapy experiments.

**Table 4**

**Measurement of Oral Activity of Cephalosporins Against**
***Streptococcus Pyogenes*[a]**

| Cephalosporin[b] | Oral ED$_{50}$ (mg/kg x 2) | MIC ($\mu$g/ml) | Peak serum conc. ($\mu$g/ml) |
|---|---|---|---|
| Cephalothin | 26 | 0.1 | 0.1 |
| Cephaloridine | 1.0 | 0.008 | 0.5 |
| Cephaloglycin | 3.9 | 0.2 | 3.8 |
| Cephalexin | 1.2 | 0.5 | 18.0 |

[a]From W. E. Wick, in E. H. Flynn, Ed., *Cephalosporins and Penicillins: Chemistry and Biology*, Academic Press, New York, 1972, p. 519.

[b]Antibiotics were administered orally to mice at 1 and 5 hours post-infection.

*D*-phenylglycine. The new compound was slightly less potent against gram-positive bacteria than other cephalosporins (see Tables 1 and 3) but was more potent than either cephalothin or cephaloridin against gram-negative bacteria. Of utmost significance was the observation that 25% of the administered oral dose was absorbed into the bloodstream. This percentage of absorbed antibiotic gave adequate levels for therapeutic cures, as shown by Brogard *et al.*[16]

Derivatives of 7-ACA share a common metabolic fate. They are deacetylated in the liver, producing deacetylcephalosporins (Figure 4). With orally administered cephaloglycin, the only antibiotic found in the urine is deacetylcephaloglycin. The metabolite was prepared and isolated in crystalline form by Kukolja.[17] It was as active as the parent drug against gram-positive bacteria and was fourfold to eightfold less active against gram-negative pathogens. Thus the excellent *in vitro* activity of the antibiotic could not be fully utilized. A significant incidence of gastrointestinal disturbances was also noted, presumably due to the unabsorbed antibiotic retained in the gut. The need existed for an improved, orally effective cephalosporin.

### 4.2   Cephalexin Development

Continued efforts to modify the acetoxyl group in the cephalosporin molecule resulted in the development of deacetoxycephalosporins. Earlier hydrogenolyses of the acetoxy group were reported by Stedman *et al.*[18] and Morin *et al.*[19] These reactions led to the formation of the 3-methyl derivative, 7-aminodeacetoxycephalosporanic acid (7-ADCA). Although it was recognized that deacetoxycephalosporins were less potent than the corresponding

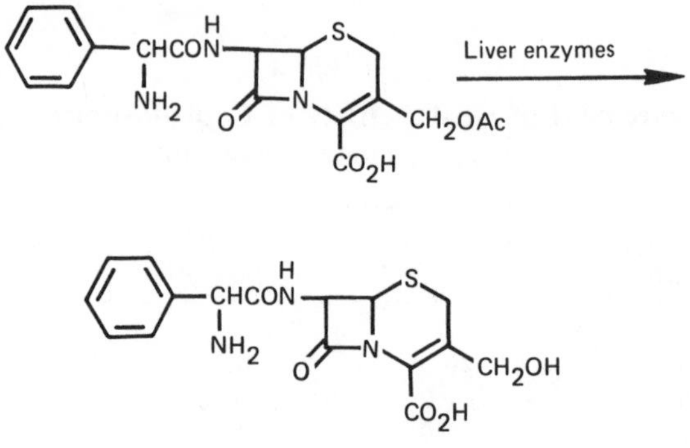

**Figure 4.**    Deacetylation of cephalosporins.

cephalosporanic acids, numerous 7-acylamino derivatives of 7-ADCA were prepared. Among such derivatives was the *D*-α-aminophenylacetamido-3-methylcephalosporin prepared by Ryan *et al.*[20] This deacetoxycephalosporin is cephalexin (Keflex, Lilly) (Figure 5). Cephalexin is the most potent of all of the 7-ADCA compounds investigated but is still significantly less active than cephaloglycin (Table 3). However, in contrast with the latter, cephalexin is: (1) essentially completely absorbed upon oral administration, (2) not metabolized and thus excreted from the body unchanged, and (3) the cause of very few side

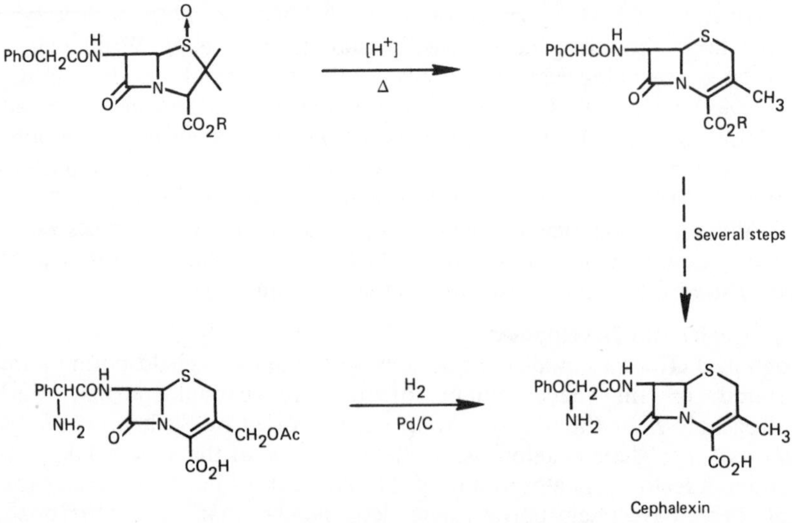

**Figure 5.**    Preparation of cephalexin.

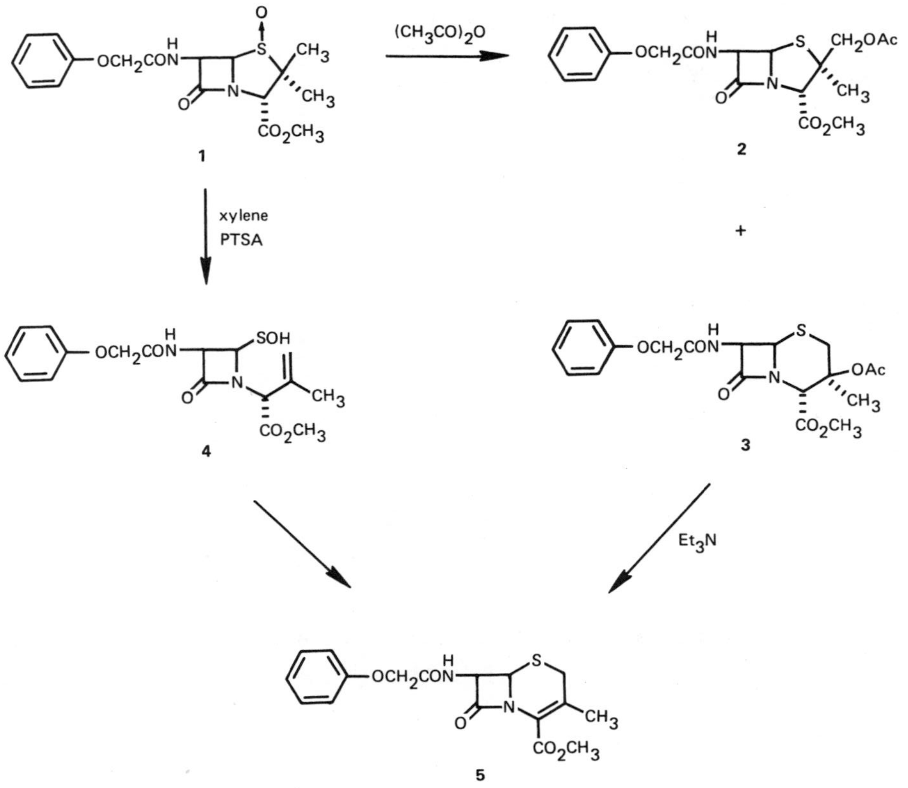

**Figure 6.** Penicillin ring expansion.

63

## Table 5

## MIC and ED$_{50}$ Values for Some Cepahlosporin Oral Candidates

| X | A | MIC ($\mu$g/ml) | | | | Mouse ED$_{50}$ (oral) vs. E. coli |
|---|---|---|---|---|---|---|
| | | S. aureus[a] | E. coli | K. pneumoniae | Enterob. aerogenes | |
| H | H | 3.1 | 6.3 | 6.3 | 13 | 20 |
| p-OH | | 3.1 | 13 | 25 | 25 | 25 |
| m-OH | | 6.3 | 6.3 | 13 | 13 | |
| o-OH (dl) | | 25 | 200 | 100 | >200 | |
| H | OAc | 6.3 | 1.6 | 3.1 | 3.1 | 18 |
| p-OH | | 6.3 | 13 | 6.3 | 6.3 | 18 |
| m-OH | | 3.1 | 3.1 | 1.6 | 3.1 | |
| o-OH (dl) | | 13 | 100 | 100 | 200 | |

| | | | | | | |
|---|---|---|---|---|---|---|
| H | | 1.6 | 3.1 | 1.6 | 3.1 | 4 |
| p-OH (cefatriazine) | | 1.6 | 1.6 | 1.6 | 1.6 | 0.5 |
| m-OH | | 3.1 | 1.6 | 1.6 | 1.6 | |
| H | | 1.6 | 1.6 | 0.8 | 1.6 | 10 |
| p-OH | | 3.1 | 1.6 | 1.6 | 3.1 | 1.4 |
| m-OH | | 3.1 | 1.6 | 1.6 | 3.1 | |
| H | | 3.1 | 6.3 | 3.1 | 6.3 | 11 |
| p-OH | | 3.1 | 6.3 | 6.3 | 25 | 2.3 |
| m-OH | | 3.1 | 6.3 | 3.1 | 13 | |

[a]Penicillin-resistant strain.

65

effects. Therapeutic levels of antibiotic are obtained in the blood despite the lower potency relative to 7-ACA-derived cephalosporins.

Cephalexin became a significant orally administered antibiotic. With its clinical acceptance, a need existed for an economical synthesis of cephalexin.

A new chemical reaction of penicillins was discovered in the Lilly Laboratories at about the same time the chemical reduction of 7-ACA became known. Morin et al.[19] were interested in a chemical model postulating that the concurrence of penicillins and cephalosporins in fermentation was a result of the bioconversion of a penicillin into a cephalosporin.* They investigated an acid-catalyzed Pummerer-like reaction on penicillin sulfoxide. Thus, as shown in Figure 6, when a penicillin sulfoxide ester 1 was heated in acetic anhydride, the compounds 2 and 3 were obtained. Compound 3 with base yielded the deacetoxylcephalosporin derivative 5. Cephalosporin 5 could be also obtained directly from 1 by heating in xylene with p-toluene sulfonic acid. These workers showed that a common intermediate in these reactions was the sulfenic acid 4. Many years later the proposed sulfenic acid intermediates were isolated in crystalline form by Chou et al.[21] These early yields of 3-methyl cephalosporins were low (10-20%). Motivated by biological interest in cephalexin, many variations in both reaction conditions and reagents were investigated by Chauvette et al.[23] Today the reaction approaches being quantitative, and cephalexin is now produced from naturally occurring penicillins.

## 4.3   Other Orally Effective Cephalosporins

The modest potency of cephalexin spurred the search for new oral cephalosporins with side chains other than D-phenylglycine. No other 7-side chain has been found that imparts significant oral absorption to these antibiotics. In attempts to overcome the problem of metabolism in cephaloglycin, the nuclei obtained by displacing the acetoxy group in 7-ACA with a variety of heterocyclic thiols were acylated with D-phenylglycine and its hydroxy derivatives. According to Dunn et al.,[24] some of the resulting compounds, listed in Table 3, possessed significant activity. One of these, cefatriazine (Table 5), is currently on clinical trial. Results published by Actor and associates[25] indicated approximately 50% oral absorption for cefatriazine. The consequence of the incomplete absorption of this potent antibiotic on the incidence of gastrointestinal side effects will be of interest in view of past experiences with cephaloglycin.

---

*Only recently, Yoshida et al.[22] have been able to show that penicillin N is converted to deacetoxy-cephalosporin C by strains of Cephalosporium fungi.

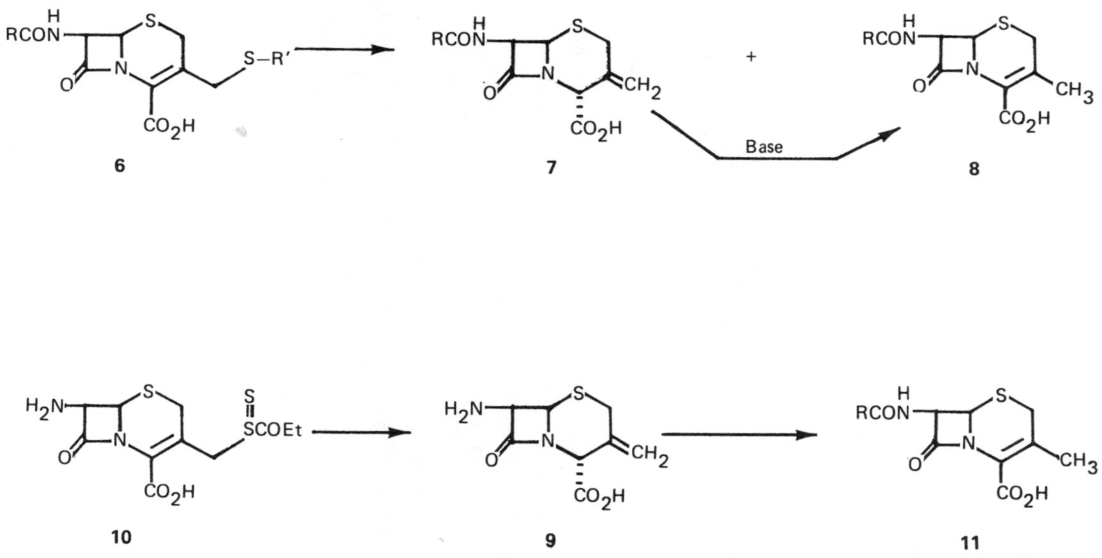

**Figure 7.** Reductive preparation of 3-exomethylenecepham.

67

**4.4   The Discovery of 3-Exomethylene Cephalosporins and their Chemistry**

Shortly after the introduction of cephalexin in clinical medicine, attention was turned to alternative methods for its synthesis, since the hydrogenolysis of the acetoxy group in 7-ACA required large quantities of a palladium catalyst and the ring expansion of penicillin sulfoxide esters was then still a conversion in only modest yield. While working on an alternative synthesis of cephalexin, Chauvette and Pennington[26] found that cephalosporins 6 (Figure 7) containing sulfur at the C-3 methylene[27] could be hydrogenolized at room temperature in aqueous ethanol solutions using Raney nickel. This reduction led to mixtures of 3-methylenecephams 7 and 7-acylamino deacetoxycephalosporins 8. In order to make the 3-methylenecepham nucleus 9, the side chain of 7-acylamino-3-methylcephams 7 was removed by the PCl$_5$/pyridine cleavage reaction either after silylation as described by Fechtig and associates[6] or with mixed anhydride protection reported by Chauvette et al.[28] The product was obtained in satisfactory yields. Alternatively, the Raney nickel reduction of the xanthate 10 afforded the zwitterionic product 9, which crystallized directly from aqueous solutions at its isoelectric point. 3-Methylenecephams 7 could be readily isomerized to 7-aminodeacetoxycephalosporanic acids 8 on treatment with pyridine.

Hall and coworkers[29] reported that electrolysis of 7-ACA in a buffered sodium bicarbonate solution, using a mercury pool cathode and a platinum sheet anode separated by a sintered glass partition, also led to 3-exomethylene derivatives. The electrolysis was carried out at 15V for 34 hours at room temperature. The course of the reduction was followed by observing the disappearance of the 258 nm cephalosporin chromaphore in the UV spectrum. The product, 7-amino-3-methylenecepham-4-carboxylic acid 9, was isolated in 64% yield. Acylation of 9 with D-phenylglycyl chloride hydrochloride and subsequent treatment with trimethylsilyl chloride and excess pyridine gave cephalexin 11 (R = phenylglycyl). Thus, though never commercialized, another convenient route to cephalexin had been established.

Spry was able to show by hydrogenation of 7 and comparison with Δ²-cephem-derived compounds of known structure[30] that the stereochemistry at C-4 of the carboxylic acid is of the α-configuration as in penicillin.

The 3-methylenecephams themselves are completely devoid of antimicrobial activity; it was recognized, however, that they had the potential for use in the preparation of new cephalosporins with electronegative substituents directly attached to the cephem ring. Although investigation of 3-methylenecephams was first directed to the production of deacetoxycephalosporins, a further exploration of their chemistry led to the preparation of 3-chloro-3-cephems and of 3-methoxy-3-cephems, which possessed marked antimicrobial activity.

Gorman and Ryan[31] proposed that the antimicrobial activity of $\beta$-lactam antibiotics was directly related to the reactivity of the $\beta$-lactam amide bond. An electron-withdrawing heteroatom at C-3 would be expected to increase the electrophilic character of the $\beta$-lactam and thereby improve biological activity. On the basis of this speculation, efforts were concentrated on the synthesis of cephalosporins bearing a halogen atom directly at C-3. A key step in this scheme was the low temperature ozonolysis of 3-methylenecephams carried out by Chauvette and Pennington.[32] The ozonolysis of 7-amino-3-methylenecepham *p*-nitro benzyl ester 12 was easily controlled to give the 3-hydroxy-3-cephem nucleus ester 13 in good purity and in high yield. An analogous ozonolysis of 3-methylenecepham benzhydryl esters was independently developed at CIBA-Geigy by Scartazzini and Bickel.[33]

The ozonolysis product of 3-methylenecephams exist largely in its enol form (Figure 8) as seen from the ultraviolet absorption in the region 268 nm typical of 3-cephem chromaphore; the infrared band at $1640^{-1}$ consistent with a strongly hydrogen-bonded ester carbonyl; the absence of an allylic proton at C-4 to accommodate the 3-keto structure in the NMR spectrum; a titratable group at 5.6 (66% DMF/water) for an enolic OH. Evidence for some 3-keto character was found in the ready-decarboxylation of the C-4 carboxyl group (Figure 8) upon removal of the ester protection. Further, the formation of *syn* and *anti* oximes resulting from the reaction of the ozonolysis product with methoxamine hydrochloride and pyridine was observed by Scartazzini and Bickel.[33]

Interest was also directed at acyl- and alkyl-substituted derivatives of the 3-hydroxycephem. While *O*-acylation (e.g., with acetic anhydride) proceeded readily on a variety of 7-substituted 3-hydroxycephem esters, upon de-esterification immediate loss of the acyl group occurred with concomitant decarboxylation to the inactive 3-keto-4,4-dihydro product. Methylation of the 3-hydroxycephem with diazomethane led to the corresponding 3-methoxy-cephem, and several amido examples were prepared and evaluated. Representative 3-methoxycephem antibiotics are shown in Table 6. In contrast with the highly active 3-chloro compounds, the activity of the 3-methoxy derivatives in general paralleled that of the 3-methyl cephalosporins. Although compound 10 (Table 6) was somewhat more active than cephalexin (7), the oral absorption properties of 10, cefaclor, and cephalexin appeared to be quite similar.

Scartazzini and Bickel[33] at the CIBA-Geigy Laboratories prepared a variety of additional 3-alkyl-substituted cephems and found that with larger alkyl groups (ethyl, butyl, and benzyl) the inhibition of gram-positive organisms

## Table 6

## Microbiological Activity of the 3-Position Direct-Substituted Cephem Derivatives

70

| | Shigella sp. N9 | E. coli N10 | K. pneumoniae X26 | E. aerogenes X68 | Sal. heidelberg X514 | Ps. aeruginosa X528 | Ser. marcescens X99 | Staph. V41[a] | Staph. V32[a] | Staph. X400[b] | Staph. V84[a] | Staph. X1.1[c] |
|---|---|---|---|---|---|---|---|---|---|---|---|---|
| 1 | 17.5[b] | 21.2 | 0.8 | 0.9 | 0.9 | >200 | >200 | 11.4 | 16.0 | >20 | 0.5 | <0.12 |
| 2 | 4.0 | 6.3 | 1.0 | 0.7 | 0.6 | >200 | >160 | 5.8 | 8.0 | >20 | 0.4 | <0.1 |
| 3 | 19.5 | 24.5 | 16.2 | 20 | 16.3 | >200 | 132 | 2.2 | 2.3 | >200 | 0.8 | 0.2 |
| 4 | 2.6 | 2.7 | 2.6 | 3.1 | 2.6 | >200 | 130 | 1.9 | 1.6 | >200 | 0.7 | <0.05 |
| 5 (Cefaclor) | 0.7 | 0.8 | 0.6 | 0.6 | 0.5 | >200 | 21.5 | 3.0 | 5.0 | >20 | 0.6 | 0.5 |
| 6 (Cephalothin) | 9.7 | 12.0 | 1.0 | 1.0 | 1.0 | >200 | >200 | 0.5 | 0.6 | >20 | <0.1 | <0.1 |
| 7 (Cephalexin) | 15.0 | 13.5 | 6.9 | 5.2 | 6.3 | >200 | >200 | 6.2 | 7.3 | >20 | 0.5 | 0.5 |
| 8 | 48.8 | 57.5 | 11.2 | 9.9 | 9.8 | >200 | >200 | >20 | >20 | | 4.0 | 0.8 |
| 9 | 8.0 | 8.6 | 4.5 | 4.3 | 4.8 | | 164 | 18.4 | >20 | | 9.4 | 0.6 |
| 10 | 4.0 | 3.8 | 3.7 | 3.3 | 3.0 | | 124 | 10.0 | 12.4 | | 3.4 | 0.5 |

[a]Penicillin-resistant strain.
[b]Methicillin-resistant strain.
[c]Non-$\beta$-lactamase-producing strain.
[d]MIC ($\mu$g/ml) by gradient plate assay.

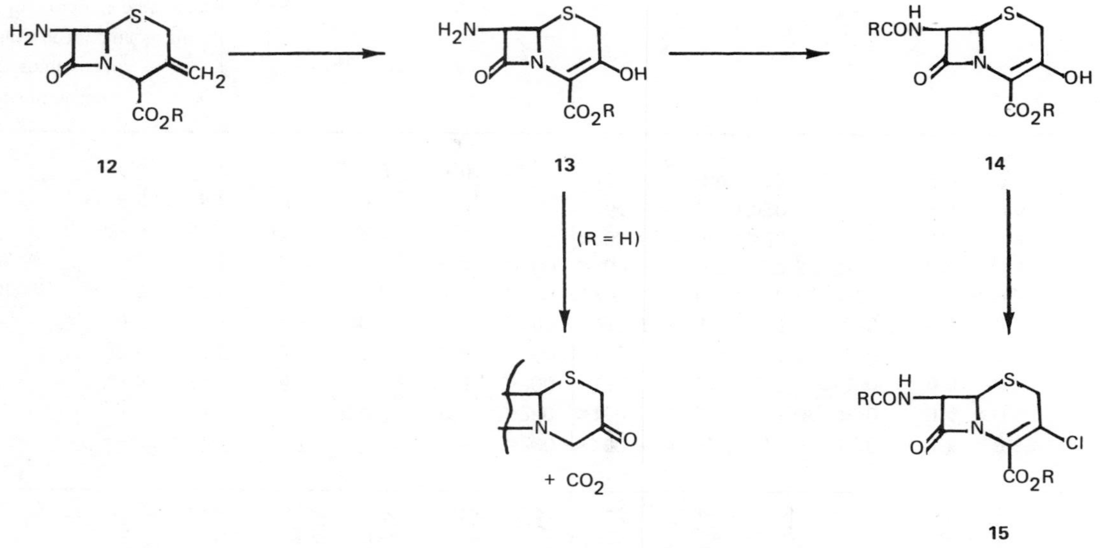

**Figure 8.** Conversion of 3-exomethylenecepham to 3-chlorocepham.

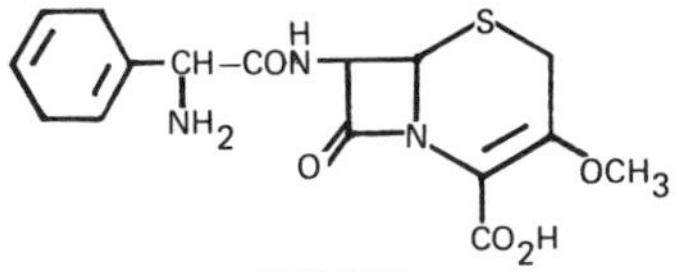

CGP 9000

**Figure 9.**   Cefroxadine

tended to improve but activity against gram-negative bacteria was drastically decreased. CGP 9000 (Figure 9) is currently being investigated clinically, and the results of these studies are reported by Zak *et al.*[34]

The reaction of 3-hydroxycephems with *p*-toluenesulfonyl chloride led to the 3-*p*-toluenesulfonate that could be converted into a number of 3-thioethers. Scartazzini and associates[33] reported that the thiomethyl ether was most active, and its activity was comparable to the 3-methoxy compounds described above. Stability of the sulfur derivatives was inferior to the oxygen series. Several 3-*N*-acyl compounds were prepared and tested. The 3-amino, like the 3-hydroxycephems, decarboxylated upon ester removal. The 3-substituted nitrogen derivatives were less active than the other series mentioned.

Spry,[35] in a series of studies, utilized the 3-aldehyde prepared from 7-ACA (Figure 10) to make the acid esters and amides at C-3. The amides could be rearranged into isocyanates and converted to 3-nitrogen-substituted compounds. Of this series, the 3-methyl esters were similar to the 7-ACA derivatives against gram-negative organisms but much less active against *Staphylococcus* species. All other derivatives in this series were much less active than the 3-methyl esters.

Reduction of a variety of 3-substituted cephalosporins, for example the 3-chloro derivative with zinc and acid, led to the 3-hydrogen cephem. While this series of compounds turned out to be as active as the 3-chlorocephems, they are too unstable in aqueous solution for practicality.

## 5.   CEFALCOR: A NEW ORALLY EFFECTIVE CEPHALOSPORIN
### 5.1   3-Position Direct-Substituted Cephalosporins
With the knowledge that 3-hydroxycephems could be obtained in reasonable laboratory yields and subsequently substituted at the 3-position with other functionality, it was of prime interest to look at the structure-activity relationships of the resulting antibiotics.

*N*-Acylation of the 3-hydroxy-3-cephem nucleus ester **13** (Figure 8) was best accomplished in aqueous media. For example, an acid chloride in dry solvent added dropwise to **13** in an aqueous-tetrahydrofuran solution containing sodium bisulfite gave good yields of the 7-aceylamido-3-hydroxy-3-cephem esters **14**.

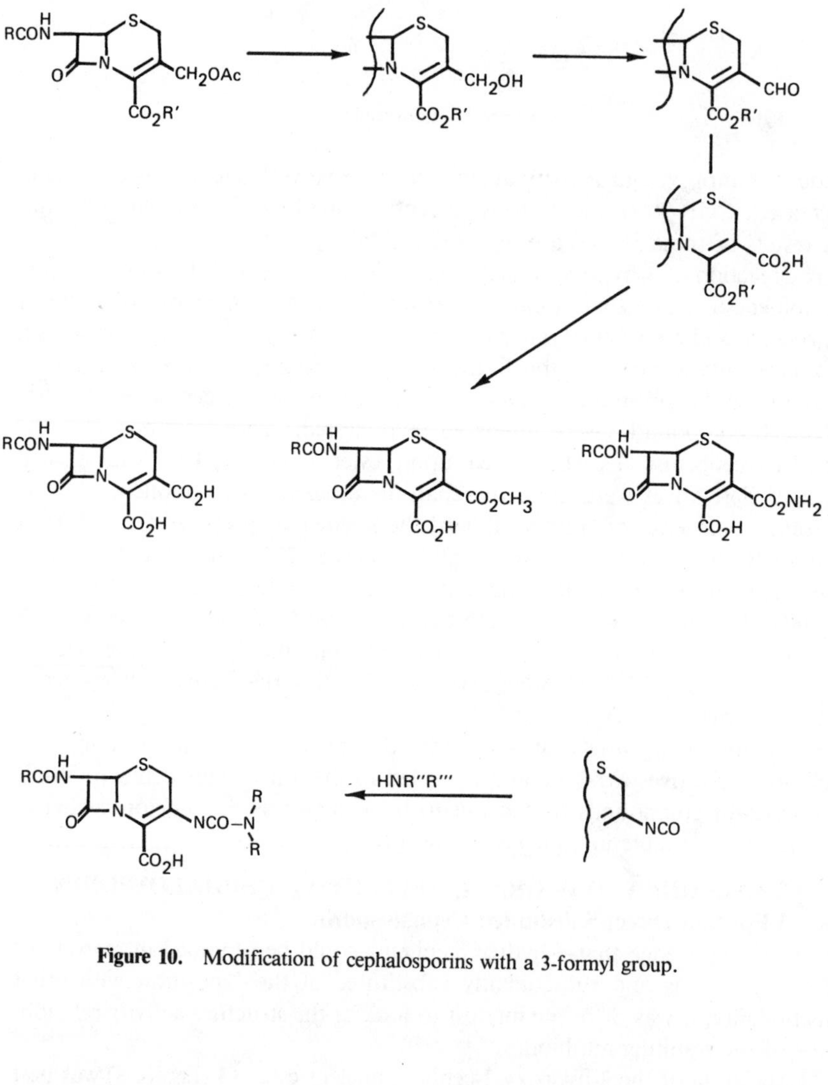

**Figure 10.** Modification of cephalosporins with a 3-formyl group.

These esters were converted to their 3-chloro derivatives under Vilsmeier conditions. Thus, 7-acylamido-3-hydroxy-3-cephem esters **14** in dry dimethylformamide with excess $PCl_3$, freshly distilled $SOCl_2$, or $COCl_2$, at room temperature for 4 hours, gave 7-aceylamido-3-chloro-3-cephem esters **15** in moderate yields.

This series of chemical transformations allowed Chauvette and Pennington[32] to prepare and evaluate a wide variety of new antibiotics containing the new 3-chloro functionality. The biological testing results for a selected group of compounds are described in the next section.

Table 6 shows the activity for a variety of 3-chlorocephem acids. With non-phenylglycyl side chains, the *in vitro* antibiotic activity appeared unimproved over that of the corresponding 7-ACA derivative (e.g., in Table 6, compare compounds **1** and **6**). In particular, activity against penicillinase-producing *Staphylococcus* strains was generally less than that for the 7-ACA derivative. Invariably, better activity was seen in the 3-chloro series than in the 3-methyl antibiotics (compare compounds **5** and **7** in Table 6). These observations indicated that if oral effectiveness was attainable with a 3-chloro compound, then an orally effective cephalosporin would be available with potency superior to that of cephalexin. This was in fact observed. Qualitatively, the pharmacokinetic properties and metabolic stability of cefaclor was equivalent to cephalexin. Thus the superior microbiology of cefaclor provided a drug with certain clinical advantages over earlier oral cephalosporins.

It is beyond the scope of this chapter to detail all the 3-position variations that have been prepared and investigated. Suffice it to mention one additional compound that has received special attention. That material, known as nitrocefin (Figure 11), was prepared at Glaxo[36] and graciously supplied by them to many investigators worldwide. It is used to detect the presence of $\beta$-lactamase enzymes. The compound is prepared from the 3-aldehyde (Figure 10). When placed in the presence of a wide variety of $\beta$-lactamase enzymes the $\beta$-lactam ring opens rapidly, giving rise to a distinct color change from yellow to red. The compound has proved to be very useful in microbiological research.

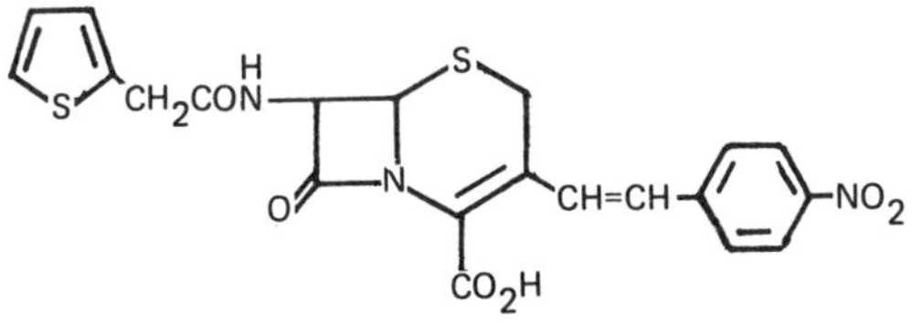

**Figure 11.**   Nitrocefin.

**Table 7**
*In Vitro* **Antibacterial Spectra**

| Bacteria | Minimal inhibitory concentration ($\mu$g/ml) | |
| --- | --- | --- |
| | Cefaclor | Cephalexin |
| *Streptococcus pyogenes* | 0.25 | 0.5 |
| *Streptococcus pneumoniae* | 2.0 | 4.0 |
| *Streptococcus* sp. (Group D) | 64.0 | >128.0 |
| *Staphylococcus aureus* (Benzylpenicillin-susceptible) | 0.5 | 1.0 |
| *Staphylococcus aureus* (Penicillinase-producing) | 2.0 | 2.0 |
| *Haemophilus influenzae* | 4.0 | 16.0 |
| *Escherichia coli* | 1.0 | 4.0 |
| *Klebsiella pneumoniae* | < 0.5 | 4.0 |
| *Proteus mirabilis* | 1.0 | 8.0 |
| *Salmonella typhosa* | < 0.5 | 2.0 |
| *Shigella flexneri* | 2.0 | 4.0 |

## 5.2  Microbiological Studies with Cefaclor

Initial studies on the 7-phenylglycyl derivative of 3-chloro cephalosporanic acid (cefaclor) were very encouraging. When a number of strains of pathogenic bacteria were used, the data shown in Table 7 were obtained and are representative of the difference in activity between cefaclor and cephalexin. Of particular interest was the improved activity against *Haemophilus influenzae,* determined by Kammer et al.[7] *H. influenzae,* a bacterium, is responsible for serious infections in very young and very old patients, and many of its strains have acquired a penicillinase enzyme that renders them resistant to penicillins previously used to treat such infections. Preston[38] found that both penicillin-resistant and penicillin-sensitive strains of this organism are sensitive to cefaclor.

During the clinical evaluation of cefaclor many studies of cefaclor vs. cephalexin were carried out. While the MIC value needed to inhibit 100% of the organisms varied with the individual clinical study, invariably cefaclor was more active, generally by two to three dilutions. A comparative study (Table 8) by Shadomy et al.[39] clearly showed the microbiological advantages of cefaclor

## Table 8
### Comparative Susceptibility of
### Gram-Positive and Gram-Negative Organisms

| Microorganism<br>(number of strains tested) | Antibiotic | Geometric mean MIC<br>($\mu$g/ml) |
|---|---|---|
| *Staphylococcus aureus* (25) | Cefaclor | 2.17 |
| | Cephalexin | 1.74 |
| | Cephradine | 1.52 |
| *Streptococcus pyogenes* (20) | Cefaclor | 0.11 |
| | Cephalexin | 0.35 |
| | Cephradine | 0.19 |
| *Streptococcus pneumoniae* (16) | Cefaclor | 0.24 |
| | Cephalexin | 0.87 |
| | Cephradine | 0.52 |
| *Escherichia coli* (25) | Cefaclor | 1.94 |
| | Cephalexin | 2.87 |
| | Cephradine | 10.8 |
| *Klebsiella pneumoniae* (21) | Cefaclor | 0.82 |
| | Cephalexin | 6.35 |
| | Cephradine | 9.43 |
| *Proteus mirabilis* (24) | Cefaclor | 2.59 |
| | Cephalexin | 16.5 |
| | Cephradine | 21.4 |

against many clinical isolates of cephalosporin-susceptible gram-negative bacteria. Thus, for 70 strains of *E. coli, K. pneumoniae,* and *P. mirabilis* (Table 8), cefaclor showed a clear microbiological superiority.

A number of studies have been carried out on the susceptibility of cefaclor to hydrolysis by different $\beta$-lactamses. It was not particularly stable to these enzymes relative to other orally effective cephalosporins; in many cases it was hydrolyzed more rapidly. This rate of hydrolysis did not appear to have an adverse effect on its minimum inhibitory concentration (MIC) when studied by Neu and Fu.[40] A similar effect against *Enterobacter* was observed by Ott *et*

Table 9
Efficacy of Orally Active Cephalosporins
in Mouse Infections

| | Strep. pyogenes | | Strep. pneumoniae | | E. coli | |
|---|---|---|---|---|---|---|
| | MIC | Oral ED$_{50}^a$ | MIC | Oral ED$_{50}$ | MIC | Oral ED$_{50}$ |
| Cefaclor | 0.25 | 0.74 | 2.0 | 17.6 | 1.0 | 5.5 |
| Cephalexin | 0.5 | 2.3 | 4.0 | 74 | 8.0 | 12.6 |
| Cephaloglycin | 0.25 | 3.6 | 1.0 | 34.0 | 1.0 | 38.0 |

[a]Median effective dose (mg/kg/dose given 1 and 5 hours after bacterial challenge).

al.,[41] using other cephalosporins such as cefamandole and cefoxitin. The reason for this apparent anomaly is obscure at present; perhaps the rate of killing or the effectiveness of inhibition of penicillin-binding proteins are involved.

The efficiency contributed by the superior potency of cefaclor in curing infections in mice was demonstrated by a comparison of cefaclor with cephalexin and cephaloglycin, reported by Preston and Wick[42] and shown in Table 9. Invariably, oral administration to mice infected with organisms of equal MIC values gave lower ED$_{50}$ values with cefaclor than with cephaloglycin. A comparison of the efficacy of cefaclor and cephalexin or ampicillin in a variety of model bacterial infections in mice is shown in Table 10, as reported by Wise,[43] Sanders,[44] and Silver et al.[45] Little difference exists in the pharmacokinetic behavior of cefaclor administered to mice orally or subcutaneously.[46] A study by Spyker et al.[47] indicated that for patients without serious renal impairment the kinetics of cefaclor and cephalexin are similar.

### 5.3  The Preparation of Cefaclor from Penicillin
Even the preliminary biological evaluation of cefaclor indicated many desirable features for this molecule and made it possible to predict that it would perform well clinically. Initially, the material for these studies was prepared, as indicated earlier, from derivatives of 7-ACA via chemical or electrochemical conversion of the acetoxylmethyl group to a 3-exomethylene functionality. In fact, several kilograms of cefaclor were prepared by this cumbersome route. About 50 kg of 7-ACA were required to prepare the first kilogram of cefaclor. The decision to proceed with a complete clinical evaluation of cefaclor was made at Eli Lilly and Company without the assurance of ever being able to produce enough of this compound at a realistic enough cost for commercial use.

**Table 10**

**Efficacy of Oral Cephalosporins in Protection of Mice
from Experimental Bacterial Infections**

| Infecting bacteria | Cefaclor | | Cephalexin | |
|---|---|---|---|---|
| | $ED_{50}{}^a$ | $MIC^b$ | $ED_{50}$ | MIC |
| *Streptococcus pyogenes* C203 | 1.3 | 0.25 | 3.3 | 0.5 |
| *Streptococcus pneumoniae* BI-343 | 2.0 | 0.25 | 22.4 | 1.0 |
| *Streptococcus pneumoniae* BI-492 | 1.7 | 0.25 | 16.5 | 1.0 |
| *Streptococcus pneumoniae* ATCC 6301 | 3.9 | 0.25 | 24.1 | 0.5 |
| *Streptococcus pneumoniae* Park I | 5.3 | 2.0 | 71 | 0.5 |
| *Staphylococcus aureus* 3055 (PS$^c$) | 0.08 | 1.0 | 0.34 | 1.0 |
| *Staphylococcus aureus* 3074 (PR$^d$) | 15.3 | 2.0 | 7.5 | 2.0 |
| *Proteus mirabilis* PR6 | 4.5 | 1.0 | 46 | 8.0 |
| *Salmonella typhi* SA12 | 4.5 | 0.5 | 11 | 2.0 |
| *Escherichia coli* EC14 | 5.5 | 1.0 | 12.6 | 8.0 |
| | Cefaclor | | Ampicillin | |
| *Haemophilus influenzae* C.L. (−) | 2.2 | 2.0 | 1.3 | 0.5 |
| *Haemophilus influenzae* R259 (+) | 8.1 | 4.0 | 242 | 64 |
| *Haemophilus influenzae* 46 (+) | 30.2 | 4.0 | 333 | 64 |

$^a$Median effective dose, mg/kg x 2.

$^b$Minimum inhibitory concentraton, $\mu g/ml$.

$^c$Penicillin G-susceptible strain.

$^d$Penicillin G-resistant strain.

In the evaluation of possible long-term approaches to this synthesis, it appeared that the best chance of success would be to follow the path that had been successful for the manufacture of cephalexin, that is, to start with a penicillin. In principle, a rearrangement of penicillin to a 3-exomethylene-cephem followed by ozonolysis and chlorination would work (Figure 12). In the early work of Morin and Jackson[48] on their penicillin rearrangement, a very minor product (<1%) was found to be the exomethylene compound. Many efforts were carried out in the Lilly Research Laboratories to increase the yield of this product, but quantities greater than 15-20% of exomethylene were not ob-

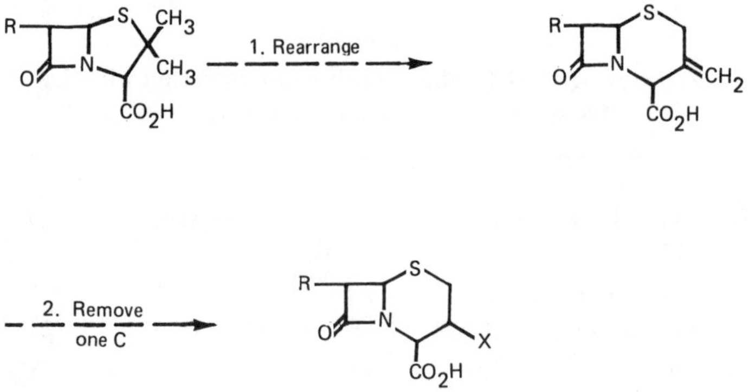

**Figure 12.** A concept for the preparation of cefaclor.

tained by a "sulfenic" acid intermediate type of ring expansion. Recently Gordon and Cimarusti[49] reported higher yields in this type of ring expansion using photochemical initiated ring closures. The decision was to look at a different ring expansion. A useful model for this chemistry was discovered by Kukolja and Lammert,[50] as shown in Figure 13. They found that the treatment of esters of phthalimido penicillin sulfoxide with sulfuryl chloride yielded the relatively stable sulfinyl chloride. With organic bases this intermediate ring closed in good yields to the deacetoxycephem sulfoxide. Subsequently,

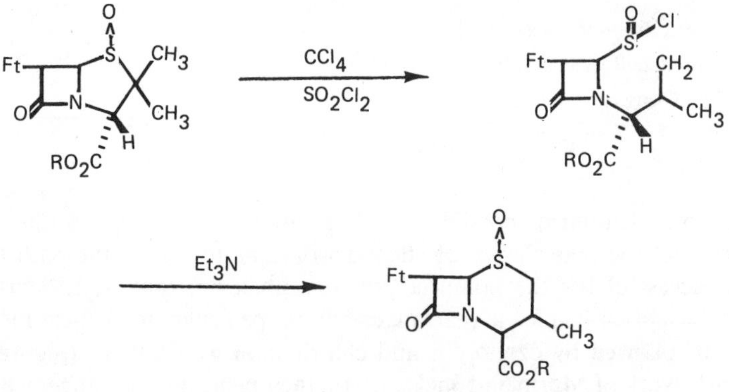

**Figure 13.** Preparation of 7-ADCA compounds by an alternative penicillin rearrangement.

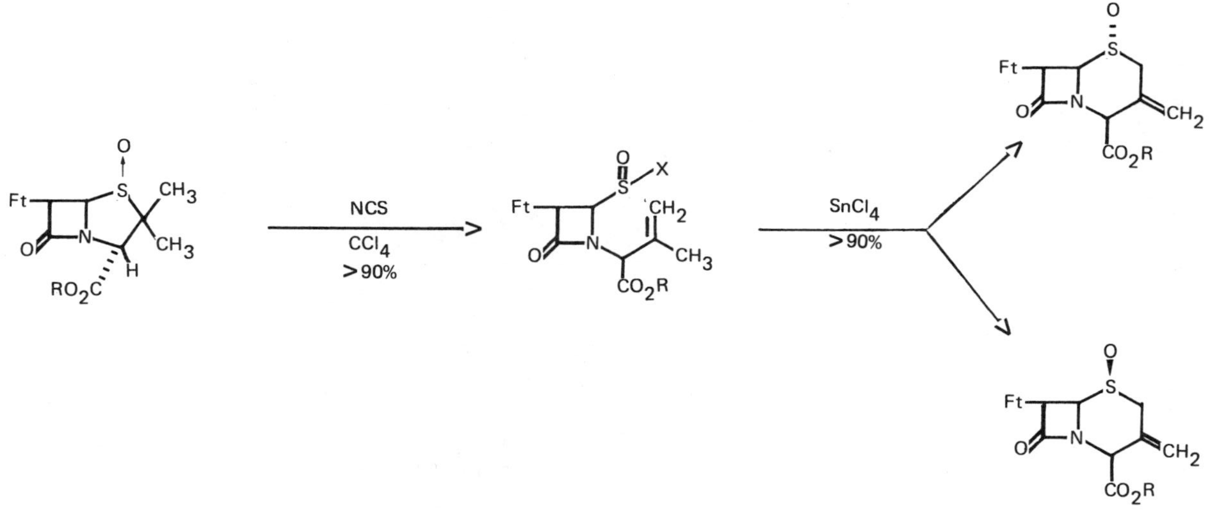

**Figure 14.** Preparation of 3-exomethylenecepham by acid ring closure of sulfinyl chlorides. Ft = phthalimido; R = CH, p-NB; X = Cl.

81

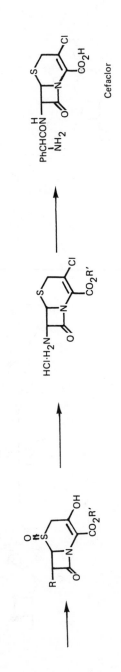

**Figure 15.** Cefaclor from penicillin. Lewis acids: TiCl₄, AlCl₃, ZnCl₂, ZnBr₂, SbCl₄, HgCl₂, FeCl₃, ZrCl₄, SnCl₄, etc. R′ = various acid-protective groups.

82

Kukolja[51] postulated that the sulfinyl group and the double bond were in the position necessary for ring closure and that perhaps with acid-catalyzed cyclization conditions the 3-exomethylene product might be obtained. Lewis acids were investigated and, as shown in Figure 14, two products were obtained. Kukolja and coworkers[52] reported both of these to be 3-exomethylenecephams with differing stereochemical arrangements of the sulfoxide.

When the reaction was tried on naturally occurring penicillin amides as their sulfoxide esters, it was found that somewhat more rigorous conditions were necessary. Higher temperatures (i.e., refluxing toluene) and an acid scavenger such as propylene oxide or calcium oxide,* to prevent side reactions, were required to obtain good yields of the 3-exomethylene sulfoxides upon ring closure (Figure 15).

The product of this new ring enlargement could be ozonized, then reduced, and chlorinated and the amide cleaved in a one-pot reaction with a variety of phosphorous halides. The hydrochloride of the 3-chloro nucleus ester was isolated and acylated with the appropriately derivatized phenylglycine derivative. Deblocking and recrystallization yielded cefaclor in an acceptable yield overall.

In addition to the successful use of 3-methylene sulfoxide in the manufacture of cefaclor, Koppel and coworkers[53] have shown that this key intermediate can be used in the preparation of other commercially important 3'-substituted cephalosporins.

Hamashima et al.,[54] Pfaendler et al.,[55] and Gosteli[56] subsequently reported several alternative methods for preparing 3-substituted cephems from penicillin.

## 6.  CONCLUSION

An extensive clinical trial of cefaclor was carried out. Overall, the compound has lived up to expectations based on animal studies. Few side effects were seen. Of more than 3,000 patients, the total percentage of side effects of any sort was only 3.9 and the drug needed to be discontinued in fewer than 2% of the patients to whom it was administered. Cefaclor is usually active against the following organisms *in vitro* and in clinical infections: *Streptococcus pyogenes, Staphylococci, S. pneumoniae, Escherichia coli, Proteus mirabilis, Klebsiella* species, and *Haemophilus influenzae.* As in the case with other orally administered β-lactam antibiotics, strains of *Pseudomonas, Acinetobacter, S. faecalis* (group D), *Enterobacter,* indole-positive *Proteus,* and *Serratia* species are resistant to cefaclor.

*T.S. Chou, U.S. Patent 4,165,316 (1979).

Thus, by a combination of factors that involved the discovery of several new chemical reactions for altering older cephalosporins and penicillins, a valuable new agent, cefaclor (CECLOR, Lilly), is available for the treatment of many infections.

## REFERENCES

1. G. Brotzu, *Lavori dell'instituto D'Igiene di Cagliari* (1948).
2. E. P. Abraham and G. G. F. Newton, *Biochem. J.,* **79,** 377 (1961).
3. B. Loder, G. G. F. Newton, and E. P. Abraham, *Biochem. J.,* **79,** 408 (1961).
4. B. Witkop, in C. B. Anfinsen, M. L. Anson, K. Bailey, and J. T. Edsall, Eds., *Advances in Protein Chemistry,* Vol. 16, 1961, p. 274.
5. R. B. Morin, B. G. Jackson, E. H. Flynn, and R. W. Roeske, *J. Am. Chem. Soc.,* **84,** 3400 (1962); R. B. Morin, B. G. Jackson, E. H. Flynn, R. W. Roeske, and S. L. Andrews, *J. Am. Chem. Soc.,* **91,** 1396 (1969).
6. B. Fechtig, H. Peter, H. Bickel, and E. Vischer, *Helv. Chim. Acta,* **51,** 1108 (1968).
7. R. R. Chauvette, E. H. Flynn, B. G. Jackson, E. R. Lavagnino, R. B. Morin, R. A. Mueller, R. P. Pioch, R. W. Roeske, C. W. Ryan, J. L. Spencer, and E. Van Heyningen, *J. Am. Chem. Soc.,* **84,** 3401 (1962).
8. E. P. Abraham and G. G. F. Newton in *Amino Acids, Peptides, Antimetabolic Activity,* Ciba Foundation Symposium, 1958, pp. 205-222, C. W. Hale, G. G. F. Newton, and E. P. Abraham, *Biochem. J.,* **79,** 403 (1961).
9. K. Kariyone, H. Harada, M. Kurita, and T. Takano, *J. Antibiot.,* **23,** 131 (1970).
10. M. Finland, D. Kaye, and M. Turck, Eds., *J. Infect. Dis.,* **128** (Suppl.) S312-S424 (1973).
11. J. L. Strominger, in T. Bucher and H. Sies, Eds., *Inhibitors: Tools in Cell Research,* Springer-Verlag, 1969, pp. 187-207.
12. D. B. Boyd and W. H. W. Lunn, *J. Med. Chem.,* **22,** 778 (1979).
13. F. P. Doyle, G. R. Fosker, J. H. C. Nayler, and H. Smith, *J. Chem. Soc.,* 1440 (1962).
14. T. Bergan, in H. Schonfeld, Ed., *Antibiotic Chemotherapy,* Vol. 25, 1978, p. 1.
15. J. L. Spencer, E. H. Flynn, R. W. Roeske, F. Y. Siu, and R. R. Chauvette, *J. Med. Chem.,* **9,** 746 (1966); R. B. Morin, U.S. Patent, 3,560,489.
16. J. M. Brogard, F. Comte, and M. Pinget, in H. Schoenfeld, Ed., *Antibiotic Chemotherapy,* Vol. 25, 1978, pp. 123-162.
17. S. Kukolja, *J. Med. Chem.,* **11,** 1067 (1968).
18. R. J. Stedman, K. Swered, and J. R. E. Hoover, *J. Med. Chem.,* **7,** 117 (1964).
19. R. B. Morin, B. G. Jackson, R. A. Mueller, E. R. Lavagnino, W. B. Scanlon, and S. L. Andrews, *J. Am. Chem. Soc.,* **91,** 1401 (1969).
20. C. W. Ryan, R. L. Simon, and E. M. Van Heyningen, *J. Med. Chem.,* **12,** 310 (1969).
21. T. S. Chou, J. R. Burgtorf, A. I. Ellis, S. R. Lammert, and S. P. Kukolja, *J. Am. Chem. Soc.,* **96,** 1609 (1974).
22. M. Yoshida, T. Konomi, M. Kohsaka, J. E. Baldwin, S. Herchen, P. Singh, N. A. Hunt, and A. L. Demain, *Proc. Natl. Acad. Sci. USA,* **75,** 6253 (1978).
23. R. R. Chauvette, P. A. Pennington, C. W. Ryan, R. D. G. Cooper, F. L. Jose, I. G. Wright, E. M. Van Heyningen, and G. W. Huffman, *J. Org. Chem.,* **36,** 1259 (1971).

24. G. L. Dunn, D. A. Berges, J. R. E. Hoover, J. J. Taggert, L. D. Davis, E. M. Dietz, D. R. Jakas, J. S. Frazee, T. Y. W. Jen, P. Actor, J. V. Uri, and J. A. Weisbach, 15th Interscience Conference on Antimicrobial Agents and Chemotherapy, September 24-26, 1975, Washington, D.C., Abstr. No. 259.
25. P. Actor, J. V. Uri, L. Phillips, C. S. Sachs, J. R. Guarini, I. Zajac, D. A. Berges, G. L. Dunn, J. R. E. Hoover, and J. A. Weisbach, *J. Antibiot.,* **28,** 594 (1975).

26.  R. R. Chauvette and P. A. Pennington, *J. Org. Chem.*, **38**, 2994 (1973).
27.  J. D. Cocker, S. Eardley, G. I. Gregory, M. E. Hall, and A. G. Long, *J. Chem. Soc., C,* 1142 (1966).
28.  R. R. Chauvette, H. B. Hayes, G. L. Huff, and P. A. Pennington, *J. Antibiot.*, **25**, 248 (1972).
29.  D. A. Hall, *J. Pharm. Sci.*, **62**, 980 (1973); D. A. Hall, D. M. Berry, and C. J. Schneider, *J. Electroanal. Chem.*, **80**, 155 (1977).
30.  D. O. Spry, *Tetrahedron Lett.*, 165 (1973).
31.  M. Gorman and C. W. Ryan, in E. H. Flynn, Ed., *Cephalosporins and Penicillins: Chemistry and Biology,* Academic Press, New York, 1972, pp. 532-582.
32.  R. R. Chauvette and P. A. Pennington, *J. Med. Chem.*, **18**, 403 (1975).
33.  R. Scartazzini and H. Bickel, *Helv. Chim. Acta,* **57**, 1919 (1974); R. Scartazzini and H. Bickel, *Heterocycles,* **7**, 1165 (1977).
34.  O. Zak, W. A. Vischer, C. Schenk, W. Tosch, W. Zimmerman, J. Regos, E. R. Suter, F. Kradolfer, and J. Gelzer, *J. Antibiot.*, **29**, 653 (1976).
35.  D. O. Spry, *J. Chem. Soc. Chem. Commun.,* 1012 (1974); D. O. Spry, *J. Org. Chem.*, **40**, 2411 (1975).
36.  C. H. O'Callaghan and P. W. Muggleton, in E. H. Flynn, Ed., *Cephalosporins and Penicillins: Chemistry and Biology,* Academic Press, New York, 1972, pp. 438-495.
37.  R. B. Kammer, D. A. Preston, J. R. Turner, and L. C. Hawley, *Antimicrob. Agents Chemother.,* **8**, 91 (1975).
38.  D. A. Preston, *Postgrad. Med. J.,* **55**, (Suppl. 4), 22 (1979); D. A. Preston, 16th Interscience Conference on Antimicrobial Agents and Chemotherapy, October 27-29, 1976, Chicago, Abstr. No. 352.
39.  S. Shadomy, C. G. Mayhall, and E. Apollo, *J. Infect. Dis.,* **136**, 697 (1977).
40.  H. C. Neu and K. P. Fu, *Antimicrob. Agents Chemother.,* **13**, 584 (1978).
41.  J. L. Ott, J. R. Turner, and D. F. Mahoney, *Antimicrob. Agents Chemother.,* **15**, 14 (1979).
42.  D. A. Preston and W. E. Wick, 14th Interscience Conference on Antimicrobial Agents and Chemotherapy, September 11-13, 1974, San Francisco, Abstr. No. 426.
43.  R. Wise, *J. Antimicrob. Chemother.,* **4**, 578 (1978).
44.  C. C. Sanders, *Antimicrob. Agents Chemother.,* **12**, 490 (1977).
45.  M. S. Silver, G. W. Counts, D. Zeleznik, and M. Turck, *Antimicrob. Agents Chemother.,* **12**, 591 (1977).
46.  W. E. Wright, unpublished work (1975).
47.  D. A. Spyker, B. L. Thomas, M. A. Sande, and W. K. Bolton, *Antimicrob. Agents Chemother.,* **14**, 172 (1978).
48.  R. B. Morin and B. G. Jackson, unpublished work (1962).
49.  E. M. Gordon and C. M. Cimarusti, *Tetrahedron Lett.,* 3425 (1977).
50.  S. Kukolja and S. R. Lammert, *Angew. Chem. Int. Ed. Engl.,* **12**, 67 (1973).
51.  S. Kukolja, in J. Elks, Ed., *Recent Advances in the Chemistry of β-Lactam Antibiotics,* The Chemical Society, London, 1977, pp. 181-188.
52.  S. Kukolja, S. R. Lammert, M. R. B. Gleissner, and A. I. Ellis, *J. Am. Chem. Soc.,* **98**, 5040 (1976).
53.  G. A. Koppel, M. D. Kinnick, and L. J. Nummy, in J. Elks, Ed., *Recent Advances in β-Lactam Antibiotics,* The Chemical Society, London, 1977, pp. 101-110.
54.  Y. Hamashima, K. Ishikura, H. Ishitobi, H. Itani, T. Kubota, K. Minami, M. Murakami, W. Nagata, M. Narisada, Y. Nishitani, T. Okada, H. Onoue, H. Satoh, Y. Sendo, T. Tsuji, and M. Yoshioka, in J. Elks, Ed., *Recent Advances in β-Lactam Antibiotics,* The Chemical Society, London, 1977, pp. 243-251.
55.  H. R. Pfaendler, P. A. Rossy, J. Gosteli, and R. B. Woodward, *Heterocycles,* **5**, 293 (1976).
56.  J. Gosteli, *Chimia,* **30**, 13 (1976).

# Pyrantel, Morantel, and Oxantel

# 4

James W. McFarland

## 1. INTRODUCTION

If one were to write a textbook example of drug discovery, none could serve better than the story of the pyrantel class of anthelmintic agents. All the elements are there: A recognized need to be filled, the development of a suitable animal disease model, the discovery of a "lead compound" through screening, the steady improvement upon the lead through analogue synthesis, the progression of the ultimate-development candidates through safety and efficacy evaluation studies, and eventual marketing. As such, the story would be straightforward and brief in the telling, but in addition there were significant challenges in formulation and manufacturing which, if not met, would have denied medical and veterinary practice the benefits of these new agents. There was the unexpected discovery of oxantel, which brought an important pathogen into the activity spectrum of this new class of anthelmintics, and there was also a subsequent exciting period of uncovering a remarkably consistent set of structure-activity relationships (SAR) that incorporated the quantitative techniques being developed at the time.

No one individual can possibly have a totally objective view of the important events and of the contributions of the many people involved in the success of a project of this scope. The difficulties in this case are compounded by an ocean separating major components of the research and development team. Therefore, in relating the details of this history, I am forced to take a personal view. As a consequence my contributions are undoubtedly magnified out of proportion while those of others may be diminished. No slight is intended. I only trust that my colleagues in this enterprise will understand that the aim is to

## Table 1
## Major Parasitic Diseases of Humans[a]

| Type | Common name | Genus | Persons afflicted (millions) |
|---|---|---|---|
| Roundworms (nematodes) | Large roundworms | *Ascaris* | 1050 |
| | Hookworms | *Ancylostoma, Necator* | 750 |
| | Whipworms | *Trichuris* | 600 |
| | | *Filarias*[b] | 500 |
| | Pinworms | *Enterobius* | 450 |
| Flatworms (trematodes, cestodes) | Blood flukes | *Schistosoma* | 200 |
| | Tapeworms | *Taenia, Hymenolepis* | 150 |
| Protozoan | Malaria | *Plasmodium* | 150 |

[a]Adapted from estimates given by: (1) O.D. Standen, *Progress in Drug Research,* **19,** 158-165 (1975); (2) L. McGinty, *New Scientist,* 1979, 649.

[b]A blood disease.

share with others the highlights of events that led this class of anthelmintics to clinical success and will forgive me if some of their efforts are unattributed in the brief space allotted here.

## 2.  THE NEED FOR MODERN ANTHELMINTIC AGENTS

Until recently the helminthiases, diseases caused by parasitic worms, have been a relatively neglected class of afflictions, yet hundreds of millions of people are adversely affected. While, in the main, the various helminthiases are not as life-threatening as bacteria-caused diseases, their debilitating effects are far-reaching and result in much human misery. People are directly affected by human parasites, such as hookworms, which cause anemia, and also indirectly by the worm parasites of their domestic animals, which reduce the supply of protein and valuable products like wool and leather. Table 1 lists some of the more important parasitic diseases of humans. Roundworms (nematodes) are by far the leading problem, although they receive less publicity than malaria and schistosomiasis.

In the mid-1950's, where our story properly begins, anthelmintic therapy was far behind that available for bacterial infections. The drug of choice at that time for the widespread human disease caused by hookworms was tetrachloroethylene (having replaced carbon tetrachloride!), while that used for the less debilitating but more prevalent disease caused by large roundworms (ascariasis) was a seven-day course of piperazine, which was only effective in little more than half the cases. Although these drugs lack the potency, breadth of spectrum, and safety that we have become accustomed to in modern drugs, additional difficulties arose from the nature of the patients at risk — mostly poor, uneducated people living in rural areas with inadequate sanitation. Such people are not equipped to pay for treatment yet they cannot afford to go untreated. The debilitating effects of their diseases result in lower productivity, hence less cash is available — clearly a vicious cycle. Compounding the problem even more is that most people with roundworm disease harbor more than one species of parasite, and in those early days with only narrow spectrum anthelmintic agents available, little benefit was to be gained by eliminating one worm species in a patient while leaving other species behind.

In the more developed countries, improved sanitation and the widespread practice of wearing shoes reduce the importance of worm diseases as direct health hazards to the populace. However, these more advanced societies depend heavily upon animals for their food supply. The practice of raising animals under crowded conditions establishes veterinary worm diseases as important factors in limiting the production of meat and other animal products. Merck introduced the first modern anthelmintic, thiabendazole, in 1961.[1] It was only then that hard evidence emerged to demonstrate the economic benefit of controlling the roundworm diseases. A farmer, for example, can recover a modest investment in drugs many times over in increased production. Thus, it became clear in the early 1960s that the development of an anthelmintic agent for veterinary applications was the surest way to enter the market. The hope was that once truly safe, effective agents were established, human applications would follow.

## 3.   DISCOVERY
### 3.1   Animal Disease Models
The search for new anthelmintic agents requires an animal disease model that reflects as accurately as possible the parasite-host relationship of interest in the human or agricultural situation. At the earliest point in our story, there were available some animal models reflecting individual worm disease states, for example the roundworm *Nippostrongylus muris* in the rat and the tapeworm *Hymenolepis nana* in the mouse, but testing compounds against several batteries of this kind is cumbersome, labor intensive, and wasteful of compounds in short supply. At this point John E. Lynch, a bacteriologist, joined Pfizer to establish a tropical disease laboratory. He realized that to make rapid progress, a more efficient screen would have to be developed. He considered first that a

mouse nematode would be preferable to *N. nuris*, whose rat host would require 10 times as much material for screening. From a suggestion in the literature he focused on developing a mouse model employing the nematode *Nematospiroides dubius*. *N dubius* establishes itself in the duodenum, a region of the mouse gastrointestinal tract unaffected by *H. nana*, which is generally found farther down in the small intestine. It occurred to Lynch that not only could both infections be established in the same mouse but there was an additional bonus of a natural infection of the pinworm *Syphacia obvelata* in the cecum. Thus, the Triple Infection Screen was created, allowing Pfizer to detect in one operation compounds active against both roundworms and tapeworms.

While it must be admitted that the presence of *H. nana* in the mouse did not lead to the discovery of clinically significant tapeworm activity, it nevertheless played a decisive role in the discovery of whipworm activity amongst pyrantel analogues. How this cestode became involved in the discovery of nematode activity will be related further on.

### 3.2 Screening: Discovery of the Lead Compound

Once the new mouse triple-infection disease model was established, the screening of compounds began. As might be expected from experience in other screening operations, the number of "hits" was exceedingly low. In fact, only one compound emerged in this initial phase that was more than marginally active. This was 2-(2-thiophenemethylthio)imidazoline hydrochloride, **1**, the adduct of 2-chloromethylthiophene and 2-imidazolidinethione (see Scheme 1).

In retrospect we were extremely lucky to have made this discovery, because animal disease models are often imperfect guides to what is to be expected in the ultimate target disease or diseases. One encounters not only false positives, compounds active in the model but not in the ultimate host, but also false negatives. As it later turned out, our screen as conducted then would not have detected thiabendazole, Merck's landmark discovery in the field of helminthiases. The moral to be drawn from these observations is that the discovery process is limited by the disease models used to screen compounds and that different systems will lead to different discoveries.

For a while it appeared that even the imidazoline **1** may have been a false positive because in the next step of evaluation it showed little activity when administered orally to sheep. However, because it is well established that isothiouronium salts, a chemical class to which **1** belongs, are unstable in aqueous solution, a ready explanation for the lack of activity in the larger host animal was at hand: **1** hydrolyzes to the inactive products 2-thiophenemethane-thiol and 2-imidazolidone (see Scheme 1). This knowledge eventually led to concepts that made pyrantel successful.

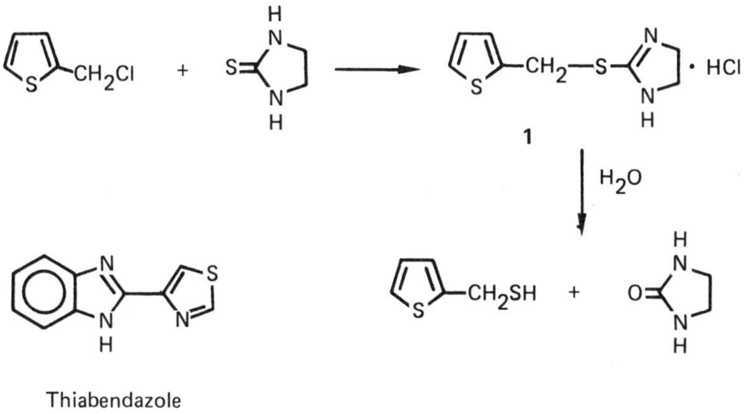

**Thiabendazole**

**Scheme 1**

### 3.3 Organization to Exploit the Lead

During this early discovery phase Pfizer was establishing two new research facilities, one at its principal U.S. manufacturing site in Groton, Connecticut, and the other at its principal overseas manufacturing site in Sandwich, U.K. The Sandwich group also had an interest in anthelmintic agents and had been proceeding along other lines. On a visit to Sandwich, a Groton chemist, Lloyd H. Conover, suggested to his British colleague William C. Austin that they also pursue the isothiouronium lead. Certainly there were plenty of ideas to follow, and an atmosphere of friendly rivalry might be just the motivation needed to achieve the goal more quickly.

It was during this period that Harold L. Howes, Jr., and I joined the project team in Groton, he as a parasitologist reporting to Lynch and I as a chemist reporting to Conover. Throughout the entire discovery phase of the work, the Groton part of the team remained basically Howes and myself as the laboratory professionals, but we received timely contributions from others at critical points. To mention two: Phillip N. Gordon, who made the initial observation on the light instability of pyrantel, and Ernest J. Bianco, who as a principal chemist in the large-scale-preparations laboratory supplied bulk amounts of pyrantel and its more interesting analogues. The Sandwich operation was more heavily manned, and thus they were able to make several key

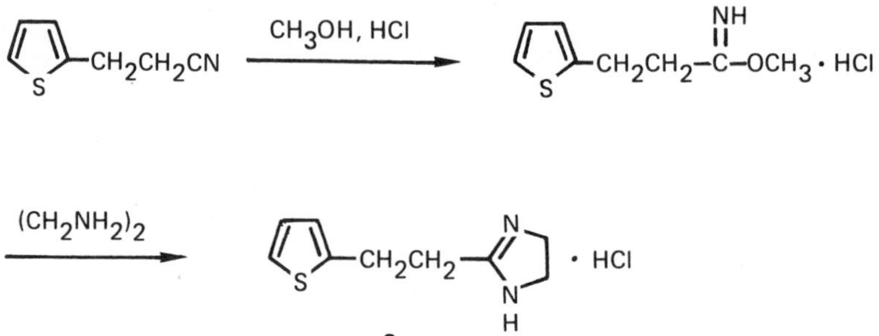

**Scheme 2**

discoveries and exploit them in a timely fashion. Besides Austin some of the principal actors were chemist John C. Danilewicz and parasitologists Rendle L. Cornwell and Mervyn Jones. From the start it was clear that Groton's role was to be secondary and mainly supportive of the Sandwich effort. Nevertheless, much of the Groton work played an important part in later discoveries and in finding the optimum manufacturing process.

### 3.4  The First Stable Analogue

As indicated earlier, one problem with **1** was its instability in aqueous solution. Therefore, the Sandwich group set out initially to determine whether a stable analogue would possess significant anthelmintic activity. Following the Pinner synthesis outlined in Scheme 2 they prepared 2-[2-(2-thienyl)ethyl]imidazoline **2**.

Cornwell and Jones then showed that not only was **2** active against *N. dubius* in mice but it was also active against a variety of roundworm parasites that simultaneously infest sheep. We were on the right track: Stable imidazolines are compatible with broad-spectrum anthelmintic activity in large animals. Unfortunately, the therapeutic index of **2** in sheep is too narrow for practical application.

### 3.5  Pyrantel

At this point we decided to explore the SAR in this series of compounds by generalizing the activity as belonging to chemical structures defined by **3** where Ar is an aromatic ring system, X a linkage of atoms to the cyclic amidine system, and R a substituent, either alkyl or phenyl. The ring could be either five-membered or six-membered ($n = 2$ or 3).

**3**

Pyrantel tartrate

What we learned was: (1) Other things being equal, the order of decreasing potency for aromatic rings (Ar) is 2-thienyl > 3-thienyl > phenyl > 2-furyl, (2) A compound in the tetrahydropyrimidine system ($n = 3$) is generally more potent than the corresponding compound in the imidazoline system ($n = 2$), (3) When the nitrogen-substituent R is methyl, a more potent analogue results than when R is hydrogen, but any other substitution results in the loss of activity, (4) For optimum potency the link X should consist of two carbon atoms, the order of potency being *trans*-vinylene > ethylene > *cis*-vinylene. The compound that incorporates the best of all these features is, of course, pyrantel. The details of this work are reported elsewhere.[2]

Having reached this stage fairly rapidly and having in hand a compound that was potentially competitive in a now lively and growing market, the project was divided between two major lines of effort. Receiving top priority was the development of pyrantel into a marketable entity. This aspect was expeditiously handled mainly by the Sandwich Research Center, but at this time Pfizer's Agricultural Research and Development facility in Terre Haute, Indiana, also became involved in the already far-flung enterprise. Parasitologist Donal P. Conway was one of the major contributors from our Midwest operation. The second line of effort had to do with exploiting pyrantel as an updated lead compound. The generalized structure **3**, while having served admirably to bring us to pyrantel, was possibly understating the scope of the discovery. Therefore, discovery research had to continue in order to assure ourselves that the most potent analogues were in our hands rather than someone else's.

One of the first extensions made at this point, and the first significant Groton discovery, was the recognition that activity does not solely reside in the imidazoline and tetrahydropyrimidine system. It was found that the simple noncyclic amidine analogue **4** is half as potent as pyrantel itself in the Triple Infection Screen.[3]

However, this hint of other possibilities was soon followed by the discovery of other types deviating significantly from the amidine system.

4                                          5

### 3.6  Dihydrothiazine Analogues

In our early consideration of analogues of the initial lead, we thought that perhaps 2-[2-(2-thienyl)ethyl]thiazoline **5** would show anthelmintic activity even though it was a weaker base than pyrantel by some six orders of magnitude.

This compound was prepared independently — a slight lapse in communication — on both sides of the Atlantic and was found to be inactive in Sandwich and marginally active in Groton. These different tests results were resolved when it was recognized that the British practice of administering test substances in peanut oil was the cause of the problem. When retested in Sandwich using 1% aqueous carboxymethylcellulose as the drug vehicle, the practice in Groton, the compound was active, and in Groton it was inactive when administered in peanut oil. Pursuit of this seemingly trivial point was in fact important because we could easily have been turned away from a major discovery.

Although the thiazolines themselves were only marginally active, we decided to at least determine if the ring homologues were better. That is, Did the same relationship as that between imidazolines and tetrahydropyrimidines hold for thiazolines and dihydrothiazines?

Indeed it did, and to a much greater degree! The first member of the dihydrothiazine series prepared was **6**, and it is twice as potent as pyrantel in the mouse test. However not all the SAR in this new system matched those of the amidines. We anticipated, by analogy, that the more direct pyrantel analog, **7** would be still more potent, but we were disappointed when tests showed it to be only half as potent as pyrantel. Details concerning the SAR of this fascinating group of compounds are published elsewhere.[4] Evaluation in sheep of the better compounds from this group showed that while they are effective, on

6                                          7

balance they offered no real advantage over pyrantel, which continued as the leading development candidate.[5]

However, one major benefit of exploring this group of compounds was the recognition of the Knoevenagel condensation in a new form that had valuable application to the tetrahydropyrimidine series of compounds. In 1954 Kuhn and Drawert[6] reported that benzaldehyde condenses with 2-methylthiazoline to furnish 2-styrylthiazoline:

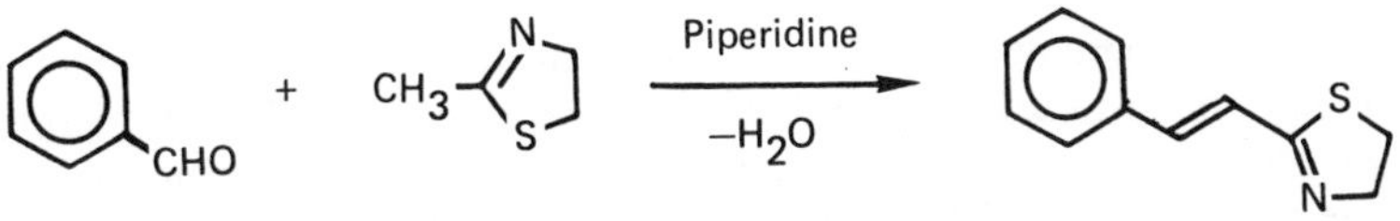

We confirmed this result and found that it works equally well with 2-methyl-1,3(4H)-dihydrothiazine; for example, with 2-thiophenecarbox-aldehyde to give **7**. This observation grew more meaningful when it became apparent that many of the desired compounds in the tetrahydropyrimidine series could not be readily prepared using the Pinner synthesis and that the alternative methods employed at that time were too brutal for some of the more sensitive compounds. Therefore, we prepared 1,4,5,6-tetrahydro-1,2-dimethyl-pyridimine (TDP) and found that it readily condenses with appropriate aldehydes to give pyrantel and its analogues:

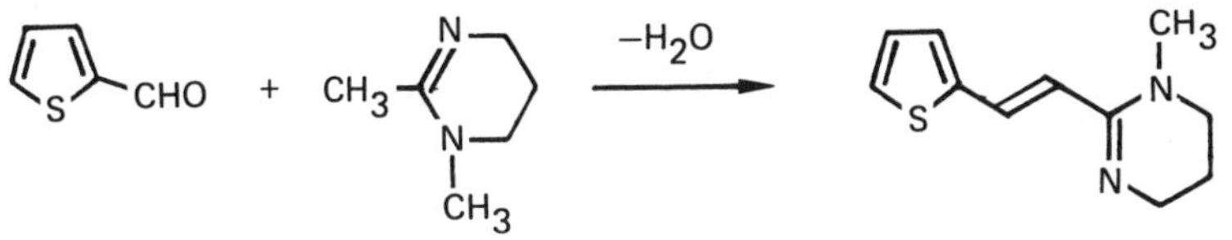

This new process greatly accelerated the discovery phase and eventually led to the ultimate process used in the manufacture of pyrantel and its congeners, morantel and oxantel.

### 3.7  1-(2-Arylvinyl)pyridinium Salts

Through my general reading of the chemical literature during this period, I became aware of a rather interesting class of compounds that bore a striking structural similarity to pyrantel. These were the 1-(2-arylvinyl)pyridinium salts, first described by Kröhnke.[7]

8                                                    9

The specific analogue of interest, **8**, had already been described by King and Brownell,[8] but there was nothing known about the anthelmintic properties of compounds in this class. These compounds are surprisingly easy to prepare, and we quickly learned that **8** is equipotent to pyrantel in the mouse test and that the SARs parallel those in the tetrahydropyrimidine series.[9]

In sheep **8** proved to be much less effective than pyrantel, but the *o*-tolyl analogue **9** was nearly as good.[5] Because there was no advantage in developing **9** at the expense of pyrantel, this series was not pursued further.

### 3.8   Hansch Analysis; Morantel

In 1964 Hansch and Fujita at Pomona College in California published the first full paper on a new method to quantitatively correlate chemical structure with biological activity.[10] This paper attracted the interest of Groton scientists, and an invitation was extended to Corwin Hansch to present a seminar on the new technique. It was a lively and stimulating session. The newness and boldness of approaching structure-activity studies in this fashion raised a great deal of skepticism but also raised hopes of conducting medicinal chemistry research in a more rational way than was prevalent at the time.

My immediate reaction to this seminar was, How ideally suited the pyrantel lead was for exploiting in this manner. We had reached the stage where it was important to understand the effect that substitution in the aromatic ring had upon activity. Here could be a tidy way of rationally selecting key substituents and plotting the course of changes in activity they effected. Twenty or 30 well-selected compounds could do the work that would otherwise require 200 or 300. Straightaway there was a benefit to the Hansch approach: One knew just which substituents to select to obtain a good correlation if there was to be one. The substituents would be those that represented a maximum spread in Hansch's new hydrophobic constant $\pi$ and in Hamett's well-known $\sigma$ constant, which reflects the electronic influences of substituent groups.

Naturally, things did not progress as smoothly as anticipated. A great deal of time had to be spent learning how to talk to computers, understanding the statistical methods employed, and making mistakes until the technique and its pitfalls were familiar to us. In those early days of quantitative structure-activity relationships (QSAR), there was no one to guide us except Hansch, who was a continent away. We quickly learned that with one important exception only "ortho" substitution in the aromatic ring is compatible with anthelmintic activity at reasonable doses. The exception was the compound that was destined to become oxantel.

Even in our earliest attempts at developing QSAR, we saw that there was a parabolic relationship between anthelmintic potency and drug hydrophobicity. At first this relationship was weak (low correlation coefficient) and not statistically significant. But as we persisted in enlarging the number of "ortho"-substituted analogues, the relationship grew stronger. We experimented with a number of electronic parameters as a means of improving the correlation and at different times thought that Hammett's $\sigma$ substituent constant and the group dipole moment ($\mu$) played a significant role in determining potency. These eventually passed away, but in the course of events we got a very good and highly significant correlation in which only the parabolic relationship with hydrophobicity and the nature of the aromatic ring, that is, whether it is benzene or thiophene, are important determinants. The following equation summarizes the results of the analysis:[11]

$$\log \frac{1}{ED_{90}} = -1.64\,\pi^2 + 1.93\,\pi + 0.66\,\delta + 0.88$$

$$n = 12 \quad r^2 = 0.962 \quad s = 0.117 \quad P < 0.0005$$

Table 2 gives the data base that was used to derive the equation and gives the potency values predicted. The analysis shows, among other things, that optimum anthelmintic potency is to be found in a 2-thiophene derivative which is substituted in the 3 ("ortho") position by a group whose $\pi$ constant is approximately 0.6 for example, a methyl group. Such a compound is morantel.

It would be nice to be able to say that the Hansch analysis led us to morantel, but in fact we already vaguely perceived a so-called "ortho methyl" effect among certain pairs of analogues prepared earlier in the synthetic program. Morantel was thus prepared initially on other grounds and was in fact a member of the set used to establish the QSAR.

Morantel hydrochloride              Oxantel hydrochloride

**Table 2**

**Relative Potencies of Some Pyrantel Analogues[a]**

| R | X | $\pi^c$ | $\delta^d$ | $\log(1/ED_{90})^b$ observed[e] | calculated[f] | $\Delta$ |
|---|---|---|---|---|---|---|
| Br | S | 0.75 | 1.0 | 2.16 | 2.07 | 0.09 |
| CH$_3$ | S | 0.68 | 1.0 | 2.08 | 2.10 | -0.02 |
| CH$_3$ | CH = CH | 0.68 | 0.0 | 1.53 | 1.44 | 0.09 |
| Cl | CH = CH | 0.59 | 0.0 | 1.49 | 1.44 | 0.05 |
| H | S | 0.0 | 1.0 | 1.46 | 1.54 | -0.08 |
| C$_2$H$_5$ | S | 1.22 | 1.0 | 1.45 | 1.45 | 0.00 |
| I | CH = CH | 0.92 | 0.0 | 1.25 | 1.26 | -0.01 |
| Br | CH = CH | 0.75 | 0.0 | 1.24 | 1.41 | -0.17 |
| H | CH = CH | 0.0 | 0.0 | 1.00 | 0.88 | 0.12 |
| C$_2$H$_5$ | CH = CH | 1.22 | 0.0 | 0.78 | 0.79 | -0.01 |
| F | CH = CH | 0.01 | 0.0 | 0.76 | 0.90 | -0.14 |
| NO$_2$ | CH = CH | -0.23 | 0.0 | 0.40 | 0.35 | 0.05 |

[a]Adapted from J. W. McFarland, *Progress in Drug Research,* **15**, 123 (1971), used by permission of Birkhaeuser Verlag, Basel.

[b]ED$_{90}$ is the dose causing a 90% reduction of the *Nematospiroides dubius* worm burden in mice. Expressed in mmol/kg.

[c]T. Fujita, J. Iwasa, and C. Hansch, *J. Am. Chem. Soc.,* **86**, 5175 (1964).

[d]Dummy variable to account for unspecified differences between 2-thienyl and phenyl systems.

[e]The values reported in this column occasionally differ from those reported originally;[2] dose response curves were determined for each compound in order to obtain more precise ED$_{90}$'s for this analysis.

[f]Calculated from the equation.

So was this exercise worthwhile? Indeed it was. In the first place even though we would not have missed morantel, we had no assurance that there were no other, more potent analogues to be discovered. The analysis told us that potency is a function of understandable properties and that all of the reasonably possible optimum compounds had been prepared. Thus, the Hansch analysis was a valuable decision tool; it told us when to go on to something else. In the second place, organization of the synthetic program with the view to doing the Hansch analysis allowed us to arrive at our conclusions with the preparation of a relatively small number of compounds. Because it was clear that the same relationships carried over into the dihydrothiazine series and into the 1-(2-arylvinyl)pyridinium salts, the efficiency was passed on to analogues in related classes. Subsequent work in other laboratories has borne out the value of approaching drug discovery in this fashion.[12]

### 3.9 Oxantel

Oxantel comes last in the list of tetrahydropyrimidine discoveries. Up to this point in our story we have been implicitly equating the anthelmintic activity of various compounds with their ability to eliminate *N. dubius* from the mouse. This roundworm serves very well as a general model for a wide variety of nematodes in animals and humans, but it is entirely inadequate for detecting activity against worms in the important genus *Trichuris,* the whipworms.

Whipworms are refractory to treatment. Only 10 years ago a hexylresorcinol enema was the typical therapy resorted to, often without success. In animals, Shell's dichlorvos-impregnated resin pellets are effective, but organophosphates have not been attractive in the treatment of human conditions. Because more than 600 million people suffer from whipworm disease, there is a need for safe, effective agents.

In the course of synthesizing various pyrantel analogues to study the effect of aromatic ring substitution upon anthelmintic potency, we prepared 3-hydroxylstyryl-1-methyl-1,4,5,6-tetrahydropyrimidine (oxantel, as it became known later). Unlike all other *meta-* and *para*-substituted analogues, this compound is active against *N. dubius* although at an $ED_{90}$ ten times that of pyrantel. From the point of view of potency this is an uninteresting compound, but there was another consideration that led Howes, the Groton parasitologist, to pursue oxantel further: Unlike pyrantel or morantel, oxantel is active against the tapeworm *H. nana* in the mouse test. Thinking that this compound might represent a significant broadening of the anthelmintic spectrum in the tetrahydropyrimidine series, Howes decided to evaluate oxantel in a group of dogs that collectively harbored several worm species among which was the tapeworm *Taenia pisiformis*. The bad news from this study was that oxantel has no practical activity against dog tapeworm; the good news was that dogs infested with whipworms were cured. Subsequently, Howes developed a mouse whipworm assay and found oxantel to be very potent. A variety of oxantel analogues have been prepared; a few of these have significant activity, but none is more potent than the parent substance.[13] Although oxantel has a very narrow activity range, it fills an important void in the anthelmintic spectrum of the tetrahydropyrimidines.

### 3.10 Competitive Climate

While pyrantel was being developed a number of other broad-spectrum anthelmintic agents appeared on the scene. One of the more novel structures is Janssen's levamisole. For a long time this was the only other major nonbenzimidazole anthelmintic, and by coincidence its discovery was announced in the same year as pyrantel's.

A number of companies followed Merck's thiabendazole lead; today there is a plethora of benzimidazole anthelmintics (see Table 3).

Pyrantel, morantel, and oxantel do not have any commercial competitors in their own class because Pfizer has pretty much preempted others by its thorough work in defining the scope of their discovery — or so I would like to think. However, there are two instances in which this present series of anthelmintic agents seemingly has influenced others.

Pfizer was exploring the 1-(2-arylvinyl)pyridinium series (see Section 3.7.) in 1966, the year the pyrantel discovery was announced in *Nature*.[14] Apparently, chemists at May and Baker in the U.K. also perceived the analogy between pyrantel and 1-[2-(2-thienyl)vinyl]pyridinium bromide[8] and independently made the same discovery. Pfizer's filing date for the patent application on this group of novel anthelmintic agents precedes that of May Baker's by only 24 days; thus we barely won a race that we did not know we were in.[15,16]

The other case is more recent. In 1977 Merck reported that 2-arylazothiazolines are active anthelmintic agents and that one of these, 2-(*o*-tolylazo)thiazoline **10** is effective against a variety of sheep nematodes.[17] Merck's stated inspiration is the known neuromuscular blocking activity of 2-aminothiazoline, but at least one SAR in this series bears a remarkable

Levamisole hydrochloride

**10**

## Table 3
### Benzimidazole Anthelmintic Agents

| Name | Company | $R_2$ | $R_5$ |
|------|---------|-------|-------|
| Thiabendazole | Merck | 4-Thiazolyl | H- |
| Cambendazole | Merck | 4-Thiazolyl | $i$-$C_3H_7OCONH$- |
| Parbendazole | Smith Kline | $NHCO_2CH_3$ | $n$-$C_4H_9$- |
| Albendazole | Smith Kline | $NHCO_2CH_3$ | $n$-$C_3H_7S$- |
| Oxibendazole | Smith Kline | $NHCO_2CH_3$ | $n$-$C_3H_7O$- |
| Mebendazole | Janssen | $NHCO_2CH_3$ | $C_6H_5CO$- |
| Flubendazole | Janssen | $NHCO_2CH_3$ | 4-$FC_6H_4CO$ |
| Cyclobendazole | Janssen | $NHCO_2CH_3$ | cyclo-$C_3H_5$-CO |
| Oxfendazole | Syntex | $NHCO_2CH_3$ | $C_6H_5S(0)$- |
| Fenbendazole | Hoechst-Roussel | $NHCO_2CH_3$ | $C_6H_5S$- |

similarity to one found in the pyrantel series, the "ortho methyl" effect which is obvious in the most potent member, **10**. The more general structural resemblance to other pyrantel analogues is also obvious, but it must be admitted that the SAR here are somewhat inverted to those found in the Pfizer thiazoline-dihydrothiazine series (see Section 3.6): (1) Among Merck's compounds the thiazolines are more potent than the corresponding dihydrothiazines, and (2) the unsaturated linkage (azo, -N = N-) results in higher potency than the saturated linkage (-NH-NH-).

## 4. Applications
In many instances the recognition of an active new chemical agent is the climax of the drug discovery process; in such cases safety evaluation, formulation, and efficacy studies proceed uneventfully, and thus are part of a familiar routine. But, this is not true of pyrantel and its congeners. As will be chronicled in these final sections, problems relating to the complex nature of parasitic worm diseases, the individual peculiarities of the various hosts of economic importance, the photoinstability of pyrantel and morantel, and palatability became

limiting as to whether a practical product could be developed. Here skills and new concepts in formulation played crucial roles in the successful elaboration of the pyrantel product line.

## 4.1 Sheep

Sheep in the field are normally treated with anthelmintics by drench: a measured dose of fluid containing the active ingredient is squirted down their throats by means of a drenching "gun." The gun has a spigot that can enter the sheep's throat and a hand-operated "trigger" that, when squeezed, pumps the drenching fluid from a large reservoir (e.g., a bucket) by means of tubing into and through the spigot.

At the time pyrantel's development phase began, it was known that the market leader, thiabendazole, is not water soluble, and its drench would of necessity be a suspension. We perceived (but really did not know) that this would result in a certain inconvenience in maintaining uniform drug concentration in the reservoir and possible clogging problems in the drenching gun, or at least necessitate some costly formulation additives to prevent these problems. Therefore, it was considered advantageous to develop pyrantel for sheep as a water-soluble drug, possible giving it an added salable feature.

A variety of acids form water-soluble salts with pyrantel base, so the ultimate choice of the tartrate rested on two practical considerations. The first was the solubility of the salt in very cold water such as might be the case in treating sheep outdoors in the Scottish Highlands on a blustery March day (as opposed to the warm offices and laboratories of the people who make decisions about salts). The second consideration was the ability to recover the salt in a reasonable yield from the production process. It was on these grounds that the tartrate salt was chosen for development.

A major problem arose when the light instability of pyrantel was recognized. A 10 percent aqueous solution of pyrantel tartrate in a standard pail loses activity uncomfortably fast when exposed to direct sunlight. The normally active *trans* isomer is transformed to the very much less potent *cis* isomer. This is one of the most facile photoisomerizations I am aware of: it can be performed in simple Pyrex glassware and does not require artificial UV light sources, filters or sensitizers. A clear laboratory demonstration of this effect has been published.[4] For development purposes this photoinstability problem was solved by packaging the pyrantel drench solution in black polyethylene containers, which are designed to serve also as the reservoirs for the drenching guns once the caps are off. Pyrantel tartrate is sold in many countries as a sheep and goat anthelmintic under the tradename Banminth; morantel tartrate (Banminth II) is the form sold in the large Australian and New Zealand markets.

## 4.2 Cattle

Cattle are quite another matter. Drenching methods can be used, but the problems of handling these larger animals is physically much more difficult. Feed incorporation is an alternative possibility, but this leads to some uncertainty whether some individual cattle are adequately dosed while others in the herd may be overdosed. Pyrantel is not active against intestinal parasites when administered by parenteral routes; therefore other approaches are needed and welcomed.

Pfizer is currently pioneering an entirely new system for controlling helminthiases in grazing cattle. This system prevents parasitic gastroenteritis by providing parasitologically safe pastures throughout the entire grazing season. The key to this system was the development of the first commercially practicable sustained-release bolus for cattle.

Morantel sustained-release bolus (morantel SRB)* is a cylindrical steel device containing morantel tartrate. The steel casing provides the device with sufficient density to prevent regurgitation or passage through the alimentary canal. The ends of the cylinder are closed with polyethylene diffusion disks that provide for the continuous release of effective amounts of morantel into the reticulum/rumen fluid of the animal for at least 60 days. The morantel SRB is administered by means of a specially designed balling gun immediately before grazing starts in the spring. The potent larvicidal action of morantel then prevents the *in vivo* multiplication of parasitic nematodes, which normally occurs after calves are infected early in the season by larvae that have survived the winter. The result is that the level of infective larvae on the pasture remains low throughout the grazing season. A series of trials conducted in Europe showed that administration of the morantel SRB at spring turnout prevented parasitic gastroenteritis through the entire grazing season and resulted in significantly superior body-weight gains over conventionally treated control animals.[18,19]

## 4.3 Swine

In the United States, large roundworm (*Ascaris suum*) is the most important intestinal parasite of swine. Its life cycle is more complex than those of other nematodes generally infesting sheep and thus presents some special problems for treatment. Eggs are ingested with the swine's food; larvae hatch in the small intestine, but instead of simply developing into adults they migrate through the intestinal walls, journey through the liver, lungs, up the trachea, only to be reswallowed. On their second visit to the small intestine the nematodes develop into sexually mature adults. The problem posed by the larvae's curious passage is that, depending on the degree of infestation, the liver becomes damaged and

---

*The trademark of Pfizer, Inc. for the morantel sustained-release bolus is Paratect bolus.

at slaughter may be condemned or may require trimming. This represents a significant economic loss.[20,21] In addition, the migration phase in the lungs results in a "pneumonia" (coughing symptoms), which in some cases weakens the pig and makes it susceptible to other infections.

The problem of ascariasis in swine is thus complex. It is not entirely satisfactory to treat swine once a large roundworm infestation has been detected (eggs in the feces); the damage to the liver has already been done. While it is good to eliminate adult worms from the swine herd to reduce the risk of infection, it is better to prevent infection in the first place. Hence, in considering swine applications, Lynch and Conover became interested in a prophylactic regimen. Early experiments conducted by Vasilios Theodorides in Terre Haute showed that pyrantel, when incorporated in feed, was the most potent by far of anthelmintic agents known at that time in preventing the migratory phase of *Ascaris* larvae. It was later shown that morantel, as might be expected, is nearly four times more potent.[22,23] Pyrantel is now sold as a feed additive for swine as a prophylactic agent to control ascariasis, both as a single agent and in combination with Pfizer's carbadox, an antibacterial agent with highly significant growth-promoting properties.

### 4.4 Horses
With several million horses in the United States alone, it became worthwhile to consider this market. With sheep, cattle, and swine the benefit of treatment must be demonstrated on economic grounds. Horses, however, are used for sport and are already clearly uneconomic. They are treated to maintain good health and appearance. While the potential number of treatments is much smaller than in meat-producing animals, the motivation for treatment is just as high.

Two forms of pyrantel are available for treating horses. The first is pyrantel tartrate (Banminth), which is sold over-the-counter as a top dressing, a dose of the drug diluted with highly nutritious grain. This ration is given to the horse at regular mealtime, and once it is consumed, the rest of the meal is provided. This is an easy way to administer an anthelmintic to a horse. For veterinarians a second form is available, pyrantel pamoate as a liquid suspension (Strongid-T). Here the drug may be administered either by drench or by intubation for more difficult cases. The very low water-solubility of the pamoate allows a more palatable formulation than the tartrate when given in very concentrated doses.

### 4.5 Dogs
Pyrantel pamoate is sold in the United States under the brand name of Nemex, as an anthelmintic agent for dogs. In numerous studies pyrantel pamoate is unequaled in effectiveness against the major intestinal hookworms: *Toxocara canis, Ancylostoma caninum,* and *Uncinaria stenocephala.*[24,25] As with horses,

the pamoate has the advantage of being more palatable than the tartrate, and there is the added bonus of greatly increased safety. In most of the animal applications discussed so far, economics of necessity dictates that excess doses not be given to the animals, so the safety margin of seven for the tartrate is sufficient to protect against an accidental double or even triple dose. However, in the hands of dog owners whose experience with or understanding of drugs may be dangerously limited, it is important to guard against possible toxicity due to overdosing. The pamoate has a built-in protection: whereas the $LD_{50}$ of the tartrate is 175 mg/kg in mice, the $LD_{50}$ of the pamoate is >5000 mg/kg. On a molar basis, however, the pamoate is just as potent against nematodes as the tartrate.

### 4.6 Humans

With the excellent results that were being achieved with pyrantel in animals, it was only natural that therapy of human parasitism should be tried. As indicated in Table 1, the four most important intestinal parasitic worms in humans are large roundworms, hookworms, whipworms, and pinworms. The first two are found in the upper small intestine, and the other two are residents of the colon. Victims are infected either with a single parasitic species or, as is often the case, with any combination. Thus for the human product, pyrantel pamoate, with its low absorption due to its low solubility, was chosen to assure that the drug would reach the colon and thereby include pinworm in the spectrum of activity. There is the additional bonus that the pamoate is easily formulated into a palatable suspension, and there is, of course, the outstanding safety margin.

Pyrantel pamoate is sold in the United States under the trade name Antiminth, and its label has indications for roundworm and pinworm infections.[26] In most other parts of the world it is sold under the trade name Combantrin and is widely recognized to be unsurpassed in treating hookworm disease as well. For these same indications pyrantel pamoate has a strong competitor in mebendazole, a drug discovered and developed by Janssen Pharmaceutica in Belgium. Various controlled studies have compared these agents[27,28] and have given one or the other a marginal degree of superiority. Because both agents are so highly effective, it is perhaps fair to simply state that they are equivalent. Two points of difference, however, should be noted. The first is that mebendazole will control whipworms against which pyrantel has no practical activity. The second is that mebendazole has been shown to be embryotoxic and teratogenic in rats and is thus contraindicated in pregnant women. Pyrantel has been evaluated in numerous animal reproduction studies and has shown no tendency to harm the fetus; nevertheless, there is no significant experience with this drug in pregnant women, so the relative benefit/risk ratio should be considered before treating such patients.

Table 4
Efficacy of Three Human Anthelmintic Products

| Days given | Worms eliminated | | |
|---|---|---|---|
| | Mebendazole[a] | Pyrantel[b] | Pyrantel-Oxantel[c] |
| 1 | pinworm | pinworm large roundworm hookworm[d] | pinworm large roundworm hookworm[d] |
| 3 | pinworm large roundworm hookworm[d] hookworm[e] whipworm | pinworm large roundworm hookworm[d] hookworm[e] | pinworm large roundworm hookworm[d] hookworm[e] whipworm |

[a]One tablet (100 mg) morning and evening each day.
[b]Oral suspension (10 mg base/kg) once each day.
[c]Oral suspension (10 mg base/kg each component) once each day.
[d]Ancylostoma duodenale.
[e]Necator americanus.

Mebendazole is effective in a single dose against pinworm, but for all other parasitic species the recommended treatment is a 100 mg tablet (for children or adults) twice daily for 3 days. Pyrantel is effective against pinworm, round-worm, and hookworm (Ancylostoma duodenale) as a single dose but must be given once a day for 3 days to control the other major human hookworm, Necator americanus. Thus, the pyrantel dosage schedule is more convenient than that of mebendazole. This situation is summarized in Table 4.

The lack of whipworm in pyrantel's activity spectrum places this drug at a competitive disadvantage in certain localities. Therefore, the discovery of oxan-tel was a welcome addition to the family of tetrahydropyrimidine anthelmintic agents. As mentioned in Section 3.9, oxantel has a very narrow activity spectrum and is, in effect, whipworm specific. Clinical studies show oxantel pamoate to be highly effective against human whipworm disease.[29,30] However, because of the high frequency of multiple worm infections, oxantel pamoate has not been developed for marketing as a single agent. Instead, a combination product of pyrantel pamoate and oxantel pamoate has been introduced as

Combantrin Compuesto in Latin America, and as Quantrel in Asia. The combination product performs as expected and acts against the same intestinal nematodes as does mebendazole (see Table 4). Again, controlled studies show these products to be indistinguishable in therapeutic results.[31] One recent controlled evaluation shows the combination product, when given as a single dose, to be as effective as mebendazole given 100 mg b.i.d. for three consecutive days against infections of large roundworm and whipworm.[32]

## REFERENCES

1. H. D. Brown, A. R. Matzuk, I. R. Ives, L. H. Peterson, S.A. Harris, L. H. Sarett, J. R. Egerton, J. J. Yakstis, W. C. Campbell, and A. C. Cuckler, *J. Am. Chem. Soc.,* **83**, 1764 (1961).
2. J. W. McFarland, L. H. Conover, H. L. Howes, Jr., J. E. Lynch, D. R. Chisholm, W. C. Austin, R. L. Cornwell, J. C. Danilewicz, W. Courtney, and D. H. Morgan, *J. Med. Chem.,* **12**, 1066 (1969).
3. J. W. McFarland and H. L. Howes, Jr., *J. Med. Chem.,* **13**, 109 (1970).
4. J. W. McFarland, H. L. Howes, Jr., L. H. Conover, J. E. Lynch, W. C. Austin, and D. H. Morgan, *J. Med. Chem.,* **13**, 113 (1970).
5. W. C. Austin, R. L. Cornwell, R. M. Jones, and M. Robinson, *J. Med. Chem.,* **15**, 281 (1972).
6. R. Kuhn and F. Drawert, *Ann.,* **590**, 55 (1954).
7. F. Kröhnke, J. Wolff, and G. Jentzsch, *Ber.,* **84**, 399 (1951).
8. L. C. King and W. B. Brownell, *J. Am. Chem. Soc.,* **72**, 2507 (1950).
9. J. W. McFarland and H. L. Howes, *Jr., J. Med. Chem.,* **12**, 1079 (1969).
10. C. Hansch and T. Fujita, *J. Am. Chem. Soc.,* **86**, 1616 (1964).
11. J. W. McFarland, *Progr. Drug Res.,* **15**, 123 (1971).
12. R. D. Cramer III, K. M. Snader, C. R. Willis, L. W. Chakrin, J. Thomas, and B. M. Sutton, *J. Med. Chem.,* **22**, 714 (1979).
13. J. W. McFarland and H. L. Howes, Jr., *J. Med. Chem.,* **15**, 365 (1972).
14. W. C. Austin, W. Courtney, J. C. Danilewicz, D. H. Morgan, R. L. Cornwell, L. H. Conover, H. L. Howes, Jr., J. E. Lynch, J. W. McFarland, and V. J. Theodorides, *Nature,* **212**, 1273 (1966).
15. Neth. Patent Application 6,800,807 (January 19, 1968) to May and Baker, Ltd.
16. Belg. Patent 700,556 (December 27, 1967) to Chas. Pfizer and Co., Inc.
17. M. T. Wu, F. S. Waksmunski, D. R. Hoff, M. H. Fisher, J. R. Egerton, and A. A. Patchett, *J. Pharm. Sci.,* **66**, 1150 (1977).
18. R. M. Jones, Vet. Parasitol., **8**, 237-251 (1981).
19. J. Armour, K. Bairden, J. L. Duncan, R. M. Jones, and D. H. Bliss, *Vet. Rec.,* **108**, 532-535 (1981).
20. K.-H. Markwardt, Inaugural Dissertation, Freie Universität, Berlin 1978 [*Vet. Bull.,* **49**, 4598 (1979)].
21. W. Haupt, E.-A. Nickel, W. Erbendruth, and H. Jacob, *Monatsh. Veterinärmed.,* **33**, 912 (1978) [*Vet. Bull.,* **49**, 5365 (1979)].
22. D. P. Conway and J. P. Raynaud, *Proceedings of the 5th World Congress of the International Pig Veterinary Society, June 13-15, 1978, Zagreb, Yugoslavia (Helminthol. Abstr.,* **48**, 4633).
23. D. P. Conway and J. P. Raynaud, *Proceedings of the 7th Congress of the International Pig Veterinary Society, June 30 to July 3, 1980, Copenhagen, Denmark.*
24. J. B. Klein, R. E. Bradley, Sr., and D. P. Conway, *Vet. Med. Small Anim. Clinic.,* **73**, 1011 (1978).

25. M. Robinson, F. G. Hooke, and K. E. Iverson, *Aust. Vet. Pract.,* **6**, 104 (1976 (*Helminthol. Abstr.,* **46**, 4498).
26. N. E. Pitts and J. R. Migliardi, *Clin. Pediatr.,* **13**, 87 (1974).
27. S. Migasena, P. Suntharasamai, and T. Harinasuta, *Ann. Trop. Med. Parasitol.,* **72**, 199 (1978) (*Helminthol. Abstr.,* **46**, 4810).
28. N. Islam and N. A. Chowdhury, *Southeast Asian J. Trop. Med. Public Health,* **7**, 81 (1976) (*Helminthol. Abstr.,* **46**, 1760).
29. E. G. Garcia, *Am. J. Trop. Med. Hyg.,* **25**, 914 (1976).
30. E. L. Lee, N. Iyngkaran, A. W. Grieve, M. J. Robinson, and A. S. Dissanaike, *Am. J. Trop. Med. Hyg.,* **25**, 563 (1976).
31. A. S. Dissanaike, *Drugs,* **15** (Suppl. 1), 11 (1978).
32. I. Farahmandian, G. H. Sahba, F. Arfaa, H. Jalali, and M. Reza, *Curr. Therap. Res.,* **26**, 114 (1979).

# Bacampicillin

# 5

## B. Ekström and B. Sjöberg

### 1. INTRODUCTION

The penicillins constitute the most widely used antibacterial group of drugs. They have achieved this position not only by virtue of their high antibacterial activity and low toxicity but also because it has been possible to find convenient and well-tolerated pharmaceutical forms, particularly for oral administration. Of the natural and biosynthetic penicillins only phenoxymethylpenicillin (Penicillin V) is absorbed well orally, whereas benzylpenicillin (Penicillin G) is so extensively destroyed by the acid of the stomach that only minor amounts of it reach the circulatory system of the body. To find derivatives that are well absorbed was thus an important objective in the development of the semisynthetic penicillins, and it was soon realized that the introduction of electron-attracting groups in the $\alpha$-position of the side chain gives penicillins with increased acid stability that are more likely to be absorbed efficiently after oral administration.[1]

1

One of the most important semisynthetic penicillins is ampicillin (**1**). It has broad-spectrum activity and in its oral form is often used as the drug of first choice for treatment of many types of bacterial infections. It is, however, only partially absorbed upon oral administration and gives urinary recoveries of 30-50% of the active compound.[2] A further drawback is a rather high incidence of diarrhea during therapy, probably caused by interaction of the unabsorbed

R-CH—CH   S   C(CH₃)(CH₃)
CO—N——CH-COOH

**2**  R= [phenyl]-CH-CO-NH-  with NH₂

**5**  R= [phenyl]-CH-CO-NH-  with N=CH₂

**3**  R= [cyclohexyl, CO-NH-, NH₂]

**6**  R= [phenyl]-CH—CO  HN   N-  H₃C  CH₃

**4**  R= HO-[phenyl]-CH-CO-NH-  with NH₂

drug with the intestinal microflora. Much work has therefore been carried out in order to find new analogues or derivatives of ampicillin with improved oral absorption properties. Epicillin (2) has antibacterial activity comparable to that of ampicillin but is not better absorbed orally,[3] whereas cyclacillin (3) is very efficiently absorbed.[4] The latter compound, however, has a reduced *in vitro* activity. Only amoxycillin (4) combines antibacterial activity comparable to that of ampicillin with clearly improved oral absorption properties.[5]

In the ampicillin molecule both the amino and the carboxyl groups are available for derivatization. Since both are essential for the antibacterial activity of the compound, it is obvious that any derivative with improved absorption must be converted back into ampicillin in the body in order to be useful, that is, the derivative must be a pro-drug of ampicillin. Condensation products between the amino group of ampicillin and aldehydes or ketones, such as metampicillin (5) and hetacillin (6), are completely hydrolyzed to ampicillin *in vivo* but their absorption properties are not better than those of ampicillin.[6,7] In contrast, pivampicillin (7), the pivaloyloxymethyl ester of ampicillin, was found to be efficiently absorbed orally and hydrolyzed *in vivo* to give improved blood levels of ampicillin,[8] showing that suitable pro-drugs can be obtained by esterification of the carboxyl group.

Esters of penicillins, particularly of Penicillin G, have been investigated repeatedly in the past, but the only compounds that have been used clinically to some extent are penethamate hydroiodide (8) and penamecillin (9). The former is slowly hydrolyzed *in vivo* and was employed as a depot preparation for intra-

7    R = –CH$_2$–O–COC(CH$_3$)$_3$

8    R=    –CH$_2$CH$_2$ N(C$_2$H$_5$)$_2$ ·H I

9    R=    –CH$_2$OCOCH$_3$

10   R = –CH–

muscular use,[9] whereas the latter compound has been found to give rather low but prolonged blood levels of Penicillin G when given orally.[10] Penamecillin and analogous acyloxyalkyl esters of some semisynthetic penicillins carrying neutral side chains have, however, limited oral absorption properties[11,12] compared with those of pivampicillin, suggesting that the basic amino group in the side chain of the ampicillin ester is essential for efficient absorption.

The improved oral absorption of an ampicillin ester should result in a reduction of the amount of active drug that can interact with the intestinal microflora. Clinical experience also indicates that pivampicillin and talampicillin (10), a more recently developed acyloxyalkyl ester of ampicillin,[13] cause less diarrhea than ampicillin. Unfortunately, both compounds appear to give upper gastrointestinal disturbances more frequently than ampicillin,[14,15] possibly due to an irritating effect on the gastrointestinal mucosa. It was thus considered of interest to investigate further types of ampicillin esters in order to find well-absorbed and well-tolerated compounds.

## 2.  CHEMISTRY

### 2.1  Potentially Useful Ester Groups

Several different types of ester groups have been investigated for transient masking of the carboxyl groups of penicillins; for a review see Hamilton-Miller.[16] The *in vivo* hydrolysis of the ester groups may occur chemically or may be catalyzed by enzymes. Simple esters are hydrolyzed too slowly *in vivo* to be of interest, and in order to achieve significant spontaneous hydrolysis activated ester groups have to be used. From a study of different activated esters of Penicillin G,[17] the β-diethylaminoethyl group of penethamate (8) emerged as a promising group in this respect. The methoxymethyl group has also been utilized in the case of hetacillin.[18] Studies indicate, however, that the hydrolysis *in vivo* of these ester groups is not complete and that unhydrolyzed ester circulates in the body. The esters have distribution properties different from those of the corresponding penicillins, which might lead to enhanced levels of antibiotic in certain tissues and organs, for example, in inflamed lung tissue as reported for penethamate hydroiodide[19] and prostatic and spinal fluid in the case of the methoxymethyl ester of hetacillin.[18] However, the incomplete hydrolysis will result in a decreased concentration of active drug.

Even more labile ester groups would result in more complete chemical hydrolysis *in vivo*. However, since the esters must be sufficiently stable to be readily manufactured and to be used in pharmaceutical preparations, it is preferable to have ester groups that are relatively stable under normal conditions but are rapidly hydrolyzed *in vivo*. This can be achieved by using ester structures that are hydrolyzed enzymatically. But humans, in contrast with small rodents for example, do not possess enzymes that can hydrolyze simple esters of penicillins.[20,21] In fact, there appears to be no record of any human enzymatic activity that readily attacks the acyl moiety derived from the carboxyl at the 3-position of the penicillin nucleus. Jansen and Russell,[22] on the other hand, showed in their work on acyloxyalkyl esters that an acyl group more distant from the penicillin ring system and situated in the alkyl group of the ester may be readily hydrolyzed by enzymes present in the human body. Most probably, the reaction proceeds in two steps where the intermediate acyldiol formed on enzymatic hydrolysis is spontaneously decomposed with the release of the carboxyl of the penicillin (Pc = penicillin moiety):

$$PcCOOCH_2OCOR \longrightarrow PcCOOCH_2OH \longrightarrow PcCOOH \qquad (eq. 1)$$

Acyloxyalkyl groups have also been used in pivampicillin (**7**) and talampicillin (**10**). It thus appeared to be interesting to explore the use of other enzymatically removable ester groups for masking the carboxyl group of ampicillin and other aminopenicillins and to prepare compounds of the general formula **11**, where the ester groups contain a carbonate structure. Carbonate structures had previously been investigated for masking hydroxyl groups, for example, trichloroethanol,[23] acetaminophen,[24] and salicylic acid.[25] These carbonate structures, derived from a halogenated alcohol or a phenolic hydroxyl, were found to be readily susceptible to hydrolysis catalyzed by enzymes present in

$R_1$ = H, CH$_3$        $R_2$ = ALKYL

**11**

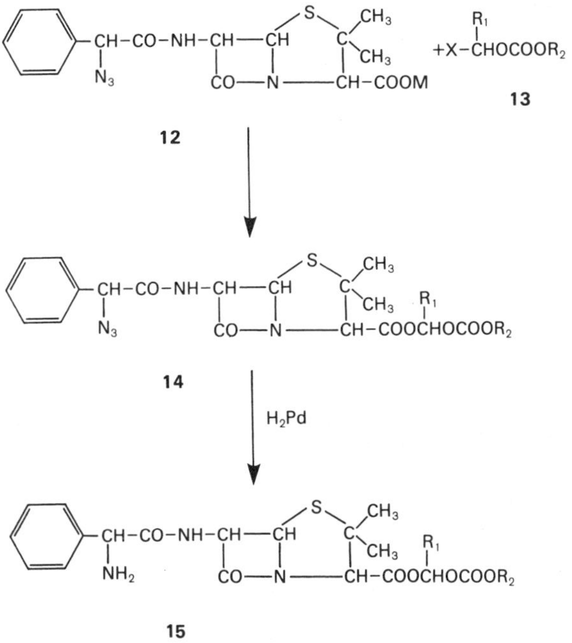

**Scheme 1.**  Method of preparation of esters of ampicillin from azidocillin.

human plasma and by a variety of isolated enzymes, including choline esterases and chymotrypsins.[24] In contrast, alkyl or cycloalkyl carbonate structures of the 2- and 7-hydroxy groups in lincomycin were found to be hydrolyzed by rat serum but not by human serum.[26] This indicates that the susceptibility of the carbonate structure to enzymatic hydrolysis may vary depending on its inherent reactivity and on the molecule carrying the carbonate moiety.

## 2.2  Synthetic Methods

Carbonate esters of ampicillin and some other aminopenicillins were prepared[27] according to two principal methods (Schemes 1 and 2). In the first a salt of a suitable azidopenicillin, for example the sodium salt of azidocillin (12), was reacted with a reactive halogenated derivative of a carbonate (13) to give an ester of azidocillin (14), which by hydrogenation over a palladium catalyst was converted to the corresponding ampicillin ester (15). The reactive precursors of the carbonate ester groups (13, X = halogen) were obtained by halogenation of carbonates or by selective alcoholysis of haloalkyl chloroformates.[28] The

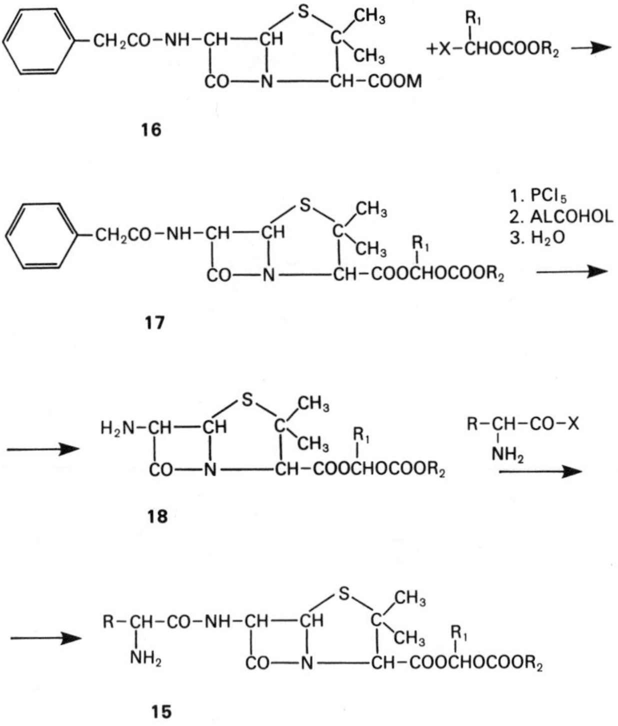

**Scheme 2.** Method of preparation of esters of aminopenicillins from benzylpenicillin.

esterification was usually carried out in dimethylformamide at room temperature or at a slightly elevated temperature or in ice-cold aqueous dioxane. The catalytic hydrogenation of the azido ester in ethyl acetate proceeded smoothly and the ampicillin ester was extracted into water as the hydrochloride, which was isolated by freeze-drying.

The other principal method involved esterification of benzylpenicillin (16) to the ester (17). The side chain in the 6-position of the penicillin was then removed by conversion into an imino chloride and subsequently to an imino ether that was hydrolyzed to give an ester of 6-aminopenicillanic acid (18). The reaction is analogous to the procedure used for chemical conversion of penicillin G into 6-aminopenicillanic acid.[29] The ester was then acylated with a suitable reactive derivative of a protected amino acid, for example, the acid chloride hydrochloride, to give the aminopenicillin ester, which was isolated as in the first method.

Both methods gave products with satisfactory yields and purities. Since azidocillin and fluoro-substituted azidocillin were readily available, the method in Scheme 1 was used in the laboratory primarily for preparation of the esters of ampicillin and some of its fluoro-substituted analogues. The second method was used primarily in cases where the azidopenicillin was not available and also where the method was found particularly suitable for production processes. Both methods have been used in similar cases[8,30] and obviously variations are possible, such as using other penicillins with a masked amino function in the side chain as starting material instead of azidocillin, or using other types of reagents for the acylation of **18**. A representative list of the carbonate esters of aminopenicillins prepared is given in Table 1.

## 3.   SCREENING

The objective of our work was to find esters that are rapidly and extensively absorbed to give markedly increased levels of aminopenicillin in the body. At the same time they had to be well tolerated, avoiding diarrhea, the main side effect of ampicillin, and upper gastric disturbances, the main side effects of available ampicillin esters. To achieve this, we considered it important to find esters that are comparatively stable chemically but that are readily susceptible to hydrolysis catalyzed by enzymes present in the body. We decided to investigate the susceptibility to hydrolysis of the ester groups in the primary screening test, and then test the absorption properties of selected compounds in animals and in volunteers. Regarding tolerance to the esters, no suitable screening method appeared to be available for investigation. However, the extent of oral absorption of the esters might be used to judge the risk of interaction with intestinal microflora of the aminopenicillin formed in the gastrointestinal tract, and the propensity of the esters to cause upper gastric disturbances had to be judged on the basis of their chemical structures and the hydrolysis products formed from the ester moieties.

### 3.1   Susceptibility of Hydrolysis

The hydrolysis of the esters to the corresponding aminopenicillins was determined in artificial gastric juice at pH 1.2, in phosphate buffer at pH 7.4, and in phosphate buffer with 10% human serum added as a source of enzyme. The esters were added to give a concentration of 10 mg/liter and the amount of aminopenicillin formed was determined after incubation for 30 min at 37 °C. For comparison the hydrolysis of pivampicillin (**7**) was measured in the same systems.

The results (Table 1) showed that all esters except the *tert*-butoxycarbonyloxymethyl compound[24] were rather stable under acidic conditions, with usually less than 2% hydrolysis taking place within 30 min. The

## Table 1
## Hydrolysis of Esters of Aminopenicillins[a]
## in Different Media at 37°C

R–CH–CO–NH–CH–CH    S    C(CH$_3$)(CH$_3$)
     |                              |
     NH$_2$        CO–N–CH–COOR'

| Compound No. | R | R' | Amount (%) of penicillin formed in 30 min. | | |
|---|---|---|---|---|---|
| | | | Artificial gastric juice (pH 1.2) | Phosphate buffer (pH 7.4) | Phosphate buffer + 10% human serum |
| 19 | C$_6$H$_5$— | —CH$_2$OCOOCH$_3$ | 0 | 27.8 | 71.4 |
| 20 | C$_6$H$_5$— | —CH$_2$OCOOC$_2$H$_5$ | 0.11 | 12.5 | 55.1 |
| 21 | C$_6$H$_5$— | —CH$_2$OCOOC$_3$H$_7$ | 2.1 | 14.5 | 53.7 |

| | | | | | |
|---|---|---|---|---|---|
| 22 | C₆H₅— | —CH₂OCOOCH(CH₃)₂ | 0.25 | 15.2 | 68.7 |
| 23 | C₆H₅— | —CH₂OCOOC₄H₉ | 1.4 | 13.0 | 41.1 |
| 24 | C₆H₅— | —CH₂OCOOC(CH₃)₃ | 17.5 | 28.2 | 27.1 |
| 25 | C₆H₅— | —CH₂OCOO(CH₂)₅CH₃ | 0.1 | 16.8 | 96.7 |
| 26 | C₆H₅— | CH₃ \ —CH-OCOOC₂H₅ | 0.15 | 3.4 | 57.3 |
| 27 | 3-F-C₆H₄— | —CH₂OCOOC₂H₅ | 0.1 | 12.3 | 81.2 |
| 28 | 3-F-C₆H₄— | CH₃ \ —CH-OCOOC₂H₅ | | 2.0 | 37.1 |
| 29 | 4-F-C₆H₄— | CH₃ \ —CH-OCOOC₂H₅ | | 1.0 | 19.8 |
| 7 | C₆H₅— | —CH₂OCOC(CH₃)₃ | 0.4 | 6.1 | 14.7 |

$^a$D-configuration at the $\alpha$-carbon of the side chain in the 6-position.

117

marked acid lability of the *tert*-butoxycarbonyloxymethyl ester is not unexpected, taking into consideration the properties of the *tert*-butoxycarbonyl group when used as a protecting group in peptide chemistry. Under neutral conditions the esters are generally much more susceptible to hydrolysis. Carbonate esters, having an unsubstituted methylene group bound to the penicillin carboxyl, were hydrolyzed to about 10-30% during 30 min at 37%C. The introduction of a methyl substituent in the methylene group reduced the degree of hydrolysis to about 1-3% (compounds 26, 28, 29), probably due to steric hindrance of the attack on the ester group. Pivampicillin (7), having a methylene group bound to the penicillin carboxyl, was somewhat less readily hydrolyzed than the corresponding carbonate esters, probably due to steric hindrance caused by the pivaloyl group.

The hydrolysis of the carbonate esters at pH 7.4 was greatly enhanced by the addition of 10% human serum to the test system, except in the case of the *tert*-butoxycarbonyloxymethyl compound (24). The introduction of a methyl substituent on the methylene group connected to the penicillin carboxyl did not affect the enzymatic hydrolysis to any great extent. The carbonate esters were appreciably more efficiently hydrolyzed than the ester groups of pivampicillin and its analogues. The results thus showed that the carbonate structure could fulfill the requirements of providing ester groups that are rapidly and extensively hydrolyzed enzymatically and are at the same time comparatively stable against chemical hydrolysis.

The mechanism of the hydrolytic reaction is most likely analogous to that given in equation 1, involving the intermediate formation of an acyldiol and a monalkyl carbonate, both of which are unstable and immediately decompose, releasing penicillin carboxyl and forming aldehyde, carbon dioxide, and alcohol (Pc = penicillin moiety):

$$Pc\text{-}CO_2\overset{R_1}{\underset{|}{C}}HOCO_2R_2 \rightarrow Pc\text{-}CO_2\overset{R_1}{\underset{|}{C}}HOH + HOCO_2R_2 \rightarrow Pc\text{-}CO_2H + \quad \text{(eq. 2)}$$
$$R_1\text{-}CHO + CO_2 + R_2OH$$

Investigations of the enzymatic and chemical hydrolysis of 26 (bacampicillin) and the corresponding ester of Penicillin G (17, $R_1 = CH_3$, $R_2 = C_2H_5$) resulted in the identification of acetaldehyde, carbon dioxide, and ethanol as hydrolysis products of the ester group. They were formed in approximately corresponding amounts, but kinetic analysis of the chemical hydrolysis of the Penicillin G ester indicated that acetaldehyde was formed slightly more rapidly than ethanol.[31] These results are compatible with the assumed mechanism (equation 2) if the intermediate acyldiol is slightly more labile than the monalkyl carbonate. The results could also be explained by a mechanism involving a primary attack on the penicillin acyl with formation of a hydroxycarbonate that subsequently decomposes in two steps into the products of hydrolysis:

$$\text{Pc-CO}_2\overset{R_1}{\underset{|}{\text{CH}}}\text{CO}_2\text{R}_2 \;\rightarrow\; \text{Pc-CO}_2\text{H} + \text{HO}\overset{R_1}{\underset{|}{\text{C}}}\text{HOCO}_2\text{R}_2 \qquad\qquad\text{(eq.3)}$$

$$\text{HO}\overset{R_1}{\underset{|}{\text{C}}}\text{HOCO}_2\text{R}_2 \;\rightarrow\; \text{R}_1\text{CHO} + \text{HOCO}_2\text{R}_2 \;\rightarrow$$

$$\text{R}_1\text{CHO} + \text{CO}_2 + \text{R}_2\text{OH} \qquad\qquad\qquad\text{(eq. 4)}$$

However, as pointed out in Section 2.1, it is not likely that the enzymatic reaction involves an attack on the penicillin acyl group of the ester moiety. Further studies on the reactivity of the ester group of bacampicillin (26) towards nucleophilic agents have indicated that the attack is exclusively on the carbonate carbonyl.[32]

### 3.2 Oral Absorption

It was thus possible to prepare esters of aminopenicillins with different susceptibilities towards chemical and enzymatic hydrolysis. The next step was to investigate whether the compounds had different oral absorption properties and whether any of them was a likely candidate for clinical use. The normal procedure in a situation like this would have been to conduct absorption experiments in animals, select those compounds that appeared to be most efficiently absorbed for further testing in volunteers, and then select the most suitable compound. A few experiments in mice verified that on oral administration the esters gave higher blood levels than ampicillin itself. But since we could expect differences between species with regard to *in vivo* hydrolysis of the carbonate esters, we decided not to include animal experiments in the selection procedure but rather to perform absorption tests with a number of the esters directly in volunteers.

Taking into consideration that a toxicity study with each compound is necessary before it could be given to human beings, it was obvious that only a restricted number of esters could be investigated. The compounds selected for the absorption experiments were the ampicillin esters 20 and 26 and the ester 27 of the 3-fluoro analogue of ampicillin. In this way compounds with different hydrolytic properties were included in the studies. The esters 20 and 27 contained the ethoxycarbonyloxymethyl group, which is rapidly cleaved enzymatically but also undergoes appreciable decomposition under nonenzymatic neutral conditions. The ester group of 26 is rapidly hydrolyzed enzymatically but is comparatively stable under nonenzymatic conditions. The *m*-fluoro-compound (27), which *in vivo* will give rise to *m*-fluoro-ampicillin, was included because previous studies in our laboratory with *m*-fluoro-azidocillin (12, side chain: 3-F-$C_6H_4$ instead of $C_6H_5$) had indicated that the fluoro substituent

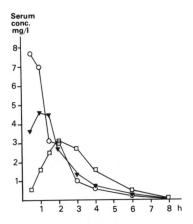

**Figure 1.** Mean serum levels of ampicillin determined in a crossover experiment in six volunteers after oral administration of 250 mg of ampicillin (□———□) or an equimolar amount of **26** (o———o). Pivampicillin (**7**, ◄———►) in a dose of 350 mg, corresponding to 244 mg of ampicillin, was included for comparison. All compounds were given in capsules. From L. Magni.[33]

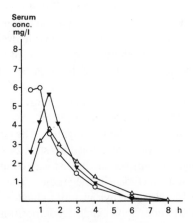

**Figure 2.** Mean serum levels of ampicillin determined in a crossover experiment in 10 volunteers after oral administration of **20** (Δ—Δ) and **26** (o———o) in doses corresponding to 250 mg of ampicillin. Pivampicillin **7**, ◄———►) in a dose of 350 mg, corresponding to 244 mg of ampicillin, was included for comparison. The latter was given in a capsule formulation, the other compounds as tablets. From L. Magni.[33]

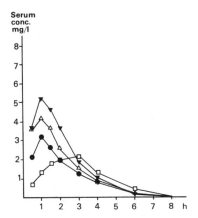

**Figure 3.** Mean serum levels of ampicillin or *m*-fluoroampicillin determined in a crossover experiment in 10 volunteers after oral administration of 250 mg of ampicillin (□——□) and equimolar amounts of **20** (Δ—Δ) and **27** (•——•). Pivampicillin (**7**, ◄——►) in a dose of 350 mg, corresponding to 244 mg of ampicillin, was included for comparison. The latter was given in a capsule formulation, the other compounds as tablets. From L. Magni.[33]

caused a slight increase in the serum half-life of the compound compared with azidocillin.

The oral absorption of the selected compounds was compared in three crossover studies with 6 to 10 volunteers, using ampicillin or pivampicillin as reference compounds. The results (Figures 1-3) showed that the two esters carrying the ethoxycarbonyloxymethyl group (**20, 27**) gave serum levels that were lower than those given by **26** and pivampicillin (**7**). Furthermore in the case of **27** there was no evidence that *m*-fluoro-ampicillin would be more slowly eliminated than ampicillin. The ethoxycarbonyloxyethyl group, on the other hand, gave an ester of ampicillin (**26**) that showed peak levels of ampicillin at least as high as those obtained with pivampicillin and considerably higher than those obtained with an equimolar amount of ampicillin. It was further evident that the peak levels of ampicillin obtained with **26** occurred earlier than those following pivampicillin or ampicillin. The urinary excretion of ampicillin during eight hours after administration was generally higher after administration of the esters **20, 26,** and **7** (50-70%) than after the ester **27** and ampicillin (35-45%).

Esterification of aminopenicillins thus leads to a marked enhancement of their oral absorption, in contrast with what has been found with esters of Penicillin G or other penicillins.[11,12] It has been suggested that the increased solubility of the aminopenicillin esters at acidic pH has a great influence on their absorption properties.[8]

**Table 2**

**Extent of Oral Absorption of $^{35}$S-Ampicillin and $^{35}$S-Bacampicillin at Different Levels of the Gastrointestinal Tract of Volunteers receiving Aqueous Solutions of the Test Compounds[a]**

| Part of gastrointestinal tract | Distance from nose to place of aspiration of sample (cm) | Cumulative percentage absorbed of given dose | |
|---|---|---|---|
| | | Ampicillin | Bacampicillin |
| Stomach | 50 | 13 | 20 |
| Duodenum | 75-100 | | 65 |
| | 90-105 | 22 | |
| Jejunum | 125-175 | | 71 |
| | 140-200 | 31 | |

[a]From Å. Swahn.[34,35]

Swahn[34] investigated the mechanism of absorption of ampicillin esters in humans, using radioactively labeled drugs. The compounds, together with unabsorbable markers, were given in aqueous solution to volunteers. Gastrointestinal probes were inserted, through which it was possible to take samples of the gastrointestinal fluid and calculate the amount of penicillin absorbed at different levels of the gastrointestinal tract. Although the experiments involved relatively few volunteers and were not done in a crossover fashion, it was apparent that the ampicillin ester (bacampicillin, **26**) is absorbed partly from the stomach and mainly from the duodenum (Table 2). Only a minor amount is absorbed from the jejunum and farther down the intestinal tract since about 82% of the radioactivity recovered in the urine (Table 3) was taken up in the stomach and the duodenum. The absorption of ampicillin,[35] determined under similar conditions, was clearly less complete than that of the ester. Only about 22% of the label given and about 50% of the radioactivity excreted into the urine was taken up from the stomach and the duodenum, thus a substantial part of the drug was absorbed from the jejunum and more distal parts of the intestinal tract.

These studies show that the ampicillin ester is more extensively and more rapidly absorbed orally than ampicillin, depending mainly on a greatly enhanced absorption from the duodenum. The ester is much more soluble than ampicillin under the acidic conditions of the stomach (Table 4), which may explain its somewhat greater absorption from this part of the gastrointestinal

### Table 3
### Urinary Recovery of Radioactive Compound after
### Oral Administraton of ³⁵S-Ampicillin and ³⁵S-Bacampicillin
### in Aqueous Solution to Volunteers[a]

| Time of Collection | Total label in urine (%) | |
|---|---|---|
| (hours) | Ampicillin | Bacampicillin |
| 0-3 | 24 | 62 |
| 0-24 | 43 | 79 |

[a]From Å. Swahn.[34,35]

### Table 4
### pH-Dependence of Aqueous Solubility and Partition
### between 1-Octanol and Water of Bacampicillin and
### Ampicillin at 37°C[a]

| | Aqueous solubility (g/liter) | | Coefficient of partition $\frac{1\text{-octanol}}{\text{water}}$ | |
|---|---|---|---|---|
| pH | Bacampicillin | Ampicillin[b] | Bacampicillin | Ampicillin[c] |
| 3 | 191 | 22.2 | 0.14 | |
| 4 | 60 | 9.0 | 0.15 | |
| 5 | 13 | 9.3 | 0.5 | 0.008 |
| 6 | 3.1 | 10.1 | 9.3 | |
| 7 | 0.5 | 19.0 | 16.9 | |

[a]Compiled from Lindquist and Svärd,[36] A. Tsuji et al.,[37] and Carney and Hurwitz.[38]
[b]Ampicillin trihydrate, from Tsuji et al.[37]
[c]From Carney and Hurwitz.[38]

system. However, at the pH of 5-6 usually found in the duodenum the solubility of the ester is much lower and not particularly greater than that of ampicillin, making it unlikely that the improved absorption is correlated primarily or solely with the solubility of the ester. Lipophilicity is, however, a very different property for ampicillin and an ester of ampicillin at the pH values found in the duodenum. Ampicillin carrying an amino and a carboxyl group will under aqueous conditions essentially be an ionized compound of a highly hydrophilic nature. By esterifying the carboxyl group, ampicillin is converted into a weak amine with a $pK_a$ of about 6.8, which at pH 5 will be partly un-ionized. The un-ionized fraction will increase with rising pH and make the compound more and more lipophilic. The partition coefficient between 1-octanol and water, which can be taken as a measure of the lipophilic properties of a compound, was for bacampicillin at pH 5 about 60 times greater and at pH 6 some 1000 times greater than for ampicillin (Table 4). Weak amines are well absorbed from the duodenum, probable *via* passive diffusion, and it is not unlikely that the extensive duodenal absorption of the ampicillin esters is due to an enhanced passive diffusion process of the un-ionized ester.

For improved ampicillin levels to be obtained in the body, the ampicillin ester must not only be rapidly and efficiently absorbed but also rapidly hydrolyzed once it has been absorbed. The screening data for the carbonate esters (Table 1) showed that the compounds were very susceptible to hydrolysis by dilute human serum. In his study on the oral absorption of ampicillin esters, Swahn[34] showed that when the compound was given to volunteers in clinical doses, the *in vivo* hydrolysis of bacampicillin (26) was so extensive and rapid that the concentration of the ester in the blood, if any, was below the detection limit of the analytical method (0.2 mg/liter). The esters were comparatively stable in gastric fluid and were hydrolyzed to varying degrees but not extensively in duodenal fluid, indicating that hydrolysis of the ester group mainly occurs in connection with or after the absorption rather than in the lumen of the gastrointestinal tract. It has been shown that intestinal villi and homogenates of intestine from various species contain enzymes that hydrolyze penicillin esters very efficiently.[34,39] It is thus likely that the hydrolysis of the ampicillin esters *in vivo* already largely occurs in the intestinal wall in connection with the absorption process.

26

## 4.   BACAMPICILLIN

Of the new aminopenicillin esters investigated, **26**, bacampicillin, appeared to have the best hydrolytic and absorption properties and it was selected for further evaluation in the clinic. As the ester group of **26** has a chiral center, resulting in the compound being a mixture of two epimeric forms, it was also necessary to study the properties of the epimers.

### 4.1   Epimeric Forms of Bacampicillin

The bacampicillin molecule contains five chiral centers. Four of these, C3, C5, and C6 of the penicillin nucleus and the alpha-carbon of the side chain at the 6-position, are sterically defined and have the same configuration as in ampicillin. The fifth center is the carbon atom of the ester group connected to the penicillin carboxyl. Since the preparation of bacampicillin proceeds via esterification of azidocillin or Penicillin G by reaction with a reactive racemic derivative of diethyl carbonate, usually $\alpha$-chlorodiethyl carbonate (Schemes 1 and 2, **13**, $R_1 = CH_3$, $R_2 = C_2H_5$), the product is a mixture of two epimers with regard to the chiral center of the ester group.

Large-scale production of either of the two epimers in pure form would have required that the enantiomers of $\alpha$-chlorodiethyl carbonate, or a method for stereoselective reaction between the penicillin salt and the racemate, be readily available, but none of these prerequisites have been fulfilled. It is possible, however, to prepare the two epimers of bacampicillin by selective crystallization of the mixture of the epimers. Another suitable method is to separate the corresponding epimeric mixture of the Penicillin G ester (**17**, $R_1 = CH_3$, $R_2 = C_2H_5$) and convert the epimers into the corresponding epimers of bacampicillin according to the method in Scheme 2. For both esters, it became evident that one of the epimers crystallizes very readily whereas the other is obtained only as an amorphous solid. The crystalline Penicillin G ester is, according to Scheme 2, converted into the crystalline bacampicillin ester, showing that the stereochemistry of the ester group is the same in the two crystalline compounds. The absolute configuration of the chiral center of the ester group of the readily crystalline epimer was determined to be $S$ by X-ray crystallographic analysis of the crystalline ester of Penicillin G and also of the corresponding ester of $p$-bromobenzylpenicillin.[40-42] In the production process, bacampicillin hydrochloride is obtained as a mixture of the two epimers with an $S/R$ ratio of about 65:35.

The hydrolytic properties of the epimers were investigated with the same test system as before. The results (Table 5) showed that the $S$-epimer is hydrolyzed enzymatically about twice as rapidly as the $R$-epimer, although there appears to be no difference between the epimers in the rate of spontaneous hydrolysis. The $R$-epimer, however, is more rapidly hydrolyzed enzymatically than pivampi-

### Table 5
### Hydrolysis of Bacampicillin and Its Epimers
### and of Pivampicillin in Various Media[a]

| | Hydrolysis to ampicillin in 30 min at 37 °C (%)[b] | | |
|---|---|---|---|
| Compound | Synthetic gastric juice (pH 1.2) | Phosphate buffer (pH 7.4) | Phosphate buffer + 10% human serum |
| Bacampicillin | 0.24 ± 0.02 | 3.2 ± 0.7 | 54.4 ± 5.8 |
| Bacampicillin, S-epimer | 0.27 ± 0.05 | 3.0 ± 0.2 | 67.6 ± 5.0 |
| Bacampicillin, R-epimer | 0.28 ± 0.03 | 2.9 ± 0.2 | 32.4 ± 2.1 |
| Pivampicillin | 0.24 ± 0.04 | 5.4 ± 0.3 | 10.2 ± 1.4 |

[a]From N. -O. Bodin et al.[43]
[b]Mean of 10 observations plus standard error of the mean.

cillin. Compared with talampicillin (10), bacampicillin is as rapidly hydrolyzed enzymatically but is more stable against spontaneous hydrolysis.[44] Oral absorption studies in volunteers demonstrated that the bioavailability of ampicillin after administration of the S-epimer of bacampicillin was comparable with that given by the R + S mixture (Figure 4). The peak levels given by the S-epimer were slightly but not significantly higher than those given by the epimeric mixture, and both gave considerably higher levels than ampicillin. The urinary recovery of ampicillin during eight hours after administration was 76.7% for the S-epimer and 75.5% for the mixture of the epimers compared with 47.8% for ampicillin. The ratio between the epimers in the production of bacampicillin has been found to be fairly constant. Should variations occur, the results of the hydrolysis and absorption experiments indicate that they should not be critical for the biological properties of the product.

### 4.2  Tolerance of Bacampicillin
One objective of our work was to find an ester of ampicillin that is well tolerated. In particular, it was considered important to have a drug that does not give a high frequency of diarrhea or upper gastric disturbances, the major

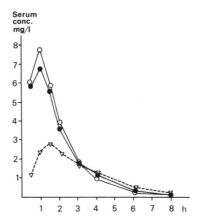

**Figure 4.** Mean serum levels of ampicillin determined in a crossover experiment in 10 volunteers receiving oral doses of 400 mg of bacampicillin (corresponding to 278 mg of ampicillin) epimeric mixture (**26**, o——o) or pure $S$-epimer (•——•), or 250 mg of ampicillin (Δ—Δ) in a crossover experiment. From Wessman and Magni.[45]

side effects of ampicillin and of the other ampicillin esters, pivampicillin and talampicillin, respectively. Oral administration of bacampicillin has been found to have very little effect on the normal bowel flora,[46] most probably because of its fast and extensive absorption from the upper gastrointestinal tract. A rather slow hydrolysis of any remaining ester to ampicillin in the intestine may also reduce the amount of antibacterial drug available for interaction with the microflora. In line with the reasoning that the frequent cases of diarrhea seen in ampicillin therapy are caused by interaction of unabsorbed drug with the bowel flora, we expected the frequency of this side effect to decrease when bacampicillin was given instead of ampicillin. Controlled clinical comparisons with ampicillin showed a significantly reduced frequency of diarrhea with bacampicillin. (Table 6).

The reasons for the upper gastric side effects found with pivampicillin and talampicillin are not clear. They may be caused by the esters as such or by their products of hydrolysis. They may also depend on the particular form and the particular pharmaceutical preparation in which the drug is given. It was recently reported that pivampicillin given as the free base in tablets is less irritating to the gastric mucosa than the hydrochloride of pivampicillin given in capsules.[48] In selecting bacampicillin for clinical evaluation it was important that the hydrolysis products of the ester group, acetaldehyde, carbon dioxide, and

**Table 6**

**Frequencies of Side Effects Recorded in Controlled
Clinical Comparisons of Ampicillin and Bacampicillin[a]**

| Side effects | Ampicillin (%) $n = 183$ | Bacampicillin (%) $n = 280$ |
|---|---|---|
| Diarrhea | 12.0 | 0.7 |
| Upper gastrointestinal disturbances | 2.7 | 0.7 |
| Rash | 5.5 | 2.1 |

[a]From A. Heimdahl et al.[46]

ethanol are innocuous substances of a physiological nature readily taken care of by the body. It seemed unlikely that the small amounts of these products produced by bacampicillin in the envisaged clinical doses would cause any adverse effects.

The increased solubility and lipophilicity of an ampicillin ester enable it to penetrate the gastrointestinal mucosa more readily than ampicillin. This might lead to increased drug concentrations in the mucosa, causing irritation and the upper gastric disturbances experienced by some patients when receiving an ampicillin ester. In the toxicity studies performed with bacampicillin hydrochloride, irritation of the gastric mucosa was provoked by very high doses of the compounds, particularly in dogs. In control groups included in the studies, the effect was not present in the animals receiving ampicillin but appeared even more pronounced in animals receiving pivampicillin hydrochloride. To investigate whether a similar effect could be seen in humans, Magnusson et al[49] measured the gastrointestinal blood loss in volunteers receiving clinical doses of bacampicillin hydrochloride (400 mg) and pivampicillin hydrochloride (350 mg) for one week in a double-blind cross-over experiment. Placebo was given for one week before and between the treatment periods with active drug. Blood loss was measured with the radiochromium method. The results (Table 7) showed that the esters caused considerably lower blood losses than those induced by a drug such as acetylsalicylic acid and below the level considered pathological. However, pivampicillin hydrochloride gave a slightly but significantly higher blood loss than bacampicillin hydrochloride. The bleeding caused by the latter did not differ significantly from that given by

**Table 7**

**Mean ( ± SEM) Daily Blood Loss (ml) During One Week
in 10 Volunteers Receiving Bacampicillin, Pivampicillin, or Placebo,
in a Controlled Crossover Experiment[a]**

| Placebo preceding pivampicillin | Pivampicillin (350 mg, 3 x daily) | Placebo preceding bacampicillin | Bacampicillin (400 mg, 3 x daily) |
|---|---|---|---|
| 0.4 ± 0.1 | 1.3 ± 0.2 | 0.4 ± 0.1 | 0.6 ± 0.2 |

[a]From B. Magnusson et al.[49]

placebo. In this investigation a commercially available capsule formulation of pivampicillin hydrochloride was used. As pointed out above, the results might have been different if a tablet formulation of pivampicillin free base had been used instead. For the development of bacampicillin hydrochloride the results were, however, of importance since they showed that the compound in a clinical dose would not be expected to give major side effects caused by an irritating effect of the compound on the gastrointestinal mucosa.

The results of the clinical trials also showed that upper gastric disturbances are an unusual side effect in bacampicillin therapy. In controlled comparisons the frequency was not higher than that found for ampicillin (Table 6). These studies and continued clinical experience have shown that bacampicillin is a well-tolerated drug that avoids side effects given by ampicillin and other ampicillin esters.[47]

### 4.3 Clinical Pharmacology
The high and rapid peak blood levels of ampicillin given by bacampicillin on oral administration are the outstanding feature of the compound with regard to clinical pharmacology. The findings in the previous absorption studies (Figures 1,2, and 4) that bacampicillin gives a peak level of ampicillin 2-3 times higher than that given by ampicillin itself and at least as high as that given by pivampicillin were corroborated by continued work.[50,51] The peak levels occur earlier than for the other two compounds. The peak levels of ampicillin obtained with bacampicillin are at least as high as those given by talampicillin.[52] Furthermore, bacampicillin gives peak levels of ampicillin at least as high as the levels of amoxycillin obtained with an equimolar amount of this drug. Here, too, bacampicillin appears to be more rapidly absorbed than the other compound.[51] The urinary excretion of ampicillin is high after bacampicillin administration,

usually corresponding to about 70% of the dose given. The oral absorption is almost complete, and the bioavailability of ampicillin after bacampicillin administration is 87-95% that of an intravenous equimolar dose of ampicillin.[53,54] Another manifestation of its efficient absorption is that the blood level of ampicillin obtained after oral bacampicillin is as high as that of an equimolar dose of intramuscular ampicillin.[54] The oral absorption of bacampicillin further appears to be unaffected by food intake and shows a good dose-response relationship.[50]

All the data obtained thus demonstrate that the oral absorption and *in vivo* hydrolysis of bacampicillin are very efficient processes resulting in high peak blood levels. Infections, on the other hand, are usually not confined to the blood but rather occur in tissues and organs of the body. Hence it was considered important during the work with bacampicillin to investigate whether the improved blood levels of ampicillin given by the compound also resulted in increased tissue levels. Several experimental studies in animals and in volunteers as well as studies in patients have verified that this is the case. The investigations included studies of the penetration of the drug into tissue compartments in rats[43] and rabbits,[55] into skin blisters produced by different techniques in volunteers,[53,56] and into purulent sputum in bronchitis patients,[57] all showing better penetration after bacampicillin than after an equimolar amount of ampicillin. Further studies in patients have shown that bacampicillin gives rise to high ampicillin levels in pleural fluid,[58] lung tissue,[59] and middle ear effusion.[55] In many of the studies it was found that the levels of antibiotic in the particular compartment studied were more sustained than in the blood, suggesting the presence of penetration barriers, and that the high serum peak levels of drug produced by bacampicillin increased the transport through such barriers into the different compartments. The results are in agreement with those of other studies suggesting that high peak serum levels of penicillins are of value for penetration of the drug into peripheral *loci*.[61]

The possibility of more sustained levels of antibiotic in the tissue compartments than in the blood can be of importance for the dosing frequency of the drug that has to be used to achieve an adequate therapeutic effect. Penicillins for oral administration have hitherto mainly been given three or four times a day. Dosing twice a day, if it could be used, should be more convenient for the patient and would probably result in better compliance with the prescribed treatment. Bacampicillin was originally documented for dosing three times a day and was found to be a highly effective antibacterial drug when used in this way. The excellent absorption properties of the drug and the data on tissue penetration made it worthwhile to investigate a twice-a-day dosage. The clinical results obtained, being as good as those achieved with dosing three times a day, have verified that such a dosage is feasible.

A detailed discussion of the clinical experience with the drug has been considered to be outside of the scope of this paper. An important observation made in our work, however, is that the actual research and development work with a drug should not be considered complete once it has been put on the market, since we are still far from being able to predict the clinical efficacy of a drug from laboratory data alone. Clinical research and experimentation are necessary to find the best way of using the drug in therapy.

## REFERENCES

1.  F. P. Doyle, J. H. C. Nayler, H. Smith, and E. R. Stove, *Nature*, **191**, 1091 (1961).
2.  G. N. Rolinson and R. Sutherland in S. Garattini, Ed., *Advan. Pharmacol. Chemother.*, Vol. 11, Academic Press, New York, 1973, p. 151.
3.  H. Gadebusch, G. Miraglia, F. Pansy, and K. Renz, *Infect. Immunol.*, **4**, 50 (1971).
4.  M. W. Hopper, J. A. Yurchenko, and G. H. Warren, *Antimicrob. Agents Chemother.*, 597, 1967.
5.  R. Sutherland, E. A. P. Croydon, and G. N. Rolinson, *Brit. Med. J.* **3**, 13 (1972).
6.  W. J. Jusko and G. P. Lewis, *J. Pharm. Sci.*, **62**, 69 (1973).
7.  R. Sutherland, S. Elson, and E. A. P. Croydon, *Chemotherapy*, **17**, 145 (1972).
8.  W. Daehne, E. Frederiksen, E. Gundersen, F. Lund, P. Morch, H. J. Petersen, K. Roholt, L. Tybring, and W. O. Godtfredsen, *J. Med. Chem.*, **13**, 607 (1970).
9.  K. A. Jensen, P. J. Dragsted, I. Kjaer, E. J. Nielsen, and E. Frederiksen, *Acta. Pathol. Microbiol. Scand.*, **28**, 407 (1951).
10  H. P. K. Agersborg, A. Batchelor, G. W. Cambridge, and A. W. Rule, *Brit. J. Pharmacol.*, **26**, 649 (1966).
11.  M. Gibaldi and M. A. Schwartz, *Brit. J. Pharmacol. Chemother.*, **28**, 360 (1966).
12.  A. B. A. Jansen and T. J. Russell, U.S. Patent 3,250,679 (1966).
13.  J. P. Clayton, M. Cole, S. W. Elson, and H. Ferres, *Antimicrob. Agents Chemother.*, **5**, 670 (1974).
14.  J. B. Wilcox, R. N. Brogden, and G. S. Avery, *Drugs*, **6**, 94 (1973).
15.  E. T. Knudsen and J. W. Harding, *Brit. J. Clin. Pract.*, **29**, 255 (1975).
16.  J. M. T. Hamilton-Miller, *Chemotherapia*, **12**, 73 (1967).
17.  R. L. Barnden, R. M. Evans, J. C. Hamlet, B. A. Hems, A. B. A. Jansen, M. E. Trevett, and G. B. Webb, *J. Chem. Soc.*, 3733 (1953).
18.  T. B. Kjaer, P. G. Welling, and P. O. Madsen, *J. Pharm. Sci.*, **66**, 345 (1977).
19.  J. Ungar and P. W. Muggleton, *Brit. Med. J.,i.*, 1211 (1952).
20.  A. P. Richardson, H. A. Walker, I. Miller, and R. Hansen, *Proc. Soc. Exp. Biol. Med.*, **60**, 272 (1945).
21.  R. M. Broh-Kahn and P. K. Smith, *Proc. Soc. Exp. Biol. Med.*, **61**, 216 (1946).
22.  A. B. A. Jansen and T. J. Russell, *J. Chem. Soc.*, 2127 (1965).
23.  H. C. Caldwell, H. J. Adams, D. E. Rivard, and J. V. Swintosky, *J. Pharm. Sci.*, **56**, 920 (1967).
24.  L. W. Dittert, G. M. Irwin, E. S. Ratte, C. W. Chong, and J. V. Swintosky, *J. Pharm. Sci.*, **58**, 557 (1969).
25.  L. W. Dittert, H. C. Caldwell, T. Ellison, G. M. Irwin, D. E. Rivard, and J. V. Swintosky, *J. Pharm. Sci.*, **57**, 828 (1968).
26.  A. A. Sinkula and C. Lewis, *J. Pharm. Sci.*, **62**, 1757 (1973).
27.  B. Å. Ekström and B. O. H. Sjöberg, Belg. Patent 772,723 (1972).
28.  E. Dahlen, to be published.

29.  H. W. O. Weissenburger and M. G. van der Hoeven, *Rec. Trav. Chim.*, **89**, 1081 (1970).
30.  J. P. Clayton, M. Cole, S. W. Elson, H. Ferres, J. C. Hanson, L. W. Mizen, and R. Sutherland, *J. Med. Chem.*, **19**, 1385 (1976).
31.  J. Hasselrot, B. Runesson, and B. Örtengren, to be published.
32.  G. Bondesson, to be published.
33.  L. Magni, unpublished results.
34.  Å. Swahn, *Eur. J. Clin. Pharmacol.*, **9** 299 (1976).
35.  Å. Swahn, *Eur. J. Clin. Pharmacol.*, **8**, 77 (1975).
36.  J. Lindquist and E. Svärd, unpublished results.
37.  A. Tsuji, E. Nakashima, S. Hamano, and T. Yamana, *J. Pharm. Sci.*, **67**, 1059 (1978).
38.  C. F. Carney and A. R. Hurwitz, *J. Pharm. Sci.*, **66**, 294 (1977).
39.  W. E. Wright and V. D. Line, *Antimicrob. Agents Chemother.*, **10**, 861 (1976).
40.  I. Csöreg and T. -B. Palm, *Chem. Commun. Univ. Stockh.*, No. 9 (1970).
41.  I. Csöregh and T. -B. Palm, *Acta Cryst.*, **B33**, 2169 (1977).
42.  Ö. Kovacs, to be published.
43.  N. -Ö. Bodin, B. Ekström, U. Forsgren, L. -P. Jalar, L. Magni, C. -H. Ramsay, and B. Sjoberg, *Antimicrob. Agents Chemother.*, **5**, 518 (1975).
44.  B. Ekström, U. Forsgren, L. -P. Jalar, B. Sjöberg, and J. Sjövall, *Drugs Exp. Clin. Res.*, **3**, 3 (1977).
45.  J. Wessman and L. Magni, unpublished results.
46.  A. Heimdahl, C.-E. Nordh, and K. Weilander, *Infection*, **7** (Suppl. 5), 446 (1979).
47.  F. Nordbring, *Infection*, **7**, (Suppl. 5), 503 (1979).
48.  H. Hey, P. Malzen, J. Thorup Andersen, E. Didriksen, and B. Nielsen, *Arch. Pharm. Chem. Sci. Ed.*, **7**, 169 (1979).
49.  B. Magnusson, L. Sölvell, and J. Wessman, *Scand. J. Infect. Dis.*, **9**, 218 (1977).
50.  L. Magni, B. Sjöberg, J. Sjövall, and J. Wessman, in J. O. Williams and A. M. Geddes, Eds., *Chemotherapy*, Vol. 5, Plenum Press, New York, 1976, p. 109.
51.  J. Sjövall, L. Magni, and T. Bergan, *Antimicrob. Agents Chemother.*, **13**, 90 (1978).
52.  J. Sjövall and L. Magni, unpublished results.
53.  C. Simon, V. Malerczyk, and M. Klaus, *Scand. J. Infect. Dis.*, (Suppl.) **14**, 228 (1978).
54.  T. Bergan, *Antimicrob. Agents Chemother.*, **13**, 971 (1978).
55.  C. Carbon, A. Contrepois, G. Beauvais, and S. Lamotte-Barrillon, *J. Antimicrob. Chemother.*, **2**, 314 (1976).
56.  K. B. Hellum, A. Schreiner, A. Digranes, and I. Bergman, in E. Siegenthaler and R. Luthy, Eds., *Current Chemotherapy I, Proceedings of the 10th International Congress of Chemotherapy, Zurich 1977*, Am. Soc. Microbiol., Washington, D.C., 1978, p. 620.
57.  F. P. V. Maesen, in *Verslag van Symposia Betreffende Luchtweginfecties*, Astra Pharmaceutica BV, Rijswijk, Holland, 1976, p. 95.
58.  W. Bronsveld, J. Stam, and D. M. MacLaren, *Scand. J. Infect. Dis.*, **14**, (Suppl.), 274 (1978).
59.  O. Hällström, O. Keyrilainen, and O. Markkula, *Infection*, **7**, (Suppl. 5), 469 (1979).
60.  S. Virtanen and E.-A. Lahikainen, *Infection*, **7** 472 (1979).
61.  M. Barza, J. Brusch, M. G. Bergeron, and L. Weinstein, *J. Infect. Dis.*, **129**, 73 (1974).

# Pivampicillin

**6**

W. O. Godtfredsen

One of the problems in connection with the medical use of penicillins and cephalosporins is that many of these valuable antibiotics are unsatisfactorily absorbed from the gastrointestinal tract. The oral absorption of penicillins like benzylpenicillin, methicillin, and carbenicillin and of most of the cephalosporins, including cephalothin and cephazolin, is so poor that these drugs have to be given by injection. Other compounds, such as the acid-stable penicillins phenoxymethylpenicillin and ampicillin, are absorbed to some extent, but the absorption is incomplete with great individual variations. The blood levels obtained after oral administration are consequently inferior to those obtained after parenteral administration of a corresponding dose.

It has therefore been a challenge for medicinal chemists to provide penicillins and cephalosporins that are well absorbed when given by mouth. One of the ways by which this problem has been approached is to adopt the pro-drug concept, that is, to synthesize derivatives of penicillins and cephalosporins that are better and more reliably absorbed than their simple salts and which after absorption are transformed into the parent penicillin or cephalosporin.

The development of pivampicillin is an example of such an effort. The story began in the summer of 1967 when I attended the 4th International Congress of Chemotherapy in Vienna. One day during this conference I had lunch with a Swedish colleague, and among the things we discussed was ampicillin, which at that time was the number-one-selling drug in Sweden. My Swedish friend told me that one disadvantage of this otherwise excellent antibiotic is that it is absorbed rather incompletely when given by mouth. This discussion encouraged me to consider ways in which the absorption of ampicillin might be improved.

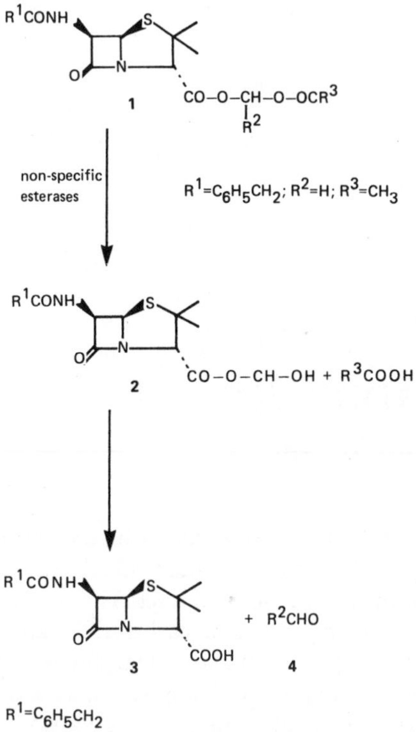

**Figure 1.**

When I returned home a few days later I found on my desk a volume of the Journal of the Chemical Society in which an article by Jansen and Russel[1] dealt with several new types of penicillin esters synthesized as potential pro-drugs. The most interesting were acyloxyalkyl esters of the general structure shown in formula 1. Such esters can be regarded as mixed esters of gem-diols (aldehyde hydrates) where one of the hydroxyl groups has been esterified with a penicillin and the other with a simple carboxylic acid.

Penicillin esters in general are devoid of antibacterial activity, and although mice and rats have esterases capable of hydrolyzing methyl and other simple alkyl or aralkyl esters of benzylpenicillin,[2] humans and higher animals lack such enzymes. It seems that the idea behind the synthesis of penicillin esters of the type shown in formula 1 has been an expectation that nonspecific esterases, which are widespread in mammals, would be able to split off the simple carboxylic acid R³COOH from **1** to leave the unstable hydroxyalkyl ester (**2**), which in turn would undergo rapid spontaneous hydrolysis to the penicillin (**3**) and the aldehyde (**4**).[3] Whatever the mechanism is, it turned out that such esters are indeed hydrolyzed in the presence of serum or various tissue homogenates, including intestinal mucosa from dogs and humans although the hydrolysis proceeds more slowly than when rat serum or rat tissues are used as enzyme sources.

Jansen and Russel[1] synthesized acyloxyalkyl esters of a number of different penicillins, including benzylpenicillin, phenoxymethylpenicillin, and methicillin. These esters are all practically insoluble in water and with one exception do not seem to be absorbed at all.[4] The exception is the acetoxymethyl ester of benzylpenicillin (**1a**), which gives rise to low but prolonged blood levels of benzylpenicillin (**3a**) when given orally to dogs or humans.[3,4] Jansen and Russel did not synthesize corresponding esters of ampicillin or other aminopenicillins. It occurred immediately to my colleague Erling Frederiksen and me after reading this article that the absorption of acyloxyalkyl esters of ampicillin might be completely different from the absorption of the esters described in the Jansen paper because the amino group in the side chain will render such esters acid-soluble and because at physiological pH they might have a lipid-water partition coefficient favorable for passage through biological membranes. We decided therefore to prepare similar esters of ampicillin.

If R² in formula **1** is different from H, a chiral center giving rise to two diastereomeric forms of the mixed esters is created, and this of course complicates the isolation and purification of such esters. To avoid this problem we decided to concentrate on mixed esters of formaldehyde hydrate.

The first ester we made was the acetoxymethyl ester (**7a**). This compound was synthesized from the potassium salt of D-α-azidobenzylpenicillin (**5**), which was converted to the corresponding acetoxymethyl ester (**6a**) by reaction with chloromethyl acetate. The azido ester (**6a**) was subsequently converted to the corresponding ampicillin ester (**7a**) by catalytic hydrogenation. The hydrogenation was carried out in ethyl acetate solution. As the amino ester **7a** formed, it was immediately extracted into an aqueous phase, which was maintained at pH 3.0 by the addition of hydrochloric acid.[5] This method was developed because it is necessary to transform the amino group into its hydrochloride as soon as it is formed in order to avoid polymerization, which would occur with the free amino β-lactam ester **7a**.

Having established a synthetic route to the acetoxymethyl ester of ampicillin (**7a**), we investigated its enzymatic hydrolysis by incubating solutions containing about 10 μg/ml of **7a** with whole blood, serum, or tissue homogenates at pH 7.4 at 37%C. At suitable intervals aliquots were extracted with ethyl acetate and the remaining aqueous phase assayed for its content of ampicillin by the

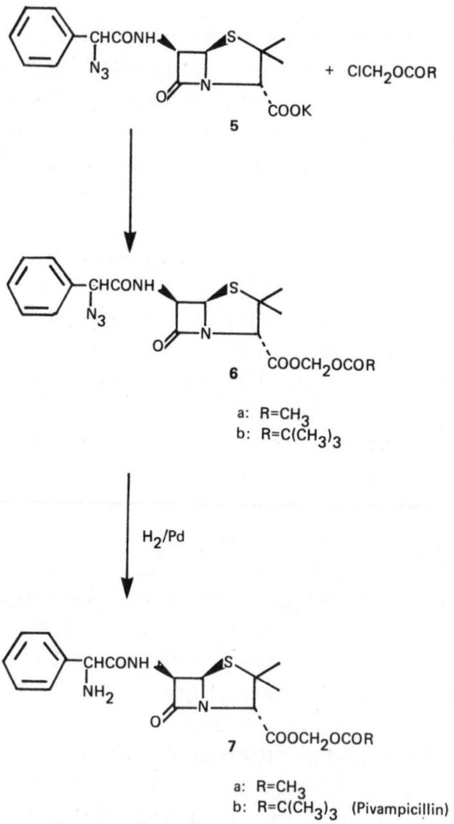

**Figure 2.**

agar-cup-plate method. By the extraction, unchanged acetoxymethyl ester of ampicillin passes into the ethyl acetate phase whereas ampicillin, formed by hydrolysis of **7a**, remains in the aqueous phase and can be determined microbiologically. By this technique we could show that **7a** was readily hydrolyzed with the liberation of ampicillin under the influence of enzymes present in human serum, dog serum, and various tissue homogenates including intestinal mucosa.[5]

The next step was to give the compound orally to rats and dogs in order to compare the resulting serum levels of ampicillin with those obtained after administration of an equimolar amount of ampicillin.*

---

*These and numerous similar absorption studies in experimental animals and human volunteers were performed by Dr. K. Roholt and his staff in Leo Pharmaceutical's biological department.

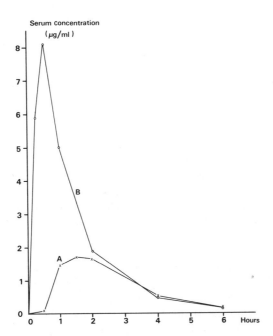

**Figure 3.** Mean concentrations of ampicillin in serum of six normal fasting volunteers after oral administration of (A) 250 mg of ampicillin and (B) 328 mg of **7a** hydrochloride (~ 250 mg of ampicillin).

The difference was dramatic. Administration of the ester (**7a**) to dogs gave rise to peak serum levels three times higher than those obtained after an equimolar dose of ampicillin, and the area under the serum level/time curve, a good measure of bioavailability, was more than twice as large. Similar results were obtained when the compound was given to rats. These results established that the pro-drug concept involving the preparation of ampicillin derivatives was well based, since a better absorption resulting in higher blood levels of ampicillin could be achieved by using acyloxymethyl esters of ampicillin rather than ampicillin itself.

After performing subacute toxicity studies, we gave the hydrochloride of **7a** and ampicillin to a group of healthy volunteers in a crossover study. It will be seen from Figure 3 that in humans the acetoxymethyl ester of ampicillin is also absorbed much better than the parent compound, as evidenced by the higher peak serum levels and the greater area under the serum level/time curve. The urinary recovery of ampicillin amounted to 56% when the ester was given but only to 29% after administration of ampicillin, also indicating a superior absorption of the ester. Encouraged by these results, we started the synthesis of a number of analogous esters in which the acetyl group was replaced by other simple acyl groups.

The enzymatic hydrolysis of all of these esters was studied in the presence of various sera and tissue homogenates by the method described above. These investigations showed that the rate of hydrolysis varied considerably with the structure of the acyloxy group. For instance, the hydrolysis of the more hindered pivaloyloxymethyl ester (7b) proceeded markedly more slowly than that of the acetoxymethyl ester (7a)[5] (cf. Table 1). This led to the idea that by choosing an ester that was hydrolyzed relatively slowly, it might be possible to achieve a further advantage in addition to an improved absorption. If the ampicillin ester remains intact in the bloodstream for a certain period of time after the absorption, it can probably be distributed in the organism in a different and perhaps more advantageous way than ampicillin because its lipid/water partition coefficient is quite different from that of the very polar drug ampicillin.*

This prospect was one of the reasons why we decided to move ahead with the pivaloyloxymethyl ester (7b), which is now called pivampicillin. Another more practical reason was that this ester forms a nicely crystalline hydrochloride whereas the hydrochloride of the acetoxymethyl ester and many of the other esters turned out to be very difficult to crystallize.

The hypothesis that pivampicillin can survive so long in the organism that a different distribution is possible turned out to be wrong. Subsequent studies indicated that hydrolysis of pivampicillin has already taken place by the time it passes through the intestinal wall. This was established by the observation that practically no unchanged pivampicillin can be detected in blood taken from the hepatic portal system of animals dosed with the compound. However, since the pivaloyloxymethyl ester was absorbed at least as well as the acetoxymethyl ester and in addition had the above-mentioned practical advantages, we decided to develop this compound further. Then began the long and painstaking development work that is necessary nowadays to bring a new drug to a point where it can be approved by the regulatory bodies and commercialized.

---

*In the early 1950s Leo developed penethamate, the 2-diethylaminoethyl ester of benzylpenicillin. This ester is a pro-drug of benzylpenicillin; after intramuscular administration it spontaneously hydrolyzes to benzylpenicillin and 2-diethylaminoethanol, the half-life at physiological conditions (pH = 7.4; t = 37 °C) being about 20 minutes.[6] Not surprisingly, penethamate is distributed differently from benzylpenicillin in the organism. For example, the lung concentrations of benzylpenicillin obtained after administration of penethamate are several times higher than those obtained after an equimolar dose of benzylpenicillin.[7] Penethamate is no longer being used in human medicine, but it still has a place in the treatment of mastitis in cattle.

## Table 1
**Hydrolysis of Acyloxymethyl Esters of Ampicillin at pH 7.4 and 37 °C in the Presence of 10% Human Serum[a]**

| Ester | % Hydrolyzed[b] after 30 min |
|---|---|
| Acetoxymethyl (**7a**) | 89 |
| Propionyloxymethyl | 80 |
| *n*-Butyryloxymethyl | 85 |
| Isobutyryloxymethyl | 89 |
| Pivaloyloxymethyl (**7b**) | 22 |
| α-Ethyl-*n*-butyryloxymethyl | 23 |
| Benzoyloxymethyl | 67 |

[a]The starting concentration of the esters was 1/35 mmol ~ 10 µg/ml of free ampicillin.

[b]The figures do not indicate the exact degree of hydrolysis since, under the applied conditions, ampicillin as well as its esters undergo transformations (probably polymerization) resulting in a loss of antibacterial activity.

## 1. SYNTHESIS

One of the first problems to confront us was the development of a synthesis of pivampicillin suitable for large-scale production that did not infringe on existing patents.

The first material we used for pharmacological and toxicological studies was synthesized by the method outlined in Figure 2. This method gave excellent results in the laboratory, but was not suitable for large-scale production because of the explosion risk for compounds containing an azido group. In addition, in 1967 D-α-azidobenzylpenicillin was covered by patents.

Another possible pathway, outlined in Figure 4, would be to convert 6-aminopenicillanic acid (6-APA) (**8**) to the corresponding pivaloyloxymethyl ester (**9**) and thereafter introduce the D-α-phenylglycyl side chain by one of the numerous methods developed for the production of ampicillin. These include among others acylation with D-α-phenylglycyl chloride hydrochloride,[8] or with a mixed anhydride (**10**) of a so-called Dane-derivative of D-α-phenylglycine followed by an acid-catalyzed removal of the protecting group in the intermediate **11**.[9]

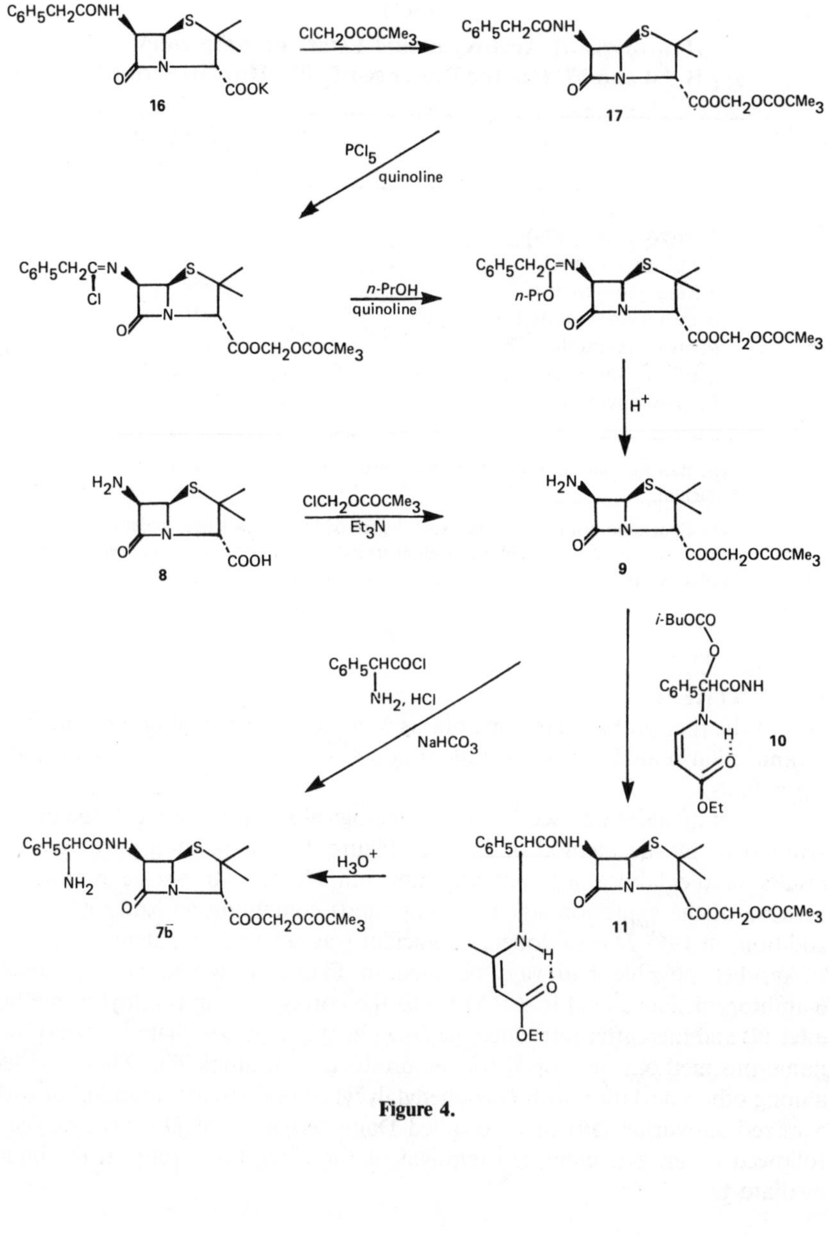
C6H5CH2CONH
COOK
16
ClCH2OCOCMe3
C6H5CH2CONH
COOCH2OCOCMe3
17
PCl5
quinoline
C6H5CH2C=N
Cl
COOCH2OCOCMe3
n-PrOH
quinoline
C6H5CH2C=N
n-PrO
COOCH2OCOCMe3
H+
H2N
COOH
8
ClCH2OCOCMe3
Et3N
H2N
COOCH2OCOCMe3
9
i-BuOCO
C6H5CHCONH
OEt
10
C6H5CHCOCl
NH2, HCl
NaHCO3
C6H5CHCONH
NH2
COOCH2OCOCMe3
7b
H3O+
C6H5CHCONH
COOCH2OCOCMe3
11
OEt

**Figure 4.**

The conversion of 6-APA (**8**) to the pivaloyloxymethyl ester (**9**) proceeded smoothly when the triethylamine salt of 6-APA was reacted with chloromethyl pivalate in DMF. Since the subsequent acylation of **9** also worked reasonably well with both of the above-mentioned acylation methods, this pathway looked promising from a technical point of view. An obstacle to commercial use of the method, however, was the existing patents covering 6-APA and the relatively high cost of this potential starting material. What we needed, therefore, was a method by which the 6-APA ester (**9**) could be synthesized without using 6-APA as a starting material.

While we were speculating on this problem a patent application was published in which a chemical method was disclosed for the removal of the side chain in benzylpenicillin or phenoxymethylpenicillin with the formation of 6-APA.[10] The principle in this method, which actually is a modification of a method for the production of 7-aminocephalosporanic acid (7-ACA) developed by Fechtig *et al.*[11] a few years earlier, is outlined in Figure 5.

A silyl ester of benzylpenicillin (**12**) is treated with $PCl_5$ in chloroform or methylene chloride in the presence of an organic base such as pyridine or quinoline to form an iminochloride (**13**), which on reaction with a suitable alcohol (ROH) is converted to an iminoether (**14**), the protecting silyl ester group being removed simultaneously. The iminoether is subsequently hydrolyzed or solvolyzed under acidic conditions to afford 6-APA and the phenylacetic ester (**15**). The overall yield by this process, which is carried out in one pot starting from benzylpenicillin, was claimed to be about 85–90%.

Having read this patent application, we of course immediately tried to determine if the method could be adapted for the synthesis of the pivaloyloxymethyl ester (**9**). As a first step, the starting material benzylpenicillin had to be converted into its pivaloyloxymethyl ester (**17**). This step presented no problems. When the potassium salt of benzylpenicillin (**16**) was reacted with chloromethyl pivalate in acetone, **17** was formed in almost quantitative yield and it turned out to be a nice, stable, crystalline compound. The removal of the side chain from **17** with the formation of **9** turned out to be a considerably more difficult process, requiring painstaking development work. It falls outside the scope of this article to detail this work. Suffice it to say that by using chloroform as solvent, quinoline as base, and *n*-propanol as the alcohol it became possible to achieve an almost quantitative conversion of **17** to **9**. The isolation of the product presented difficulties because of its physicochemical properties, but these were also overcome, and in the end yields of about 90% of the hydrochloride of **9** could be obtained.

The process of converting the pivaloyloxymethyl ester of benzylpenicillin (**17**) to the corresponding 6-APA ester (**9**) was developed by Frantz J. Lund, who thereby generated an interest in penicillin chemistry that later led to the

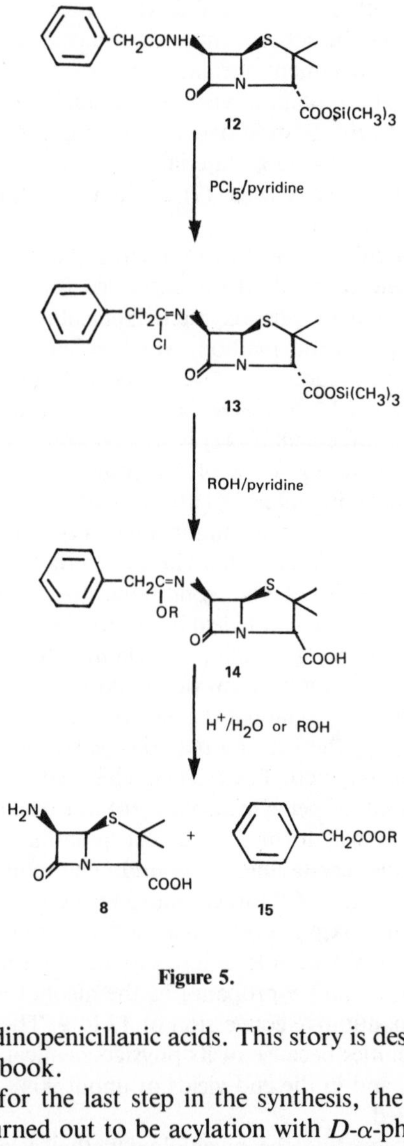

**Figure 5.**

discovery of the amidinopenicillanic acids. This story is described by Dr. Lund in Chapter 7 of this book.

The best method for the last step in the synthesis, the conversion of **9** to pivampicillin **(7b)**, turned out to be acylation with *D*-α-phenylglycyl chloride. By this method a yield of about 85-90% of pivampicillin could be obtained,[5] but the upscaling of the process required a considerable amount of development work.

**Table 2**
**Enzymatic Hydrolysis of Pivampicillin**

| Enzyme source | Half-life[a] (min) |
|---|---|
| None | 103 |
| Mouse serum 1% | < 1 |
| Rat serum, 1% | < 1 |
| Dog serum, 5% | 50 |
| Dog serum, 10% | 23 |
| Human serum, 10% | 50 |
| Homogenate of dog gastric mucosa, 10% | 10 |
| Homogenate of dog intestinal mucosa, 10% | 5 |
| Homogenate of dog liver, 10% | < 5 |
| Homogenate of human gastric mucosa, 10% | 5 |
| Homogenate of human duodenal mucosa, 10% | 5 |
| Human whole blood | 5 |
| Dog whole blood | 3-4 |

[a]In all experiments, the starting concentration of pivampicillin hydrochloride was 14.3 $\mu$g/ml. Determinations were made at pH 7.4 and 37°C.

## 2.  BIOLOGICAL STUDIES

Parallel with the efforts of developing a suitable method for the synthesis of pivampicillin, a number of biological studies were performed.

### 2.1  Hydrolysis *in vitro* and *in vivo*

It has already been mentioned that pivampicillin is readily hydrolyzed, with the liberation of ampicillin, in the presence of whole blood, serum, and various tissue homogenates.[5] Table 2 shows, for example that in the presence of human whole blood the half-life of pivampicillin is approximately 5 min. It was important to show that pivampicillin is also hydrolyzed rapidly *in vivo* because the interpretation of the absorption studies is based upon the assumption that all of the pivampicillin that has been absorbed is present in the organism in the form of ampicillin. In order to show that this is really what happens, we worked out a method that allows the determination in blood of ampicillin as well as intact ester.[12] By using this method it was possible to show that even in blood drawn as early as 15 min after the administration of pivampicillin more than 99% was present as ampicillin. Later on it became possible to analyze portal vein blood from a few patients treated with pivampicillin.[13] Since these samples contained traces of unchanged pivampicillin only, it can be concluded that practically all the pivampicillin is already being hydrolyzed during the passage through the intestinal wall.

## 2.2   Toxicology

The toxicological studies of pivampicillin included, in addition to the acute studies, three-month studies in rats and dogs. These showed nothing abnormal in doses up to 630 mg/kg/day.[12] Since the reproduction studies also were clean, there was no hindrance for initiating clinical studies.

## 2.3   Pharmacokinetics

It falls outside the scope of this article to review the numerous studies performed in healthy volunteers and patients[5,12-22] to compare the pharmacokinetic properties of pivampicillin with those of ampicillin and related drugs like amoxycillin. Suffice it to say that these studies consentaneously have confirmed the first impression that pivampicillin is absorbed much more efficiently and also more reliably than the parent drug ampicillin.

A typical result of such a comparative study is illustrated in Figure 6, which shows mean serum levels of ampicillin after oral administration of equimolar amounts of ampicillin and pivampicillin hydrochloride to a group of healthy volunteers in a crossover study. Comparing the two curves, it is obvious that the bioavailability of pivampicillin is much better than that of ampicillin. The area under the serum level/time curve (AUC) in this particular study was 2.37 times greater for pivampicillin than for ampicillin, and the urinary recovery was increased by a factor of 2.05.

That the absorption of pivampicillin is virtually complete follows from the observation that oral administration of pivampicillin gives rise to AUC values and urinary recoveries that are almost identical with the values obtained after parenteral administration of an equimolar amount of ampicillin.[15,18]

## 3.   FORMULATION

During the clinical studies pivampicillin was used in the form of capsules containing its hydrochloride, and this formulation was also used in the first years after marketing. But the need for a pediatric suspension presented a problem. The hydrochloride was unsuitable for this purpose because of its ready solubility in water combined with the instability and intense bitter taste of aqueous solutions. At first we tried to overcome these problems by preparing sparingly soluble salts such as the pamoate and the tosylate. However, such salts turned out to be absorbed rather inefficiently, and another approach had to be followed.

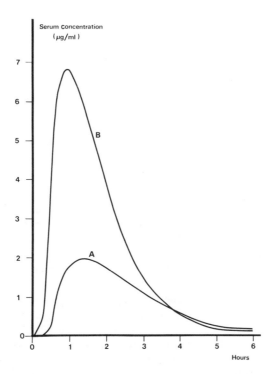

**Figure 6.** Mean concentrations of ampicillin in serum of eight normal fasting volunteers after oral administration of (A) 250 mg of ampicillin and (B) 358 mg of pivampicillin hydrochloride (~250 mg of ampicillin).

The solution to the problem came when we succeeded in obtaining the free base of pivampicillin (which used to be an oil) in the crystalline state. In contrast with the hydrochloride, pivampicillin base is practically insoluble in water and when mixed with suitable auxiliary agents it can be made up to aqueous suspensions that are sufficiently stable for practical purposes and have an acceptable taste. Absorption studies carried out with such suspensions revealed that pivampicillin base is absorbed as well as the hydrochloride, even in patients with a decreased production of gastric acid.[16,19]

Shortly after the introduction of pivampicillin it became clear that in some patients the drug gave rise to upper gastrointestinal side effects such as nausea, heartburn, and vomiting. Although these side effects were mild in most cases, they were nevertheless disturbing and we began to look for means to overcome them. Here again the free base of pivampicillin turned out to be the solution to the problem.

We reasoned that these side effects were due to a local irritating effect of pivampicillin. When the drug is given in the form of capsules containing the hydrochloride, a small part of the gastric mucosa is exposed to a strong aqueous solution of pivampicillin hydrochloride when the capsule releases its contents. With the sparingly soluble pivampicillin base, it is possible to make tablets that rapidly disintegrate in such a way that the content is spread over a large area of the gastric mucosa. Several studies [20-22] revealed that these tablets are much better tolerated than capsules containing the hydrochloride, and as a consequence of these results the capsules were abandoned in favor of the tablets.

### Epilogue

The sucessful application of the pro-drug principle to improve the oral absorption of ampicillin represented by pivampicillin has been followed by the development of two similar ampicillin esters, the ethoxycarbonyloxyethyl ester called bacampicillin[23] and the phthalidyl ester talampicillin.[24,25] Both bacampicillin and talampicillin contain a chiral center in the ester moiety and therefore two diastereomeric forms exist. The commercial preparations are mixtures of the two diastereomers.

Using the same principle it has been possible to improve the oral absorption of other $\beta$-lactam antibiotics containing an amino function in the side chain, such as cephaloglycin and mecillinam. Both these antibiotics are absorbed poorly when given by mouth whereas absorption of the corresponding pivaloyloxymethyl esters is excellent.[26,27]

That the absorption of $\beta$-lactams that do not contain amino functions in the side chain also can be enhanced by conversion to the corresponding pivaloyloxymethyl ester is illustrated by the $\beta$-lactamase inhibitor penicillanic acid sulfone. This drug is poorly absorbed when given by mouth, but its pivaloyloxymethyl ester seems to be absorbed very well.[28]

### Acknowledgment

Many of my colleagues, in particular the chemists W. v. Daehne, F. Lund, H. J. Petersen, and S. Vangedal, the analysts the late P. Mörch and Mrs. E. Gundersen, as well as the biologists K. Roholt and L. Tybring, took active part in the development of pivampicillin. It is a pleasure to acknowledge their most valuable contributions.

### REFERENCES

1. A. B. A. Jansen and T. J. Russell, *J. Chem. Soc.,* 2127 (1965).
2. A. R. Richardson, H. A. Walker, I. Miller, and R. Hanson, *Proc. Soc. Exp. Biol. (N.Y.),* **60**, 272 (1945).
3. H. P. K. Agersborg, A. Batchelor, G.W. Cambridge, and A. W. Rule, *Brit. J. Pharmacol.,* **26**, 649 (1966).
4. A. B. A. Jansen and T. J. Russell, *Brit. Patent 1,003,479.*

5.  W. v. Daehne, E. Frederiksen, E. Gundersen, F. Lund, P. Mörch, H. J. Petersen, K. Roholt, L. Tybring, and W. O. Godtfredsen, *J. Med. Chem.*, **13**, 607 (1970).

6.  K. A. Jensen, P. J. Dragsted, I. Kjär, E. Juhl Nielsen, and E. Frederiksen, *Ugeskr. Laeg.*, **113**, 1035 (1951).

7.  J. Ungar and P. W. Muggleton, *Brit. Med. J.*, 1211 (1952).

8.  G. A. Hardcastle, Jr., D. A. Johnson, and C. A. Panetta, *J. Org. Chem*, **31**, 897 (1966).

9.  E. Dane and T. Dockner, *Chem. Ber.*, **98**, 789 (1965).

10. H. W. O. Weissenburger and M. G. van der Hoeven, *U.S. Patent 3,499,909.*

11. B. Fechtig, H. Peter, H. Bickel, and E. Vischer, *Helv. Chim. Acta*, **51** 1108 (1968).

12. W. v. Daehne, W. O. Godtfredsen, K. Roholt, and L. Tybring., *Antimicrob. Agents Chemother. 1970,* 431 (1971).

13. B. Lund, J. P. Kampmann, F. Lindahl, and J. Mölholm Hansen, *Clin. Pharm. Ther.*, **19**, 587 (1976).

14. E. L. Foltz, J. W. West, and H. Wallich, *Antimicrob. Agents Chemother. 1970,* 442 (1971).

15. M. C. Jordan, J. B. de Maine, and W. M. M. Kirby, *Antimicrob. Agents Chemother. 1970,* 438 (1971).

16. K. Roholt, B. Nielsen, and E. Kristensen, *Antimicrob. Agents Chemother,* **6**, 563 (1974).

17. H. Knothe, B. Lauer, and K. Fabricius, *Arzneimittelforschung,* **24**, 951 (1974).

18. M. Ehrnebo, S. Nilsson, and L. O. Boreus, *J. Pharmacokin. Biopharmaceutics,* **7**, 429 (1979).

19. J. M. T. Hamilton-Miller, J. Kosmidis, and W. Brumfitt, *Infection,* **2**, 193 (1974).

20. H. Hey, T. J. Medalen, P. M. Moelstad, and K. Stokholm, *Infection,* **5**, 22 (1977).

21. H. Hey, P. Matzen, J. Thorup Andersen, E. Didriksen, and B. Nielsen, *Br. J. Clin. Pharmacol.,* **8** 237 (1979).

22. H. Hey, P. Matzen, J. Thorup Andersen, E. Didriksen, and B. Nielsen, *Arch. Pharm. Chem. Sci. Ed.,* **7**, 169 (1979).

23. N. O. Bodin, B. Eckström, U. Forsgren, L. P. Jalar, L. Magni, C. H. Ramsay, and B. Sjöberg, *Antimicrob. Agents Chemother.,* **8** 518 (1975).

24. J. P. Clayton, M. Cole, S. W. Elson, and H. Ferres, *Antimicrob. Agents Chemother.,* **6**, 670 (1974).

25. Y. Shiobara, A. Tachibana, H. Sasaki, T. Watanabe, and T. Sado, *J. Antibiotics,* **27**, 665 (1974).

26. E. Binderup, W. O. Godtfredsen, and K. Roholt, *J. Antibiotics,* **24**, 767 (1971).

27. K. Roholt, B. Nielsen, and E. Kristensen, *Chemotherapy,* **21**, 146 (1975).

28. G. Foulds, W. E. Barth, J. R. Bianchine, A. R. English, D. Girard, S. L. Hayes, M. M. O'Brien, and P. Somani, *Abstr. 11th Internal. Congr. Chemother,* 312 (1979).

# Pivmecillinam

# 7

## Frantz J. Lund

The pro-drug pivmecillinam with the chemical name pivaloyloxymethyl 6$\beta$-[(hexahydro-1H-azepin-1-yl)methyleneamino]penicillanate (Figure 1) is converted to the slightly absorbable true antimicrobial agent mecillinam after oral administration.[1] It is therapeutically efficient mainly in the treatment of urinary-tract infections caused by gram-negative bacteria.[2-4] Compared with penicillins and cephalosporins, mecillinam shows an unusual antibacterial spectrum[5] and mode of action.[5-8] This difference is attributed to its chemical structure, which is quite unlike that of all other $\beta$-lactam antibiotics. Mecillinam shows synergy with penicillins and cephalosporins.[9,10] It is the objective of this chapter to give an account of how the unconventional structure of pivmecillinam emerged.

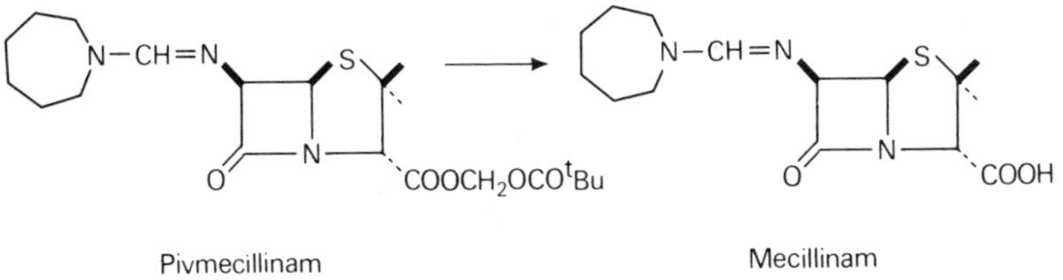

|  Pivmecillinam | Mecillinam |

**Figure 1.**

## 1. INTRODUCTION

The history of medicinal chemistry is abundantly spiced with examples of drugs developed on more or less perfect biological misconceptions! It was not the colored azo dye prontosil that killed the bacteria but rather the sulfanilamide

**149**

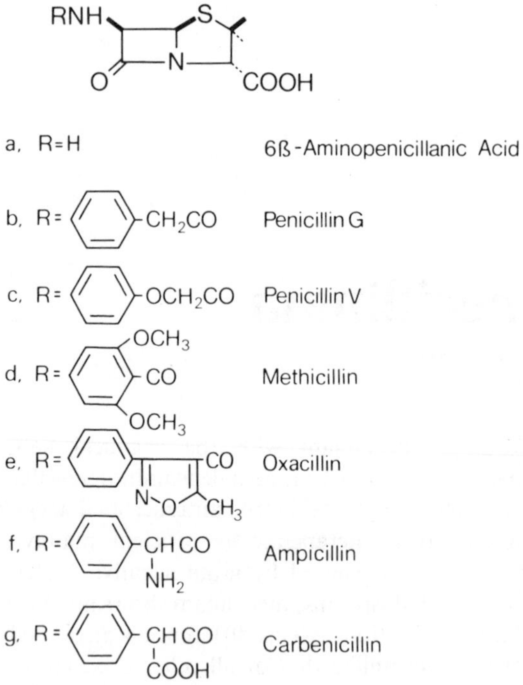

| | | |
|---|---|---|
| a, | R=H | 6ß-Aminopenicillanic Acid |
| b, | R= ⬡—CH₂CO | Penicillin G |
| c, | R= ⬡—OCH₂CO | Penicillin V |
| d, | R= ⬡ (OCH₃, OCH₃) —CO | Methicillin |
| e, | R= ⬡—isoxazole—CO | Oxacillin |
| f, | R= ⬡—CHCO (NH₂) | Ampicillin |
| g, | R= ⬡—CHCO (COOH) | Carbenicillin |

**Figure 2.**

generated from it by biotransformation.[11] Phenylbutazone was introduced as a solubilizing agent for amidopyrine before its antirheumatic effect was discovered.[12] The hypotensive methyldopa was originally invented as a dopa decarboxylase inhibitor. Later its activity was explained by the false-transmitter theory,[13] and now it is associated with a central effect.[14] These few prominent examples from different areas of medicine should not be construed as limiting my statement. The list could easily be extended with more examples and by future developments.

Chemical misconceptions resulting in useful drugs are more unusual. Nevertheless, it was actually an intermediate in an unsuccessful synthetic program initiated at the beginning of 1969 that provided the "lead compound" to the antibiotic pivmecillinam. Its constitution was not in accord with time-honored concepts concerning structure-activity relationships among β-lactam antibiotics.

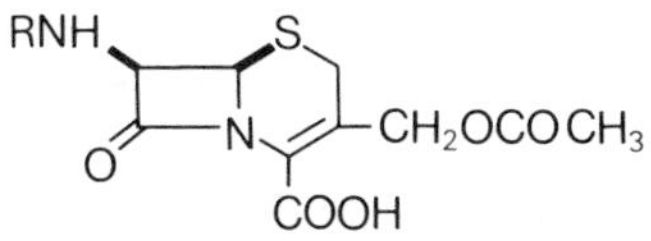

a, R=H: $7\beta$ – Aminocephalosporanic Acid

b, $HOOCCH(CH_2)_3CO$ : Cephalosporin C
   $\quad$ |
   $\quad$ $NH_2$

**Figure 3.**

## 2. THE BIRTH OF A MYTH

Until 1969, useful $\beta$-lactam antibiotics could be characterized chemically as amides substituted at the nitrogen atom by a highly reactive bicyclic $\beta$-lactam ring system. In penicillins, a $\beta$-lactam and a thiazolidine ring are fused to form the penam nucleus (Figure 2) whereas in the cephalosporins the latter has been replaced by a dihydrothiazine ring (Figure 3).

This amide structure is present in the natural $\beta$-lactam antibiotics and in the semisynthetic variants produced and marketed by the pharmaceutical industry when the requisite amino-substituted nuclei, 6$\beta$-aminopenicillanic and 7$\beta$-aminocephalosporanic acids (Figures 2a and 3a), became available as starting materials for the synthetic chemist in 1959 and 1962, respectively. In addition, the amide group was preserved in most of the numerous derivatives of these key compounds that were prepared but that never appeared outside the laboratories.

The organic chemist certainly knows many other ways to substitute an amino group, but all attempts to replace the amide configuration by other nitrogen-containing structures invariably led to compounds with inferior antibiotic activity.[15] Oddly enough, the amidino group was not included in these early efforts to explore other types of nitrogen substitution, so medicinal chemists working with $\beta$-lactam antibiotics were convinced that God had thought it over carefully when designing these compounds as amides, and to the medicinal chemist's treasure of delusions was added the myth of the amide side chain as a prerequisite for useful activity in $\beta$-lactam antibiotics. Considerable advances were achieved on this basis. By following the amide approach, scientists in the pharmaceutical industry succeeded in improving on the established wonder drug penicillin G (Figure 2b) in several respects. The answer to the instability to acid of penicillin G was found in penicillin V (Figure 2c). The threat from $\beta$-lactamase-producing staphylococci was met with methicillin (Figure 2d) and the isoxalylpenicillins (Figure 2e). The rather poor performance of the older penicillins against several gram-negative organisms was to some extent remedied by the discovery of ampicillin (Figure 2f) and carbenicillin (Figure 2g).

### 3.  THE BACKGROUND AT LEO FOR MORE WORK ON PENICILLINS

This raises the intriguing question why a medicinal chemist was encouraged to take an interest in the synthesis of a new type of *N*-substituted 6β-aminopenicillanic acid derivative such as the 6β-amidinopenicillanic acids when it seemed most likely that they should be antibiotically inactive.

My interest in work on β-lactam antibiotics originated from a fortunate combination of tradition and recent events in these laboratories. As the first company outside Great Britain and the United States to produce penicillins, Leo Pharmaceutical Products had already been able to produce and market penicillin G during the Second World War. This was achieved without access to outside information because of the German occupation of Denmark. Ever since then, work on penicillins has continued in our research laboratories. By the end of 1967, this work had led to the novel recognition of the utility of the easily hydrolyzable acyloxymethyl esters of ampicillin. After oral administration this special type of ester is rapidly absorbed and hydrolyzed, giving rise to higher blood concentrations of ampicillin than are obtainable directly with an equivalent oral dosage of ampicillin. The story of the selected ester (Figure 4) is recorded by Godtfredsen in Chapter 6 on pivampicillin.

Pivaloyloxymethyl 6β-aminopenicillanate hydrochloride is a key intermediate in the synthesis of pivampicillin, and I became involved in the development of production methods for this compound. In consonance with the liberal research policy of these laboratories, when the synthetic problems had been

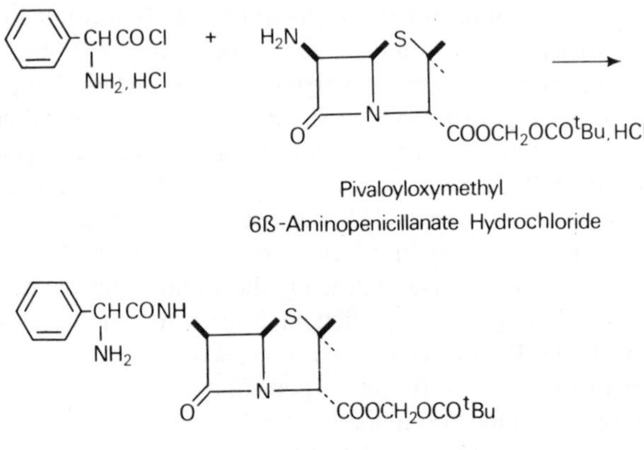

Pivaloyloxymethyl
6ß-Aminopenicillanate Hydrochloride

**Figure 4.**  Preparation of pivampicillin.

solved it was natural to speculate on other possible uses of this valuable
6β-aminopenicillanic acid derivative that offered the following advantages:

1. It was easily accessible and relatively cheap.
2. In contrast with 6β-aminopenicillanic acid, as the free base the ester was soluble in most organic solvents.
3. The ester grouping was sufficiently stable to allow further chemical transformations elsewhere in the molecule.
4. Presumably, the esters resulting from such syntheses could be tested for antibiotic activity following enzymatic hydrolysis. This avoided the need for chemical removal of the carboxylic acid protective group with the inherent danger of damage to other parts of the molecule.
5. Such esters might be absorbed orally.

## 4. REJECTION OF A BACTERIOLOGICAL MISCONCEPTION BY MEANS OF A CHEMICAL MISCONCEPTION

Since the prospects for obtaining new valuable penicillins by traditional modification of the side chain seemed to be poor, I decided to explore the feasibility of replacing the thiazolidine part of the penam system with other heterocyclic rings.

A contributing factor to this decision was my aversion for work on penicillins! Many years ago when I first came to these laboratories, I spent my time producing intractable smears instead of the beautifully crystallizing penicillin esters imagined by my boss. Since then, I had avoided that kind of chemistry as much as possible, so I was not too familiar with the traditional thinking and respect for the fragility of the penicillin molecule that dominated the thoughts of the more experienced penicillin chemists.

More important was that I recalled my pleasure in reading Woodward's Nobel Lecture[16] a few years earlier, with its description of an elegant synthesis of cephalosporin C (Figure 3b). The synthetic route involved the key intermediate shown in Figure 5, and this was obtained by the Woodward team in

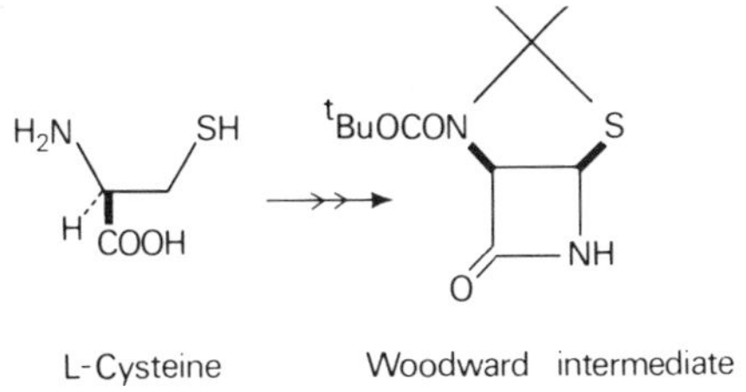

L-Cysteine          Woodward intermediate

**Figure 5.**

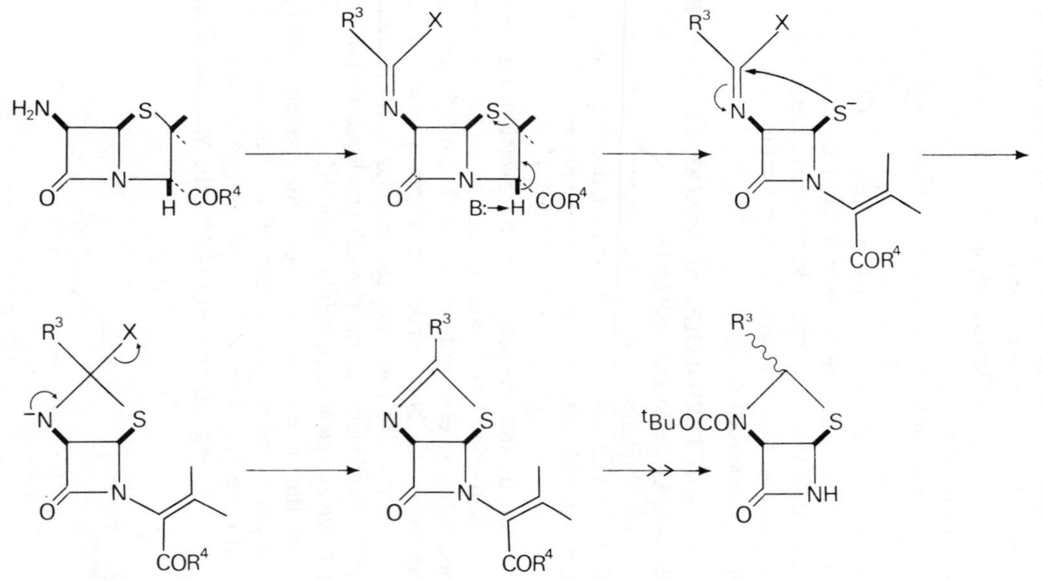

R³ = H; R⁴ = OCH₂OCOᵗBu; X = NMe₂.

**Figure 6.**

nine steps. I envisaged an analogous intermediate that might also be obtained more directly from our cheap 6β-aminopenicillanic acid ester through the reactions outlined in Figure 6. If this could be achieved in an economically feasible way, it would then be possible to explore its potential for the synthesis of other β-lactams and their evaluation as new antibacterials.

The crucial step in the projected synthesis was an initial base-catalyzed cleavage of the thiazolidine ring between the sulfur and the quaternary carbon atom, with simultaneous formation of a thiazoline ring and the elimination of the leaving group X as HX. Removal of dimethylpyruvic ester from the derived enamide by hydrolysis, followed by reduction with aluminum amalgam and protection of the nitrogen atom in the resulting thiazolidine derivative, would afford the desired key intermediate with correct stereochemistry.

Among several leaving groups we considered, X = $(CH_3)_2N$ was selected in the first attempt to achieve our goal because the requisite starting material was expected to be easily accessible. We further hoped that the basic amidino group in the molecule would catalyze the opening of the thiazolidine ring and the formation of a thiazoline ring with the elimination of the volatile dimethylamine, despite the poor ability of $(CH_3)_2N$ as a leaving group. $R^3$ was H to minimize steric effects.

Our first assumption was correct. A vigorous exothermic reaction took place when chlorodimethylformiminium chloride in anhydrous chloroform was added to a stirred solution of an equivalent amount of pivaloyloxymethyl 6β-aminopenicillanate and two equivalents of triethylamine in anhydrous chloroform at -30°C. After stirring at 0°C for 1 hour and a work up, pivaloyloxymethyl 6β-dimethylaminomethyleneaminopenicillanate crystallized nicely, either as such or as its hydrochloride (Figure 7).

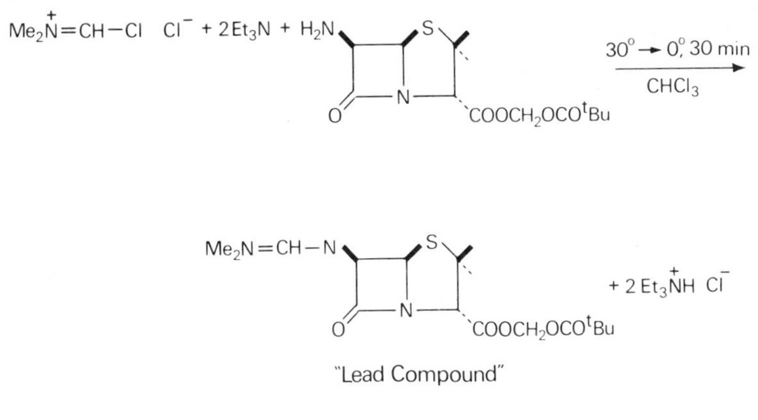

"Lead Compound"

Figure 7. Preparation of the "lead compound."

Our second expectation was wrong. All attempts to achieve the desired transformation failed.

Meanwhile our noncooperative starting material was sent to our microbiological department for routine testing. This department is headed by the very competent microbiologist L. Tybring, and he deserves much credit for the successful conclusion of the pivmecillinam story.

*In vitro* antibacterial screening of new compounds against a standard selection of gram-positive and gram-negative bacteria was at that time performed by the usual serial dilution technique with NIH broth. The results were evaluated by comparison with a number of known antimicrobial agents including penicillin G and ampicillin. In our case, the tests were preceded by an enzymatic hydrolysis with 25% mouse serum for 1½ hours at 37 °C and pH 7.4 to obtain the corresponding 6$\beta$-formamidinopenicillanic acid.

The results were amazing. Contrary to the ideas of orthodox medicinal chemists and our own expectations, this "deformed" $\beta$-lactam was able to kill bacteria, although gram-positive bacteria behaved as expected. The activity against *Staphylococcus aureus* was 135 times less than that of penicillin G. However, our compound was definitely active, only 1.5 to 4.5 times less potent than ampicillin, against a number of gram-negative organisms, including *Salmonella, Shigella, Klebsiella,* and *Proteus* species. It equaled ampicillin in potency against *Escherichia coli.* The old doctrine that determined how $\beta$-lactam antibiotics should be constructed was refuted by a compound with far more pronounced activity against gram-negative than gram-positive bacteria although the side chain had been profoundly modified.

Good fortune lent us a hand during the screening. NIH broth was our customary test medium; later experience has shown that the *in vitro* activity of mecillinam formed from the selected drug pivmecillinam,[9,17] and presumably all its relatives, is seriously reduced in media with high sodium chloride content. For example, increasing the 0.25% sodium chloride content of NIH agar medium fourfold completely protected highly sensitive *E. coli* and *Salmonella typhimurium* strains from the lytic action of mecillinam. Among all commercially available media, NIH broth was subsequently found to contain the least sodium chloride.

As soon as the results of the screening appeared, a rather excited Dr. Tybring reported his findings on the telephone. This conversation initiated a close and very inspiring cooperation between microbiologist and chemist. Needless to say, the chemist's interest was immediately turned away from new $\beta$-lactam nuclei to the old honorable penicillin nucleus carrying the new type of amidine side chain.

## 5. SYNTHESIS OF 6β-AMIDINOPENICILLANIC ACIDS AND THEIR DERIVATIVES[18]

The amidino group has not enjoyed the same popularity among medicinal and synthetic chemists as has the amide group. Whereas a variety of synthetic methods exist for the formation of the amide linkage by condensation between an activated carboxylic acid and an amine, the number of available methods for condensing an activated acid amide with an amine to form an amidine is limited. The presence of the reactive β-lactam ring in the molecule prevents the use of severe reaction conditions, and the obvious requirement of producing fully *N*-substituted amidines restricts the number of useful methods even further.

The 6β-amidinopenicillanic acid derivatives were, in principle, synthesized by two complementary routes, A and B (Figure 8). Most of the compounds could be obtained in satisfactory yield and purity by treatment of a reactive derivative of a tertiary amide or thioamide with a 6β-aminopenicillanic acid derivative (Route A). For activation, the amides were converted either to iminium chlorides, iminium ethers, thioiminium ethers, or amide acetals. The choice of activation method was of minor importance for simple amides, but activation of more complex amides required the careful selection of reactive derivatives and optimum conditions for their preparation.

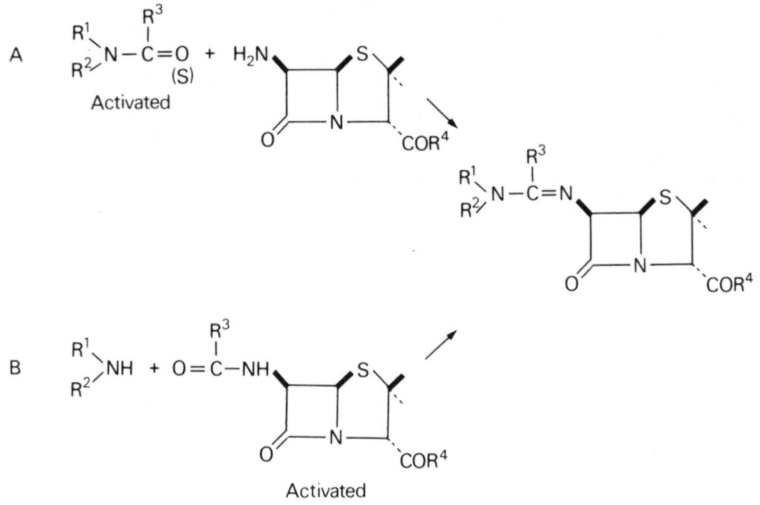

R¹, R² = (substituted) alkyl or aryl; R³ = H, (substituted) alkyl or aryl;
COR⁴ = carboxylic acid derivative.

**Figure 8.** Preparation of 6β-amidinopenicillanic acid derivatives.

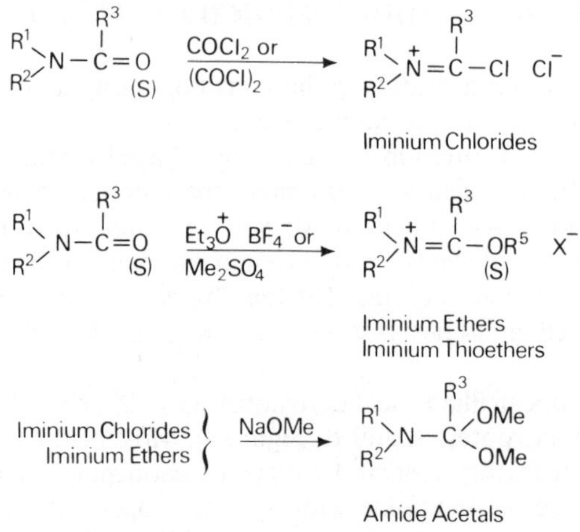

$$\begin{array}{c} R^1 \\ R^2 \end{array}\!\!\!>\!\!N - \overset{\overset{\displaystyle R^3}{|}}{C} = O \quad \xrightarrow{\;COCl_2 \text{ or}\;(COCl)_2\;} \quad \begin{array}{c} R^1 \\ R^2 \end{array}\!\!\!>\!\!\overset{+}{N} = \overset{\overset{\displaystyle R^3}{|}}{C} - Cl \quad Cl^-$$

(S)

Iminium Chlorides

$$\begin{array}{c} R^1 \\ R^2 \end{array}\!\!\!>\!\!N - \overset{\overset{\displaystyle R^3}{|}}{C} = O \quad \xrightarrow{\;Et_3\overset{+}{O}\;\;BF_4^- \text{ or}\;Me_2SO_4\;} \quad \begin{array}{c} R^1 \\ R^2 \end{array}\!\!\!>\!\!\overset{+}{N} = \overset{\overset{\displaystyle R^3}{|}}{C} - OR^5 \quad X^-$$

(S)                                                                    (S)

Iminium Ethers
Iminium Thioethers

Iminium Chlorides $\Big\{$  $\xrightarrow{\;NaOMe\;}$  $\begin{array}{c} R^1 \\ R^2 \end{array}\!\!\!>\!\!N - \overset{\overset{\displaystyle R^3}{|}}{C}\!\!\!<\!\!\begin{array}{c} OMe \\ OMe \end{array}$
Iminium Ethers $\Big($

Amide Acetals

$R^1$, $R^2$ = (substituted) alkyl or aryl; $R^3$ = H, (substituted) alkyl or aryl; $R^5$ = Me, Et;
$X^-$ = $BR_4^-$, $MeSO_4^-$.

**Figure 9.** Activation of tertiary amides and thioamides.

Iminium chlorides (Figure 9) were the preferred activated derivatives of tertiary amides. They are almost comparable with acid chlorides in reactivity and are generally precipitated as hygroscopic solids when tertiary amides or their more reactive sulfur analogues are treated with reagents like phosgene or oxalyl chloride in anhydrous ether. A disadvantage of iminium chlorides is that they cannot be purified. This is unimportant with the simple amides because they generally afford the corresponding iminium chlorides in high yield and purity. But purity and yield are adversely affected in heavily substituted amides or amides containing other functional groups. Oily, ill-defined products usually result from such amides owing to sluggish reaction with the reagent, or further transformation of the iminium chlorides once formed, or both.

The reaction of iminium chlorides with 6β-aminopenicillanic acid derivatives was performed in inert solvents in the presence of a tertiary amine at low temperature. Excellent yields (75-85%) of the desired 6β-amidinopenicillanic acid derivatives could be obtained when pure iminium chlorides and optimal conditions were used.

Iminium and thioiminium ethers (Figure 9) are less reactive, but they are useful alternatives to iminium chlorides, especially when the preparation of the latter is troublesome. They are obtained by alkylation of amides or thioamides, respectively, and the thioiminium salts can usually be purified by recrystallization.

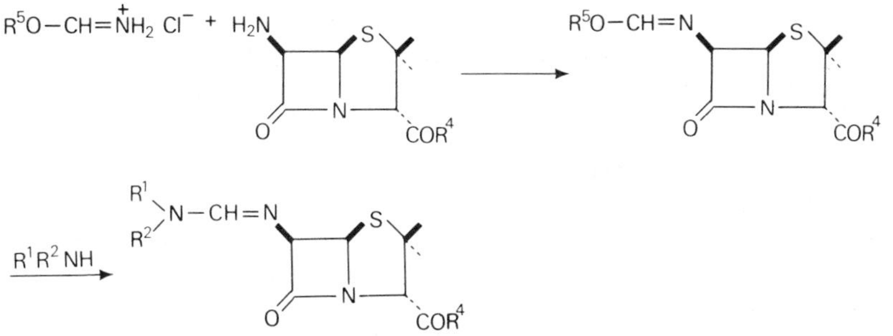

R[1], R[2] = (substituted) alkyl or aryl; COR[4] = carboxylic acid derivative; R[5] = alkyl.

**Figure 10.** Preparation of 6$\beta$-formamidinopenicillanic acid derivatives (Route B).

Although the preparation of amide acetals (Figure 9) from the corresponding iminium salts by reaction with alkali alkoxides requires an extra step, they have two advantages over their precursors. They can usually be purified by distillation, and during their reaction with amines, alcohols instead of ammonium salts are formed in addition to the desired amidines. The use of amide acetals was particularly advantageous for the preparation of the water-soluble zwitterionic 6$\beta$-amidinopenicillanic acids, since the absence of other salts greatly facilitated purification.

In Method B (Figure 8), only elaborated at a later stage of the project, the 6$\beta$-amidinopenicillanic acid derivatives were obtained by treatment of a reactive penicillin derivative with a secondary amine. Starting from 6N-alkoxymethylene-6$\beta$-aminopenicillanic acid derivatives (Figure 10), this approach proved especially suitable for the preparation of several 6$\beta$-formamidinopenicillanic acid derivatives that contain additional functional groups incompatible with the activating reagents used in Method A. Based upon analogy with $\alpha$-aminocarboxylic acid esters,[19] a convenient synthesis of the starting material could be devised. When an ethereal solution of the requisite 6$\beta$-aminopenicillanic acid derivative was stirred with formimidic ester hydrochloride, ammonium chloride precipitated, leaving an ethereal solution of the desired starting material in high yield.

Only pivaloyloxymethyl esters of the 6$\beta$-amidinopenicillanic acids were prepared during the first phase of our efforts to correlate the structure of the 6-side chain with *in vitro* antimicrobial activity, because these esters were generally easily crystallized and methods for the synthesis of the acids had yet to be developed. Before antibacterial testing, the esters were enzymatically hydrolyzed to the acids.

A weakness of this test procedure was the inherent risk of reduced yields of the acids due to side reactions and incomplete hydrolysis of the esters. In later experiments, acids prepared chemically have sometimes shown higher anti-bacterial activity than those formed *in situ* by enzymatic hydrolysis of the corresponding esters.

## 6.  FROM "LEAD" TO OPTIMUM COMPOUND

In consequence of the "ester approach" with the *in situ* formation of the actual antimicrobial agents, no relevant physicochemical data were obtainable for mathematical analysis of test results à la Hansch. We could therefore head for the optimum compound without delay.

What was our position at the start of developing 6$\beta$-amidinopenicillanic acids from a chance observation to a useful drug? A close and friendly relationship had long existed between the bacteriological and chemical research departments, with an open exchange of ideas. Both sides were experienced and not yet senile, at least according to our own judgment. None of us suffered from self-distrust! These assets more than counterbalanced the liabilities owing to the limited resources that could be allocated this project. Two other drugs, bumetanide and pivampicillin were under development in the research laboratories at the same time. Only one technician, later on two, took part in the first phase of the synthetic work that led to the preparation of pivmecillinam as the 19th compound of the series in less than four months.

At the beginning, we were confronted with an exciting and complicated problem, in a sense even larger than that faced when the development of the semisynthetic penicillins began. The side chain R³CO (Figure 11) constitutes the only site for structural variation in the penicillins when the unmodified penicillanic acid residue is retained. In contrast, the substituted 6$\beta$-amidinopenicillanic acids contain in principle three independent variables

R³-Penicillin

R¹R²R³ – Substituted
6ß-Amidinopenicillanic Acid

R¹, R² = (substituted) alkyl or aryl; R³ = H, (substituted) alkyl or aryl.

**Figure 11.**

$R^1$, $R^2$, and $R^3$. A further complication resulted from the assumed special mode of action of the "lead compound,"[5] which implied that structure-activity relationships found in penicillins would most likely not be valid in the new type of antibiotic. In addition, it was imaginable that our active amidine belonged to a subgroup of the much larger group of basic compounds containing the structural element N=C-N. Chemically, amidines differ from amides by their basic properties, and the peculiar antibacterial activity of our "lead compound" was quite naturally ascribed to this character. Consequently, other types of 6N-substituted penicillanic acids containing this subunit, such as guanidines and imidic esters, might be more profitably explored than simple amidines.

The preparation of pure imidic esters was expected to be troublesome and their stability poor, so the synthesis of the simplest stable guanidine, $R^1 = R^2 = CH_3$, $R^3 = N(CH_3)_2$ (compound **9**, Table 2), and another amidine, $R^1 = R^2 = C_2H_5$, $R^3 = H$ (compound **2**, Table 1), was initiated from the requisite substituted urea and amide through the derived chloroformamidine (Figure 12)

$$Me_2N\,CO\,N\,Me_2 \xrightarrow{\;COCl_2\;} Me_2\overset{+}{N}=C-N\,Me_2$$
$$\underset{Cl\ \ Cl^-}{|}$$

Chloroformamidine

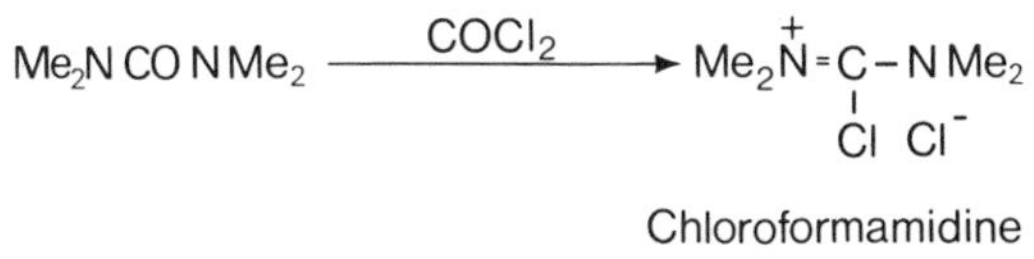

**Figure 12.** Activation of tetramethylurea.

and iminium chloride, respectively. The amidine, only slightly modified, was expected to be antibacterially active (after hydrolysis). It could at the same time meet the microbiologists' demand for more material and suggest whether the activity could be increased by enlargement of the $R^1$ and $R^2$ alkyls. Among the numerous conceivable members of these series, our "lead compound" with $R^1 = R^2 = CH_3$ and $R^3 = H$ occupies the unique position as an ester of the smallest stable 6β-amidinopenicillanic acid. Compounds containing $R^1 = H$ would be expected to be converted to imidazol-4-one derivatives through intramolecular acylation of the $R^2NH$ group by the reactive β-lactam carbonyl group. Besides, the synthesis of compound **2** would be straightforward, giving me time to increase my knowledge of amidine chemistry.

Retrospectively, the development from "lead" to optimum compound seems to have taken place in three almost clear-cut and systematic sections. This is demonstrated in Tables 1-3. The tables list the compounds in chronological order as they were obtained analytically pure and tested. In the first phase (Table 1), the influence of chiefly aliphatic $R^1R^2$-variations on activity was studied in formamidines with compound **3** as the only exception. In the second

**Table 1**

**Antibacterial Activity of**
**Substituted β-Amidinopenicillanic Acids**

$$R^1_{R^2}\!\!>\!\!N\text{--}\overset{\overset{\displaystyle R^3}{|}}{C}\!\!=\!\!N\text{---}$$

(penicillanic acid ring structure with S, N, COOH, O)

| Compound | $R^1_{R^2}\!\!>\!\!N\text{--}$ | $R^3$ | IC$_{50}$ ($\mu$g/ml) | | |
|---|---|---|---|---|---|
| | | | | | *S. aureus* |
| | | | *S. aureus* | *E. coli* | *E. coli* |
| 1 | $CH_3$ $CH_3$ $>$N-- | H | 1.6 | 0.5 | 3 |
| 2 | $C_2H_5$ $C_2H_5$ $>$N-- | H | 5.0 | 0.1 | 50 |
| 3 | $CH_3$ $CH_3$ $>$N-- | (phenyl)-- | 10 | > 100 | < 0.1 |
| 4 | (benzyl) -CH$_2$ $CH_3$ $>$N-- | H | 1 | 0.5 | 2 |
| 5 | $n-C_3H_7$ $n-C_3H_7$ $>$N-- | H | 7.9 | 0.16 | 50 |
| 6 | $i-C_3H_7$ $i-C_3H_7$ $>$N-- | H | 50 | 0.2 | 250 |
| 7 | (morpholino) O$\bigcirc$N-- | H | 0.63 | 5.0 | 0.13 |
| 8 | (piperidino) $\bigcirc$N-- | H | 2.0 | 0.05 | 40 |
| Ampicillin | | | 0.025 | 1.3 | 0.02 |

**Table 2**

**Antibacterial Activity of**
**Trisubstituted β-Amidinopenicillanic Acids**

| Compound | $\begin{array}{c}R^1\\R^2\end{array}$>N– | $R^3$ | IC$_{50}$ ($\mu$g/ml) | | S. aureus |
|---|---|---|---|---|---|
| | | | S. aureus | E. coli | E. coli |
| 9 | $\begin{array}{c}CH_3\\CH_3\end{array}$>N– | $\begin{array}{c}CH_3\\CH_3\end{array}$>N– | >100 | >100 | — |
| 10 | $\begin{array}{c}CH_3\\CH_3\end{array}$>N– | $CH_3$- | 10 | 13 | 0.8 |
| 11 | $\begin{array}{c}CH_3\\CH_3\end{array}$>N– | n-C$_3$H$_7$- | 2.0 | >100 | <0.02 |
| 12 | | | 79 | 13 | 6 |
| 13 | $\begin{array}{c}CH_3\\CH_3\end{array}$>N– | ⬡-CH$_2^-$ | 0.25 | >100 | <0.0025 |
| Ampicillin | | | 0.025 | 1.3 | 0.02 |

phase (Table 2), the consequences of R$^3$-variations were examined in trisubstituted amidines with fixed R$^1$R$^2$-substituent except in the special compound **12**. Finally, the third phase comprises mainly the study of formamidines containing various rings (Table 3.)

The reality was quite different. The tables don't reflect the *starting* order of synthesis of the tabulated compounds. This is partly because of initial synthetic difficulties and partly because of changes in the perceived importance of compounds in progress concurrently with the latest results from the microbiologists.

**Table 3**

**Antibacterial Activity of**
**Substituted β-Formamidinopenicillanic Acids**

$$\begin{array}{c} R^1 \\ {}^{R^2}\!\!>\!N\!-\!C=\!N\!- \\ \text{(penicillanic acid core with S, N, COOH)} \end{array}$$

| Compound | $\overset{R^1}{\underset{R^2}{>}}N-$ | $R^3$ | IC$_{50}$ ($\mu$g/ml) | | |
|---|---|---|---|---|---|
| | | | | | S. aureus |
| | | | S. aureus | E. coli | E. coli |
| 14 | CH$_2$=CH–CH$_2$, CH$_2$=CH–CH$_2$ >N– | H | 1.6 | 0.5 | 3 |
| 15 | ⬡N– (azetidine) | H | 2.5 | 0.2 | 13 |
| 16 | (2,6-dimethylpiperidine) N– CH$_3$/CH$_3$ | H | 13 | 0.08 | 160 |
| 17 | CH$_3$ (methyl-phenyl) N– | H | 1.3 | 10 | 0.13 |
| 18 | CH$_3$ (methyl-cyclohexyl) N– | H | 5.0 | 0.2 | 25 |
| 19 | (azepane) N– | H | 6.3 | 0.016 | 400 |
| Ampicillin | | | 0.025 | 1.3 | 0.02 |

Returning to 1969 and compound **2**, the exploration of the amidine series was extended in two directions during the following weeks. The influence of the R$^3$-substituent was examined while keeping R$^1$R$^2$N constant as (CH$_3$)$_2$N, and by the preparation of some formamidines (R$^3$ = H), information could be obtained about the effect of R$^1$R$^2$-variations. The synthesis of compounds **10, 13** (Table 2), and **3** (Table 1) was begun in order to learn how the replacement of hydrogen in compound **1** (Table 1) by the smallest possible alkyl, arylalkyl, and aryl R$^3$-groups, respectively, would influence the activity. Though not unjustifiable the incorporation of a benzyl-substituted amidine (and later the form-amidine compound **4**) among the first few projected compounds reflects the conservatism of a medicinal chemist. It was hard to enter the new antibiotic field with an unbiased mind and ignore the presence of the benzyl group in certain of the most important penicillins. In the formamidine series, the preparation of compound **7** (Table 1) containing the weakly basic morpholine moiety would indicate the influence of base strength on activity. Compound **17** (Table 3) represented the smallest aromatic member of this series, and compound **15** (Table 3) was a ring-closed analogue of compound **2**.

The tables summarize our test results by reproducing the *in vitro* activities of the compounds against a typical gram-positive organism, *S. aureus,* and a typical gram-negative one, *E. coli,* (*E. coli* is the most common pathogenic organism in urinary tract-infections.) As is usual in our laboratories, the activities are expressed as $IC_{50}$ values, that is, the concentrations of the test compounds that cause 50% inhibition of growth. In addition, for reasons that will appear from the further development of the $6\beta$-amidinopenicillanic acids, in the last column of the tables the ratio between the two $IC_{50}$ values is taken as a measure of the relative predominance of the gram-negative component of the antibacterial activity. A large figure of the ratio indicates a relatively higher gram-negative activity, and conversely a low figure indicates a relatively higher gram-positive activity. For comparison, the activities of ampicillin as we determined them are given at the bottom of the tables.

In the meantime, testing of compound **2** had shown very encouraging results, as shown in Table 1. The drastic increase of the "gram-negative selectivity" to 50 from a modest figure of three with the lead compound results from a marked improvement of gram-negative potency and a simultaneous decrease in performance against gram-positive bacteria. This progress, and the appearance of discouraging antibacterial data for compounds **3** and **4** (Table 1) at almost the same time, prompted the immediate syntheses of compounds **5** and **6** (Table 1) in which the ethyl groups of compound **2** were replaced by propyl and isopropyl groups, respectively. In addition, the preparation of the homologue containing $R^1 = R^2 = n$-butyl was initiated because we intuitively expected this compound to limit the increase of activity in this series. But the testing of compounds **5** and **6** (Table 1) already suggested that other lines of development should be sought during the first rough screening of the numerous possibilities, and the synthesis of the butyl-containing derivative with an activity indistinguishable from that of compounds **5** and **6** was not completed until later.

During these weeks, compound **2** (after enzymatic hydrolysis) underwent a closer bacteriological examination. The unusual antibacterial spectrum of the first formamidines suggested that their mode of action was different from that of penicillins.[5] Consequently, they might potentiate the effect of penicillins.

Indeed, *in vitro* synergy was found between ampicillin and the acid resulting from the hydrolysis of compound **2**.

A lessening of base strength, as in compound **7** (Table 1) apparently would not increase the gram-negative potency, although the increased effect against gram-positive bacteria was interesting and unexpected. The obvious question to ask next was, How would increasing the base strength influence the activity? The preparation of the earlier projected pyrrolidine compound **15** (Table 3) might provide the answer, but because of inexperience with the preparation of iminium chlorides, we had met with difficulties in synthesizing the requisite starting material.

To save time, a synthesis of compound **8** (Table 1) containing the six-membered strongly basic piperidine ring was carried through without problems. Comparison of the bacteriological results of compounds **8** and **5** immediately suggested that a closer look at ring-closed compounds was warranted.

In the meantime, we had finally prepared our first guanidine derivative, compound **9** (Table 2) and a number of long planned R³-substituted amidines, compounds **10-13** (Table 2). We had wasted much time trying to avoid using the most suitable reagent, phosgene, for the preparation of iminium chlorides and chloroformamidines because my previous mishandling of this toxic gas several years before had sent a number of my colleagues to the hospital for 24 hours! Eventually I overcame my concern and resumed work with phosgene.

The inactivity of compound **9** (Table 2) was not quite unexpected in view of the known inferior activity of related substituted ureas.[20] In contrast, the high gram-positive activity and simultaneously low gram-negative activity displayed by compound **13** was very exciting as it demonstrated the presence of at least two types of antibacterial activity inside the 6$\beta$-amidinopenicillanic acid group. Work that had already started, aiming at the investigation into other types of N-C = N-substituted penicillanic acids such as amidrazones and amidoximes containing the structural elements N-C = N-N and N-C = N-O, respectively, was therefore intensified. But owing to the lack of useful synthetic methods, such derivatives (which, incidentally, did not have an encouraging antibacterial activity) were not obtained until much later by replacing the secondary amines of Method B (Figure 8) with the appropriate hydrazines and hydroxylamines.

Compounds **14** and **17** (Table 3) were stragglers from the earlier exploration of the influence of R¹R² substitution on activity in the formamidine series. They had not been obtainable until phosgene was tried for the preparation of the requisite iminium chlorides. The antibacterial properties of the unsaturated derivative **14** were depressing, as were those of the aromatic compound **17** that appeared shortly afterwards.

The increased importance of ring compounds indicated by the piperidine derivative **8** resulted in a reexamination of the unsuccessful attempts to prepare the long-requested pyrrolidine compound **15** (Table 3) and the speedy accomplishment of its synthesis and antibacterial evaluation. The results clearly indicated that inferior activity was associated with the reduction of ring size. Preparation of the next higher homologue was the logical consequence. The necessary starting material hexamethyleneimine was fortunately available and cheap, so we could immediately bring about the synthesis of the intermediary formamide derivative. Following conversion to the derived iminium chloride, this was treated with pivaloyloxymethyl $6\beta$-aminopenicillanate in the usual way to yield compound **19** (Table 3).

Meanwhile, two other compounds (**16** and **18**, Table 3) appeared as offshoots of our saturated ring program. The main reason for the preparation of compound **16** was to find out whether the steric hindrance provided by the two methyl groups around the amidine bond would increase resistance to $\beta$-lactamases. This was prompted of course, by the effect it can have of shielding the $\beta$-lactam carbonyl group in penicillins from attack by these enzymes. In addition, compound **16** might give us some clue to the possibility of increasing the potency of compound **8** by methyl substitution. Neither of these hopes was fulfilled, nor did the replacement of an alkyl by a cyclohexyl group in the aliphatic open-chain formamidines provide any improvement, as evidenced by compound **18**.

Compound **19** met our expectations, showing an 80 times higher *in vitro* activity (after enzymatic hydrolysis) than ampicillin against *E. coli*. In other words, this compound demonstrates essentially the same potency against the gram-negative bacillus as does penicillin G against the gram-positive *S. aureus*. Compound **19**, in the form of its hydrochloride, named FL 1039, proved to be the optimum candidate for further extensive evaluation despite our increased efforts in the following years to find even better compounds. The outcome of the slow procedure of meeting regulatory requirements was the approval and marketing of the drug pivmecillinam, mainly for the treatment of urinary-tract infections, in Denmark at the beginning of 1978 and afterwards in a number of other countries.

## 7. EFFECT OF SIDE CHAIN MODIFICATIONS ON ACTIVITY

During this first phase of the search for the optimum compound within the substituted $6\beta$-amidinopenicillanic acids, we had additionally achieved a general view of the most important structure-activity relationships of the side chain. Two main types of antibacterially active compounds are discernible:
1.  Those containing $R^3 = H$ (Figure 11) have predominantly gram-negative activity. The already considerable activity of compounds having small

alkyl or cycloalkyl $R^1$,$R^2$-substituents (compounds **2**, **5**, **6**, and **18**, Tables 1 and 3) may be further increased by closing the alkyl chains to rings, as exemplified by compounds **8** and **19**.

2.   Among those containing $R^3$ = H, $R^1$ and $R^2$ = small alkyls, marked grampositive activity is displayed when $R^3$ is benzyl (compound **13**, Table 2).

Between these extremes are a number of compounds with low to moderate gram-positive and gram-negative activity in varying ratios (compounds **1**, **4**, **7**, and **17**).

Thus the substituted 6β-amidinopenicillanic acids cover a broader spectrum of activity in terms of *in vitro* potency than do the penicillins.

Several hundred representatives of this class of β-lactam antibiotics containing more or less elaborate side chains have been prepared and evaluated in these laboratories and elsewhere. The more detailed knowledge thus obtained of the influence of side chain variations on activity has been recorded elsewhere,[18] except for the interesting finding of Binderup[21] that certain formamidines containing aminoalkyl-substituted rings display antipseudomonas activity. Maximum gram-negative activity was found in formamidines with six or seven carbon atoms in a monocyclic or bicyclic ring, and the highest gram-positive activity was shown by trisubstituted amidines when $R^3$ is benzyl or phenoxymethyl, irrespective of the meaning of $R^1$ and $R^2$.

Amidines are generally hydrolyzed more easily than amides, and this explains the striking similarity between trisubstituted 6β-amidinopenicillanic acids and penicillins with respect to structure-activity relationships. The "grampositive" amidines are hydrolyzed to the derived $R^3$-penicillins (Figure 11) with simultaneous liberation of the $R^1R^2$-substituted amines. This observation has been shown to be well-based by the investigations of Baltzer and Rastrup-Andersen.[22]

Incidentally, the degradation of the formamidines by hydrolysis is more complex, especially at pH $\geqslant 7$.[23] As luck would have it, the side chain of pivmecillinam appears to be more stable to hydrolysis than most of those contained in its analogues; for example, the rate of hydrolysis is increased by a factor of three at pH $\geqslant 7.4$ and 37 °C when the seven-membered ring of mecillinam is replaced by the six-membered ring of the highly active 6β-formamidinopenicillanic acid derived from compound **8**.[22]

## 8.   COMMENT

Accumulated knowledge tends to generate doctrines. These may be useful but they can also be detrimental to further progress. A time-honored doctrine determined that β-lactam antibiotics should be constructed as 6β-acylaminopenicillanic acids. This was overturned by the discovery of the substituted 6β-formamidinopenicillanic acids with their high activity against gram-negative organisms. It is possible that challenges to other doctrines in medicinal chemistry would result in the discovery of new drugs.

## ACKNOWLEDGMENTS

I am greatly indebted to my colleagues of the Chemical, Analytical, and Bacteriological Departments of Leo Pharmaceutical Products for their contributions to the pivmecillinam project. I also express my gratitude to Mr. G. Andersen, my assistant for more than 20 years, and to Professor W. D. Ollis for helpful suggestions during the preparation of the manuscript.

## REFERENCES

1.  K. Roholt, B. Nielsen, and E. Kristensen, *Chemotherapy,* **21,** 146 (1975).
2.  J. C. Christoffersen, H.-G. Iversen, J. Jacobsen, B. Korner, H. K. Petersen, F. Rasmussen, and L. Tybring, *Scand. J. Urol. Nephrol.,* **8,** 185 (1974).
3.  E. R. Verrier Jones and A. W. Asscher, *J. Antimicrob. Chem.,* **1,** 193 (1975).
4.  B. Bresky, *J. Antimicrob. Chem.,* **3** (Suppl. B), 121 (1977).
5.  F. Lund and L. Tybring, *Nature New Biol.,* **236,** 135 (1972).
6.  J. T. Park and L. Burman, *Biochem. Biophys. Res. Comm.,* **51,** 863 (1973).
7.  S. Matsuhashi, T. Kamiryo, P. M. Blumberg, P. Linnett, E. Willoughby, and J. L. Strominger, *J. Bacteriol.,* **117,** 578 (1974).
8.  B. G. Spratt, *J. Antimicrob. Chem.,* **3,** (Suppl. B), 13 (1977).
9.  L. Tybring and N. H. Melchior, *Antimicrob. Agents Chemother.,* **8,** 271 (1975).
10. E. Grunberg, R. Cleeland, G. Beskid, and W. F. Delorenzo, *Antimicrob. Agents Chemother.,* **9,** 589 (1976).
11. R. G. Shepherd, "Sulfanilamides and other *p*-Aminobenzoic Acid Antagonists," in A. Burger, Ed., *Medicinal Chemistry,* 3rd ed., Wiley-Interscience, New York, 1970, p. 255.
12. M. W. Whitehouse, "Some Biochemical and Pharmacological Properties of Anti-Inflammatory Drugs," in E. Jucker, Ed., *Progress in Drug Research,* Vol. 8, Birkhauser, Basel, 1965, p. 321.
13. W. T. Comer and A. W. Gomoll, "Antihypertensive Agents," in A. Burger, Ed., *Medicinal Chemistry,* 3rd ed., Wiley-Interscience, New York, 1970, p. 1019.
14. R. J. Frankel, I. A. Reid, and W. F. Ganong, *J. Pharmacol. Exp. Ther.,* **201,** 400 (1977).
15. J. R. E. Hoover and R. J. Stedman, "The $\beta$-Lactam Antibiotics," in A. Burger, Ed., *Medicinal Chemistry,* 3rd ed., Wiley-Interscience, New York, 1970, p. 371.
16. R. B. Woodward, *Science,* **153,** 487 (1966).
17. L. Tybring, *Antimicrob. Agents Chemother.,* **8,** 266 (1975).
18. F. J. Lund, "6$\beta$-Amidinopenicillanic Acids: Synthesis and Antibacterial Properties," in J. Elks, Ed., *Recent Advances in the Chemistry of $\beta$-Lactam Antibiotics,* The Chemical Society, London, 1977, p. 25.
19. E. Schmidt, *Ber.,* **47,** 2545 (1914).
20. Y. G. Perron, W. F. Minor, L. B. Crast, and L. C. Cheney, *J. Org. Chem.,* **26,** 3365 (1961).
21. E. T. Binderup (Loevens kemiske Fabrik Produktionsaktieselskab), Ger. Offen. 2,728,588; *Chem. Abstr.,* **88,** 152,610d (1978).
22. B. Baltzer and N. Rastrup-Andersen, unpublished data.
23. B. Baltzer, F. Lund, and N. Rastrup-Andersen, *J. Pharm. Sci.,* **68,** 1207 (1979).

# Doxorubicin

8

Frederico Arcamone

## 1. INTRODUCTION

Twenty years ago no one would have predicted that a member of the then well-known family of anthracycline pigments would become an important chemotherapeutic agent for the treatment of human cancer. Nor could it have been predicted that its introduction would arouse renewed interest in cancer chemotherapy. This development changed cancer chemotherapy from the character of a mere palliative to that of a major treatment for this disease.

This chapter deals with the discovery of doxorubicin (Adriamycin) and with the further chemical synthesis of related compounds showing the promise of becoming second-generation drugs in this class. The account presented here is restricted to work done in my laboratory. A detailed review of work reported in the scientific and patent literature up to June 1979 has recently been published.

## 2. THE CLASSICAL ANTHRACYCLINES (1950-1960)

The accumulated knowledge concerning the anthracycline antibiotics at the beginning of the 1960s was exhaustively reviewed by Hans Brockmann in 1963.[2] The generic name was derived from the presence of an anthraquinone chromophore and from the similarity of the polycyclic ring system to that of the well-known tetracyclines. The biologically active compounds were red or yellow glycosides whose aglycones, the anthracyclinones, originated biogenetically from acetate via polyketide intermediates. Different dehydration, deoxygenation, and hydroxylation reactions give rise to the various final tetracyclic hydroxyanthraquinone chromophores. A single terminal propionate unit was included, leading to the two-carbon-atom side chain present in most anthraquinones. Typical aglycones were $\beta$-rhodomycinone (1), $\epsilon$-rhodomycinone (2), $\epsilon$-pyrromycinone (3), and aklavinone (4). The main carbohydrate component, rhodosamine (5), was attached to position 7 (and/or 10, in 1); other sugars, namely 2-deoxy-$L$-fucose and rhodinose (6), are also present in some glycosides. The anthracyclines exhibited antibacterial activity (mainly towards gram-positive microorganisms), but toxicity in laboratory animals precluded their clinical use for the treatment of bacterial infections.

## 3. ANTITUMOR ANTIBIOTICS AND THE FARMITALIA SCREENING PROGRAM (1955-1960)

Strong interest had been aroused in the search of fermentation products as potential antitumor agents starting from the recognition in 1952 of the activity of actinomycins against certain experimental neoplasms.[3] This led to clinical investigations of mitomycin C and, in our laboratories, to the study in the late 1950s of the antibiotic distamycin A.[5] By 1966, some 50 compounds of microbial origin that showed some kind of antitumor activity had been described[6] but the toxicity of actinomycin D and mitomycin C, as well as the subsequently developed chromomycin $A_3$,[6] greatly limited the use of the corresponding commercial preparations.

I began work on the chemistry of new (or presumably new) constituents of microbial cultures mainly belonging to the genus *Streptomyces*, in the section of Chemotherapy and Microbiology of Farmitalia Research Institute in 1954. As head of the department, Professor Aurelio Di Marco (himself having come from the renowned school of pathology of Professor Rondoni at the Istituto Nazionale per lo Studio e le Cura dei Tumori, Milan) was personally interested in cancer chemotherapy. New chemical species, either in the pure or crude state, were tested in experimental systems in order to evaluate the presence of antitumor properties. The program of research on antitumor anthracyclines had become well established at Farmitalia by the 1960s. Strong support from Dr. Giulio Bertini, the Scientific Director and General Manager of Farmitalia, assured continuation of the program when, in 1964, Professor Di Marco left to take the position of Head of the Department of Experimental Oncology at Istituto Nazionale Tumori.

## 4.  ANTITUMOR ANTHRACYCLINES

In 1957, biological activity in the murine Ehrlich carcinoma and sarcoma 180 test systems shown by different isolates (laboratory codes X-27, X-28, X-45 through X-47, X-52 through X-63, X-87 through X-92, X-101) derived from strain 1683 (isolated from a sample of soil collected in India) aroused our interest in the corresponding active principles. The presence of red pigments containing a hydroxyanthraquinone chromophore had been deduced on the basis of the characteristic ultraviolet and visible absorption spectrum of the active preparations. Isolation of the pigments by a countercurrent extraction procedure afforded a material showing properties (spectroscopic and indicator-like behavior) similar to those of the rhodomycin complex[7] and endowed with a marked inhibitory effect on the growth of the above experimental tumors.[8] Although the toxicity of the substance precluded further development of these products, the results suggested that antitumor activity was associated with the anthracycline structure. The possibility of developing a useful drug from this family of antibiotics was not considered very likely at the time. A similar observation had been made by Swiss authors regarding the cinerubins.[9] The main component of active preparations extracted from strain 1683 was eventually identified at my laboratory with rhodomycin B (7) (unpublished work).

A year later our interest in anthracycline-like substances was reawakened when the presence of related compounds was detected in new preparations (laboratory codes X-80 to X-82 of December 15, 1958, and X-105, X-106 of February 16, 1959) that also showed antitumor properties in the Ehrlich ascite tumor. Those substances were obtained by solvent extraction of both the mycelium and the filtered media of a new *Streptomyces* species isolated from a soil sample collected in Apulia near the ancient Swabian manor of Castel del Monte. The names of the pre-Roman peoples living in the region, the *Peucetii* and the *Daunii*, were used to derive the names respectively of the microorganism (*S. peucetius*) and the main active substance (daunomycin). Although the presence of different bioactive compounds, including antifungal polyenes, somewhat hampered the identification of the component responsible for the observed antitumor (cytotoxic) activity, the component was eventually obtained in pure form by chromatography on buffered cellulose and was crystallized as the hydrochloride in January 1962.[10] The new antibiotic daunomycin inhibited the growth of the test tumor and prolonged survival of tumor-bearing animals to a greater extent than the known antitumor antibiotics mitomycin C and actinomycin C.[11]

These results, extended to other biological systems,[12] stimulated the investigation of the chemical structure of daunomycin with the objective of ascertaining structural differences from the "classical" anthracyclines that were responsible for the improved pharmacological properties. The chemical studies were carried out in collaboration with G. Cassinelli, G. Franceschi, and P. Orezzi, great assistance being provided by NMR specialist Rosanna Mondelli of Politecnico, Milan. By 1964, the structures of the aglycone and sugar moieties of daunomycin (8) were established and published.[13,14] In brief, acid hydrolysis of daunomycin afforded the aglycone daunomycinone, and the aminosugar daunosamine, both fragments corresponding to previously unknown compounds. Analytical and spectroscopic measurements, together with the formation of naphthacene upon zinc dust distillation, allowed the establishment of the tetracyclic system and of functionalities of daunomycinone. The latter was also converted to a bisanhydro derivative in a variety of conditions and to a 6-deoxy derivative upon hydrogenolysis. Other important derivatives were the trimethyl ether and the tetraacetate. Alkaline fusion gave salicylic acid whereas oxidative fission of bisanhydrodaunomycinone gave 3-methoxyphthalic and trimellitic acid. The presence of the methylketone side chain on a carbon bearing a hydroxyl group was proved by the formation of acetaldehyde by borohydride reduction followed by periodate oxidation of daunomycinone. These results were consistent with the structure assigned to daunomycinone, although the position of the methoxy group, either at C-1 or at C-4, was not ascertained. At the same time the structure and stereochemistry of daunosamine were determined on the basis of periodate oxidation studies (particularly important was the oxidation of *N*-benzoyldaunosamine yielding a nonvolatile aldehyde that was converted to *N*-benzoyl-*L*-aspartic acid upon treatment with hypoiodite), NMR measurements, and conformational arguments.

The comparison of daunomycin (8) with rhodomycin B (7) indicated that minor differences in anthracycline structure could give rise to improved biological activity, and we were therefore encouraged to proceed further in the investigation of *S. peucetius* metabolites. We were also encouraged by the observation that preparations containing different related pigmented components exhibited variations with respect to the increase of survival of tumor-bearing mice. (Other important reasons for the continuation of our efforts to select the "best" candidate for cancer treatment are outlined in the following section.) Structural studies to clarify the details of the daunomycin structure were completed in subsequent years.[15,16] The position of the methoxyl group was determined by aromatization and demethylation of 9, which was obtained by chromic oxidation of daunomycinone to 10a or 10b the latter resulting when the demethylation reaction was carried out with aluminum chloride in benzene. The pattern of hydroxylation in 10a and 10b was established on the basis of their visible spectra in different solvents and the absence of the nonchelated quinone bond in the infrared spectra of the corresponding pericarbonates. The site of attachment of the glycosidic linkage was determined by hydrogenolysis to 7-deoxydaunomycinone and daunosamine, and the $\alpha$-configuration was determined by PMR measurements. The absolute configuration of the aglycone moiety was established by converting daunomycinone trimethyl ether to 11, followed by oxidation of the latter with lead tetraacetate to a diquinone

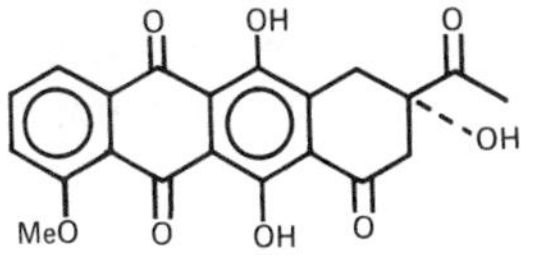

9

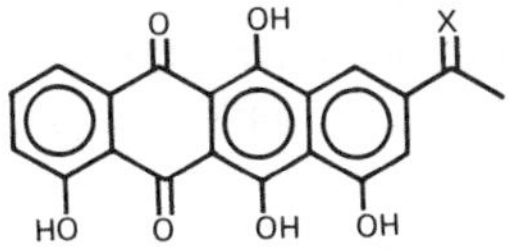

10a: X = O
10b: X = H, Ph

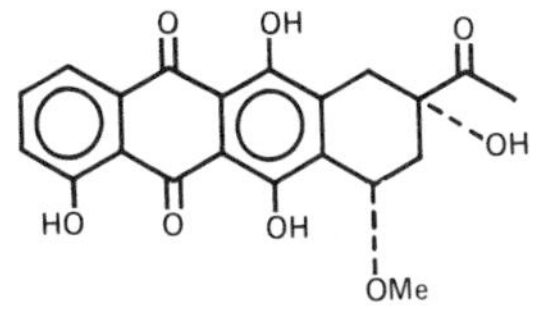

11

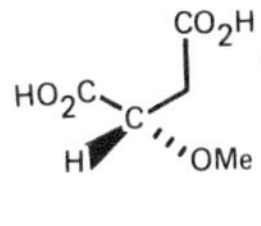

12

whose fission with the Lemieux reagent afforded $S(-)$-methoxy-succinic acid
(12) (for a further review of structural-determination studies see reference 17;
for experimental details see reference 18).

The significance of the establishment of aglycone stereochemistry went
beyond simply the structural determination of daunomycin. The absolute configuration of all other known anthracyclinones could be derived from that of
daunomycinone through the comparison of circular dichroism curves.[19] In
addition, knowledge of the absolute configuration of daunomycin was a prerequisite for subsequent studies concerning the structure of the complex between the antibiotic and its biological receptor.[20] Confirmation of the structure
and stereochemistry of daunomycin was obtained by X-ray analysis of the
$N$-bromoacetyl derivative.[21]

## 5.   DAUNOMYCIN IS PROVED CLINICALLY EFFECTIVE AND BECOMES "DAUNORUBICIN"

The first clinical report confirming the therapeutic efficacy of daunomycin in
the treatment of acute leukemias was presented by C. Tan and A. Di Marco.[22]
This study was the consequence of the prompt delivery in 1963 of a pure sample
of the antibiotic by A. Di Marco to the late Professor Karnofsky of Memorial
Hospital, New York. In that year, however, we became aware that the priority
of the daunomycin patent[23] was seriously affected by a patent issued by Rhone-
Poulenc in which what appeared to be a very similar substance (13.057 RP) was
described and claimed.[24] The new antibiotic, named rubidomycin, was also
reported by the French group in a scientific publication;[25] prompt exchange of
samples proved the two substances to be identical.[10] Preclinical and clinical
studies performed with the drug independently prepared by the two groups
were presented in an international meeting held in Paris at Hopital Saint-Louis
on March 11, 1967. The antibiotic was described as a powerful inducer of
remission in acute lymphoblastic leukemia (60% complete response rate) and
acute myeloblastic leukemia (35-55% complete response rate), improved results
being obtained through the use of drug combinations. On the other hand, low
response rates were reported in other tumor diseases.

A joint announcement by the two companies, Rhone-Poulenc and Farmitalia, stated that the two antibiotics called *rubidomycin* and *daunomycin* had
been shown to be the same product and to have the same physicochemical and
biological properties.[26,27] In order to clearly take account of the dual origin, the
generic name proposed and then adopted by WHO was *daunorubicin*. The two
producing strains *S. peucetius* and *S. coeruleorubidus* are notably different,
and although direct comparison showing the two microorganisms to belong to
unequivocally different species (A. Grein, personal communication) has never
been published, the same conclusion can be drawn from the reported com-

parison of *S. peucetius* strain F-106, itself differing only in pigmentation from the original *S. peucetius* isolate,[28] with *S. coeruleorubidus.* The morphological and cultural characteristics of the two microorganisms allowed a clear differentiation.[29]

## 6. THE ISOLATION OF DOXORUBICIN

It was evident from the early investigations on *S. peucetius* metabolites that a series of other anthracycline-like compounds, either glycosides or aglycones, was present in variable amounts in the cultures of the original microorganism and in new strains derived from it by spontaneous or induced mutation. The most interesting appeared to be a component of crude extracts characterized as a daunorubicin-related glycoside showing higher polarity than daunorubicin in different chromatographic systems. Preparations in which this component was present in high amounts behaved better than daunorubicin itself in the animal tests. The recovery of this compound in the pure state and in sufficient amounts to allow chemical characterization was difficult, however, because of (1) the small amount, about a few micrograms per ml present in the culture fluids, and (2) the presence of a second compound, namely 13-dihydrodaunorubicin (now also known as daunorubicinol), which behaved identically in the chromatographic systems used routinely at the time. Isolation of the new compound was complicated by the greater stability of daunorubicinol through the extraction procedure involving alkalinization steps for the recovery of the free bases into a solvent phase from their aqueous solution. However, once obtained in pure form by G. Cassinelli in 1967, the structure of doxorubicin (Adriamycin) was promptly established as **13**.[29,30] Acid hydrolysis of the antibiotic gave daunosamine and a new aglycone, adriamycinone, whose structure was elucidated on the basis, *inter alia,* of the PMR spectrum of the corresponding

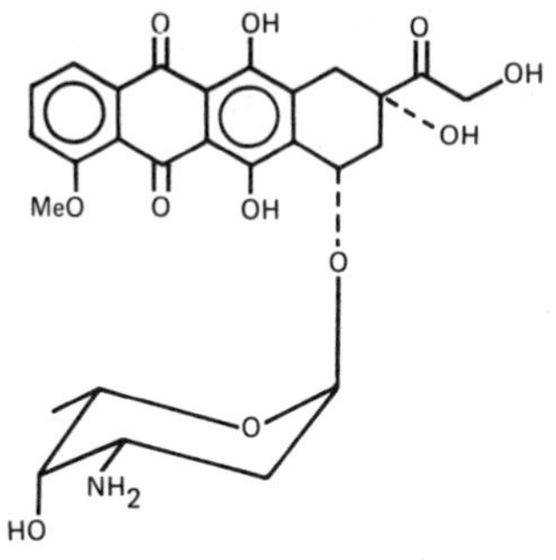

13

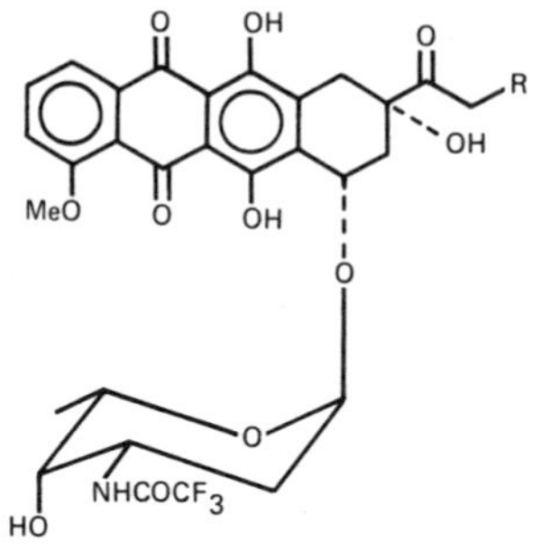

14a: R = I
14b: R = OAc
14c: R = OH

penta-O-acetyl derivative, clearly showing the presence of a pair of doublets at 4.66 and 5.00 δ ($J_{gem}$ = 16.5 Hz) due to the $COCH_2OAc$ group, whereas other signals were in close analogy with those shown by already known dauno-mycinone derivatives. Doxorubicin was chemically correlated with daunorubicin according to the following sequence: Photohalogenation of N-trifluoroacetyldaunorubicin gave **14a**, which was then converted to **14b** with sodium acetate. Compound **14b** gave, upon mild alkaline treatment, N-tri-fluoroacetyldoxorubicin **14c**, also obtained from doxorubicin by N-trifluor-acetylation. Conversion of **14c** to doxorubicin itself was carried out by protec-tion of the side chain ketol function as a cyclic orthoformate followed by alkaline removal of the N-acyl group and acid hydrolysis of the orthoester.[31]

## 7.  THE DEVELOPMENT OF DOXORUBICIN
The activity of doxorubicin in different experimental animal tumors was readily demonstrated by Di Marco et al. at the Istituo Nazionale Tumori, Milan. The antibiotic markedly inhibited the proliferation of murine Ehrlich ascites and solid Sarcoma 180, affording a greater increase of survival time than did daunorubicin, induced a noticeable increase in the survival of mice inoculated with a transplantable lymphosarcoma, and inhibited the growth of OGG myeloma in rats. Doxorubicin also displayed a more favorable therapeutic index when compared directly with daunorubicin.[32]

It was clear at this point that we had in our hands a valuable compound, potentially superior to the already clinically useful daunorubicin. However, quantities of the biosynthetic material available from fermentation procedures on a pilot-plant scale, although of a high level of purity, were too limited to satisfy the anticipated needs even for early preclinical and clinical development. Here again, the know-how gained in the chemical manipulation of the anthra-cyclines in our laboratory (mainly due to the contributions of G. Francheschi and S. Penco) came to our aid. It had already been observed that dauno-mycinone could be quantitatively brominated at C-14 and that the 14-bromo compound was a good substrate for nucleophilic substitution. A procedure was therefore developed, starting from the more easily available daunorubicin, that involved electrophilic bromination to give 14-bromodaunorubicin followed by substitution of the halogen with a hydroxyl group by means of a mild alkaline treatment.[33] A 50 g batch of doxorubicin hydrochloride was prepared in the laboratory in 1968 in different runs, allowing the start of doxorubicin develop-ment with minimum delay.

Further data coming from Di Marco's laboratory confirmed the outstanding antitumor properties of doxorubicin. The activity on murine sarcoma virus-induced tumors (Moloney virus) was without inhibition of spontaneous regres-sion (as was the case with daunorubicin). Activity on transplantable and spon-taneous mouse mammary carcinoma[35] suggested a potential for doxorubicin in the treatment of solid tumors in humans. However, it was the publication of a clinical paper by Bonadonna et al.[36] in 1969 indicating that doxorubicin was a wide-spectrum anticancer agent, that aroused international interest in the new drug. Worldwide investigations both at the preclinical and clinical level soon followed. At the same time, the production of doxorubicin hydrochloride was transferred to a pilot plant in the Farmitalia plant near Turin. As a result, an International Symposium on Adriamycin was held in Milan on September 9 and 10, 1971, to analyze and discuss the findings emerging from work performed by different groups in different countries. On this occasion a large representation of the peerage of internationally known clinical oncologists, including G. Bonadonna, E. Frei III, Y. Kenis, I. H. Krakoff, G. Mathe, C. Praga, M. Pavone-Macaluso, C. Rozman, J. F. Holland, C. Tan, J. M. A. Whitehouse, K. Kimura, and K. Ota, generally concluded that Adriamycin was an outstandingly effective drug giving, either alone or in combination, remarkable response rates in acute leukemias, in malignant lymphomas, in pediatric solid tumors such as neuroblastoma, Wilms's tumor, and Ewing sarcoma, and in other solid tumors such as soft-tissue sarcomas, testicular tumors, lung carcinoma, bladder carcinoma, and breast tumors. An account of further developments of Adriamycin after registration in all major countries for the medical treatment of cancer diseases lies outside the scope of this chapter. This history was, however, far from being at an end.

## 8.   NEW DERIVATIVES AND ANALOGUES

In applied research, one of the consequences of a success, be it a product or a process, is its obligatory exploitation as a starting point for further improvements. This seems obvious, but it is not as widely accepted a practice as might be expected. In our case, despite some intramural and extramural skepticism, I eventually obtained authorization in 1972 to use an adequate portion of available resources to proceed further with the antitumor anthracycline work.

Doxorubicin is not devoid of serious toxic side effects. Important but reversible toxicity that frequently limits the size of individual doses includes myelosuppression, stomatitis, nausea and vomiting, alopecia, and ECG abnormalities. Less frequent but usually fatal is the cardiac failure that intervenes in approximately 1% of patients and limits the total cumulative dose to a value in the range from 450 to 550 mg/m$^2$. Drug extravasation, which can occur accidentally during the intravenous treatment, is also currently considered a problem because of the ulcerative properties exhibited by the drug in this condition. In addition, a number of cancer types of the utmost clinical importance, such as colorectal cancer, malignant melanoma, and renal carcinoma (to cite only a few) are not responsive to doxorubicin treatment. It appeared therefore that a considerable improvement would have been represented by the development of

new agents possessing the following characteristics:
1. Lower acute toxicity, thus allowing a reduction of side effects and possibly higher dosages with enhanced anticancer activity.
2. Activity by the oral route.
3. Lower cardiotoxicity, thus allowing a prolongation of treatment when desirable.
4. A wider spectrum of activity, allowing treatment of tumors on which doxorubicin shows a low response rate or no response.

In drawing up the program for analogue development, the available knowledge of the mode of action of doxorubicin was taken into account along with a consideration of structure-activity relationships. Binding to cell DNA with consequent impairment of DNA structure and function were accepted as the main mode of action of the antitumor anthracyclines. Therefore, only structures possessing the planar, electron-deficient anthraquinone chromophore linked to a sugar residue at C-7 were taken into consideration. The presence of an amino group at C-3' was also required on the basis of the stabilization that this group was thought to bring to the drug-DNA intercalation complex. Moreover, because of the pivotal nature of aglycone ring A in determining the spatial orientation of the different parts of the molecule, it was predicted that most useful and least risky modifications would have been those involving the sugar moiety and aglycone ring D. Modification of the sugar residue was also of interest in connection with the known dependence of enzymic reactions and biological transport processes on the structure and stereochemistry of carbohydrate derivatives. Because of the limited number of new chemical species that one could presumably get by strain mutation and/or cultural modifications, we placed emphasis on the development of semi-synthetic and entirely synthetic procedures.

Three main difficulties would have to be overcome for the success of the synthetic program. First, high yield preparative methods for the 3-amino-2,3,6-trideoxy-L-hexoses were not readily available. Second, literature information concerning the stereoselective glycosidation of complex aglycones was scant, mostly restricted to the Koenigs-Knorr type of condensation of limited preparative value. Third, although anthracycline antibiotics had been known for 20 years, no obvious approach for the total synthesis of fully functionalized anthracyclinones was available at the beginning of the 1970s (the synthetic studies actually started towards the end of 1972).

Synthesis of daunosamine analogues was carried out by starting either from daunosamine itself, as was the case for acosamine[37] and 4-deoxydaunosamine[38] derivatives, and more recently for the 4-O-methyl[39] and 4-C-methyl[40] analogues, or from commercially available L-arabinose and L-glucose, as was the case for the L-ribo, the L-xylo and 6'-hydroxylated analogues.[41,42] The synthesis of the glycosidic linkage was carefully investigated in our laboratory. Different methods were used: the Koenigs-Knorr reaction,[43,44,45] the Fischer procedure,[46] the acid-catalyzed glycosidation of glycals,[47,48] and glycosidation with soluble silver salts.[38,49,50]

As to the total synthesis of new daunomycinone derivatives, we had already addressed ourselves to the classical approach based on the reaction of a substituted tetralin with a phthalic acid derivative,[51,52] a scheme also used by some American researchers for the preparation of a simplified analogue.[53] However, in 1971 Professor Chiu Ming Wong of University of Manitoba published what was the first synthesis of a fully functionalized anthracyclinone derivative,[54] and the report of the total synthesis of racemic daunomycinone followed two years later.[55] Using improved versions of Wong's scheme, we were able to synthetize different daunomycinone analogues showing modifications in the substitution of ring D. The new aglycones were glycosidated to afford a group of compounds endowed with strong antitumor activity.[50]

In addition to the above-mentioned lines, two others were opened in connection with two research contracts granted by the U.S. National Cancer Institute. These were (1) the synthesis of doxorubicin analogues starting from the biosynthetic glycosides, and (2) the synthesis of doxorubicin analogues starting from biosynthetic aglycones (daunomycinone). Fulfillment of these latter programs raised the total number of new derivatives and analogues obtained by the end of the 1970's to more than 200 compounds, among which quite a few showed distinct potential as candidates for further development. Many others are still under evaluation. By 1982, three compounds had reached the clinical stage, 4'-epidoxorubicin, 4'-deoxydoxorubicin, and 4-demethoxydaunorubicin.

## 9. 4'-EPIDOXORUBICIN AND 4'-DEOXYDOXORUBICIN

Synthesis of these analogues, formerly carried out by glycosidation of daunomycinone with the corresponding aminosugar followed by functionalization at C-14, has been recently considerably improved. In fact, daunorubicin is now directly converted to these compounds, as shown in Scheme 1.[56]

Both 4'-epi and 4'-deoxydoxorubicin display affinity for native double-stranded DNA comparable with that shown by the parent drug, and they behave similarly to the latter in a range of experimental mouse tumor systems.[1] 4'-Epidoxorubicin appears to be less toxic to the animals, thus showing a more favorable therapeutic index or a higher efficacy at highest tolerated doses when compared with doxorubicin. The results of distribution studies suggest that this different pharmacological behavior might be related to a lower concentration in certain tissues, such as the heart, the kidneys, and the spleen. Clinical evaluation, based on 265 patients from different studies,[57,62] indicates that 4'-epidoxorubicin is endowed with a wide spectrum of activity and that the side effects are less marked than with doxorubicin.

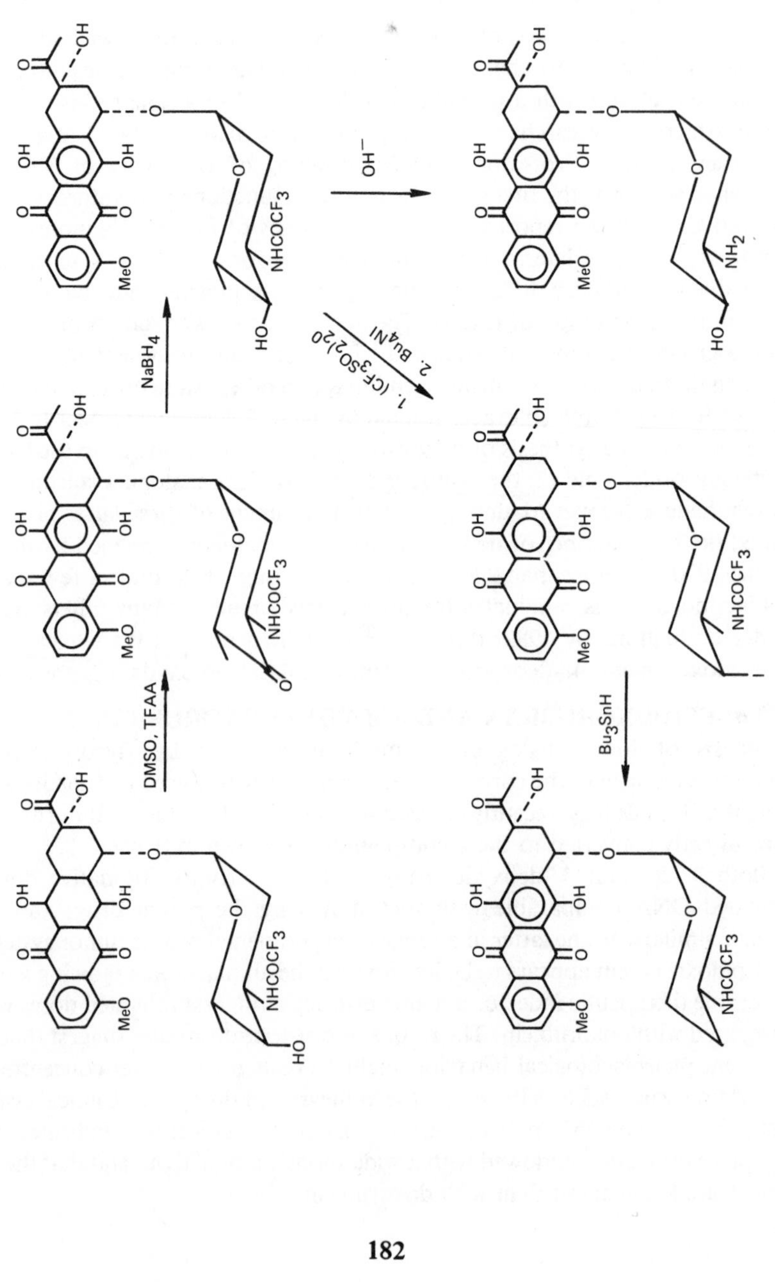
DMSO, TFAA
NaBH$_4$
1. $(CF_3SO_2)_2O$
2. $Bu_4NI$
$OH^-$
$Bu_3SnH$
MeO
NHCOCF$_3$
NH$_2$

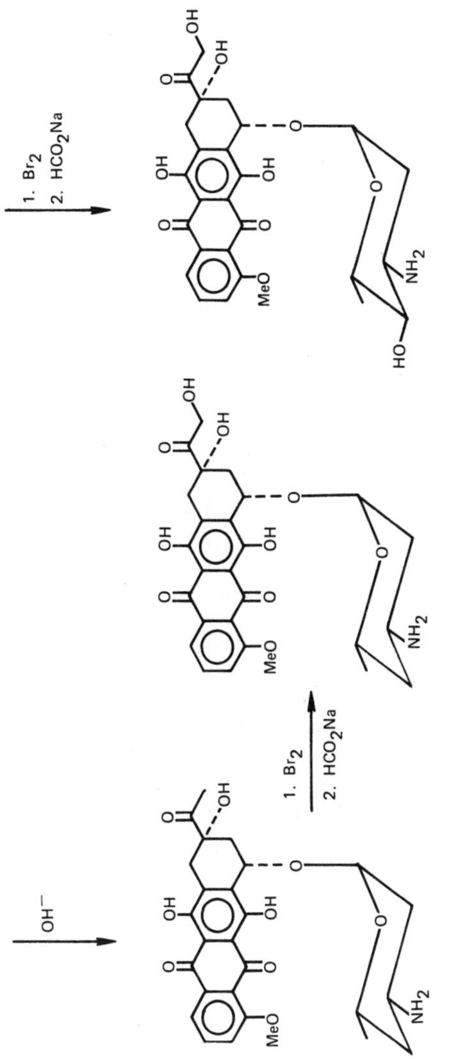

**Scheme 1.**

183

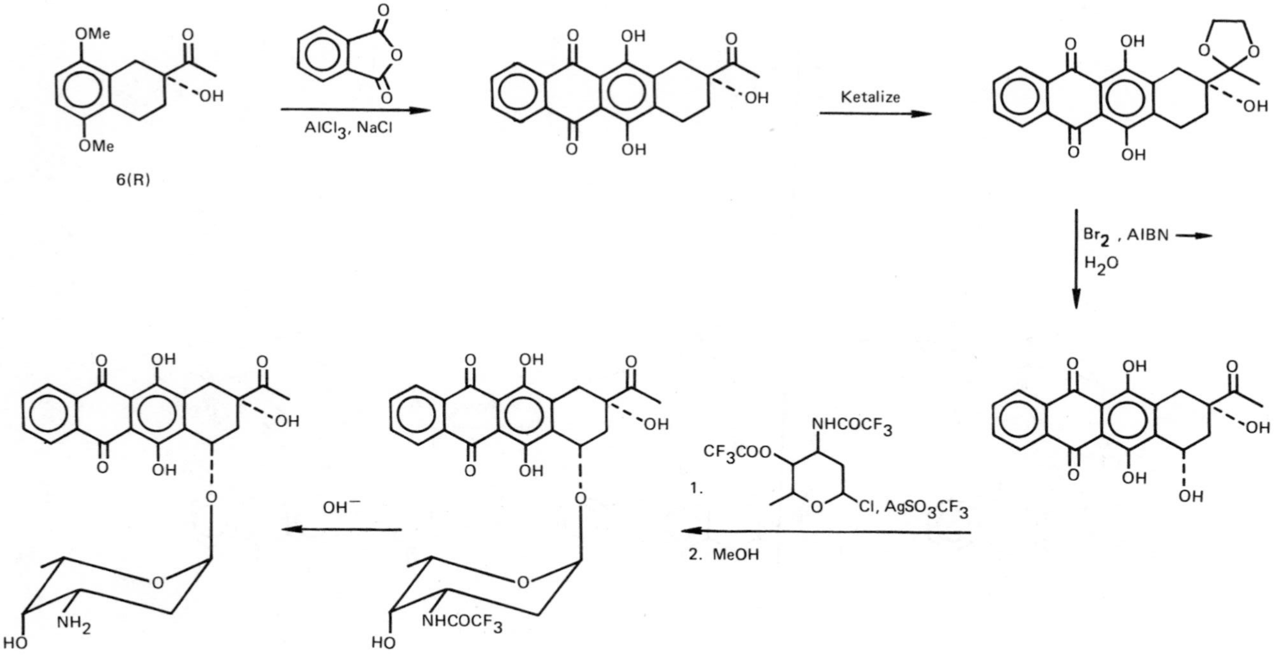

Scheme 2.

184

4'-Deoxydoxorubicin has aroused considerable interest in our laboratory because of the absence of cardiotoxicity at tolerated doses in different experimental models coupled with outstanding antitumor properties in transplantable murine tumors.[63] The compound also exhibits activity against nine human colorectal tumors transplanted in athymic (nude) mice.[64]

## 10.   4-DEMETHOXYDAUNORUBICIN

The synthesis of 4-demethoxydaunorubicin is presented in Scheme 2. The sequence proceeds through five reaction steps starting from the levorotatory enantiomer of Wong's tetralin. The same route has been used for the preparation of different analogues, including 4-demethoxydoxorubicin, 4-demethoxy-4'-epidoxorubicin, and 4-demethoxy-2,3-dimethoxydoxorubicin, compounds endowed with remarkable antitumor properties.[1]

4-Demethoxydaunorubicin has been selected for clinical evaluation because of its activity on oral administration against experimental mouse leukemias and its reduced cardiotoxicity when compared with doxorubicin in experimental systems.[65] Phase 1 trials have established recommended dosages for both i.v. and oral treatments.[66,67]

## CONCLUSIONS

The history of the antitumor anthracyclines represents an important contribution of the chemistry of natural products and medicinal chemistry to the field of medicine. Starting from the early chemical studies concerned with the elucidation of daunorubicin structure and stereochemistry, and progressing through the discovery of doxorubicin to the development of the semisynthetic and totally synthetic analogues, we have covered in the period of 20 years a substantial portion of the working life of the chemists involved. However, recent results strongly indicate that the full potential of the anthracyclines as useful anticancer agents leaves room for further exploitation and improvements in the years to come.

## ACKNOWLEDGMENTS

In addition to the main contributors whose names appear in the text, the patent literature records also the names of F. Angelucci, A. Bargiotti, L. Bernardi, G. Canevazzi, A. M. Casazza, F. Forenza, G. Franchi, M. Gaetani, P. Giardino, F. Gozzi, E. Lazzari, P. Masi, S. Merli, B. Patelli, M. C. Ripamonti, G. Rivola, D. Ruggieri, O. Sapini, A. Suarato, and G. P. Vicario. Thanks are also given to other colleagues who have participated at various stages of the developments reported here and whose names appear in the relevant scientific literature. I also thank Professor Steve Hanessian of the University of Montreal for his helpful cooperation in clarifying some important aspects of the chemistry of new semisynthetic glycosides.

## REFERENCES

1.  F. Arcamone, *Doxorubicin,* Medicinal Chemistry Series, Vol. 17, Academic Press, New York (1981).
2.  H. Brockmann, "Anthracyclinone und Anthracycline" in L. Zechmeister, Ed., *Fortschritte der Chimie Organischer Naturstoffe,* Vol. 21, Springer Verlag, Vienna, 1963, p. 121-128.
3.  C. Hackmann, *Z. Krebsforch.,* **58**, 607 (1952).
4.  A. E. Evans, *Cancer Chemother. Rep.,* **14**, 1 (1961).
5.  A. Di Marco, M. Gaetani, P. Orezzi, and F. Arcamone, *Cancer Chemother. Rep.,* **18**, 15 (1962).
6.  J. A. Stock, *Exp. Chemother.,* **4**, 239 (1966).
7.  H. Brockmann, "Pyrromycins and Pyrromycinones, Rhodomycins and Rhodomycinones" in *Sostanze Naturali,* Roma Acc. dei Lincei, 33 (1961).
8.  F. Arcamone, A. Di Marco, M. Gaetani, and T. Scotti, *Giorn. Microciol.,* **9**, 83 (1961).
9.  L. Ettlinger, E. Gaumann, R. Hutter, W. Keller-Schierlein, F. Kradolfer, L. Neipp, V. Prelog, P. Reusser, and H. Zahner, *Chem. Ber.,* **92**, 1867 (1959).
10. G. Cassinelli and P. Orezzi, Giorn. Microbiol., **11**, 167 (1963).
11. A. Di Marco, *Path. Biol.,* **15**, 897 (1967).
12. A. Di Marco, M. Gaetani, L. Dorigotti, M. Soldati, and O. Bellini, *Tumori,* **49**, 203 (1963).
13. F. Arcamone, G. Franceschi, P. Orezzi, G. Cassinelli, W. Barbieri, and R. Mondelli, *J. Amer. Chem. Soc.,* **86**, 5334 (1964).
14. F. Arcamone, G. Cassinelli, P. Orezzi, G. Franceschi, and R. Mondelli, *J. Amer. Chem. Soc.,* **86**, 5335 (1964).
15. F. Arcamone, G. Franceschi, P. Orezzi, and S. Panco, *Tetrahedron Lett.,* **30**, 3349 (1968).
16. F. Arcamone, G. Cassinelli, G. Franceschi, P. Orezzi, and R. Mondelli, *Tetrahedron Lett.,* **30**, 3353 (1968).
17. F. Arcamone, "Daunomycin and Related Antibiotics," in P. G. Sammes, Ed., *Topics in Antibiotic Chemistry, Vol. 2, Ellis Horwood, Chichester, 1978, pp. 100-239.*
18. *F. Arcamone, G. Cassinelli, G. Franceschi, R. Mondelli, P. Orezzi, and S. Panco, Gazz. Chim. Ital., 100, 949 (1970).*
19. H. Brockmann, H. Brockmann, Jr., and J. Niemeyer, *Tetrahedron Lett.,* **45**, 4719 (1968).
20. W. J. Pigram, W. Fuller, and L. D. Hamilton, *Nature New Biol.,* **235** (1972).
21. R. Angiuli, E. Foresti, L. Riva di Sanseverino, N. W. Isaacs, O. Kennard, W. Motherwell, D. L. Wampler, and F. Arcamone, *Nature New Biol.,* **234**, 78 (1971).
22. C. Tan and A. Di Marco, *Proc. Amer. Assoc. Cancer Res,* **6** 64, Abstr. 253 (1965).
23. A. Di Marco, G. Canevazzi, A. Grein, P. Orezzi, and M. Gaetani, "Daunomycin, an "Antibiotic for Tumor Treatment," Belg. Patent 639,897 (Mar. 2, 1964); *Chem. Abstr.* **62**, 16922a (1965).
24. Rhone-Poulenc S. A., Belg. Patent 632,391 (Nov. 18, 1963); *Chem. Abstr.,* **61** 11296f (1964).
25. R. Despois, R. Dubost, D. Mancy, R. Maral, L. Ninet, S. Pinnert, J. Preud'Homme, Y. Charpentie, A. Belloc, N. de Chezelles, J. Lunel, and J. Renaut, *Arzneim.-Forsch.,* **17**, 934 (1967).
26. Anonymous, *Arzneim.-Forsch.,* **17**, 1338 (1967).
27. J. Bernard, P. Paul, M. Boiron, A. Jacquillat, and R. Maral, Eds., *Recent Results in Cancer Research: Rubidomycin,* Springer-Verlag, Berlin, 1969, p. 5.
28. F. Arcamone, G. Cassinelli, G. Fantini, A. Grein, P. Orezzi, C. Pol, and C. Spalla, *Biotechnol. Bioeng.,* **11**, 1101 (1969).
29. F. Arcamone, G. Cassinelli, A. Di Marco, and M. Gaetani, U.S. Patent 3,590,028 (June 29, 1971).

30. F. Arcamone, G. Franceschi, S. Penco, and A. Selva, *Tetrahedron Lett.,* **13**, 1007 (1969).
31. F. Arcamone, W. Barbieri, G. Franceschi, and S. Penco, *Chim. Ind.,* **51**, 834 (1969).
32. A. Di Marco, M. Gaetani, and B. M. Scarpinato, *Cancer Chemother. Rep.,* **53**, 33 (1969).
33. F. Arcamone, G. Franceschi, and S. Penco, U.S. Patent 3,803,124 (Apr. 9, 1974).
34. A. M. Casazza, A. Di Marco, and G. Cuonzo, *Cancer Res.,* **31**, 1971 (1971).
35. A. Di Marco, L. Lenaz, A. M. Casazza, and B. M. Scarpinato, *Cancer Chemother. Rep.,* **56**, 153 (1972).
36. G. Bonadonna, S. Monfardini, M. de Lena, and F. Fossati-Bellani, *Brit. Med. J.,* **3**, 503 (1969).
37. F. Arcamone, S. Penco, A. Vigevani, S. Redaelli, G. Franchi, A. Di Marco, A. M. Casazza, T. Dasdia, F. Formelli, A. Necco, and C. Soranzo, *J. Med. Chem.,* **18**, 703 (1975).
38. F. Arcamone, S. Penco, S. Radelli, and S. Hanessian, *J. Med. Chem.,* **19**, 1424 (1976).
39. G. Cassinelli, D. Ruggieri, and F. Arcamone, *J. Med. Chem.,* **22**, 121 (1979).
40. A. Bargiotti, G. Cassinelli, F. Arcamone, and A. Di Marco, Ger. Offen. 2,942,818 (May 8, 1980).
41. F. Arcamone, A. Bargiotti, G. Cassinelli, S. Penco, and S. Hanessian, *Carbohy. Res.,* **46**, C3-C5 (1976).
42. A. Bargiotti, G. Cassinelli, G. Franchi, B. Gioia, E. Lazzari, S. Redaelli, A. Vigevani, F. Arcamone, and S. Hanessian, *Carbohyd. Res.,* **58**, 353 (1977).
43. S. Penco, *Chim. Ind.,* **50**. 908 (1968).
44. F. Arcamone, S. Penco, and A. Vigevani, *Cancer Chemother. Rep.,* **6**, 123 (1975).
45. F. Arcamone, L. Bernardi, P. Giardino, B. Patelli, A. Di Marco, A. M. Casazza, G. Pratesi, and P. Reggiani, *Cancer Treat. Rep.,* **60**, 829 (1976).
46. G. Cassinelli, French Patent 2,183,710 (Dec. 21, 1972).
47. F. Arcamone and G. Cassinelli, U.S. Patent 4,020,270 (Apr. 26, 1977).
48. F. Arcamone, A. Bargiotti, G. Cassinelli, S. Redaelli, S. Hanessian, A. Di Marco, A. M. Casazza, T. Dasdia, A. Necco, P. Reggiani, and R. Supino, *J. Med. Chem.,* **19**, 733 (1976).
49. F. Arcamone, A. Bargiotti, A. Di Marco, and S. Penco, Ger. Offen. 2,618,822 (Nov. 11, 1976); *Chem. Abstr.* **86**., 140416 (1977).
50. F. Arcamone, L. Bernardi, B. Patelli, P. Giardino, A. Di Marco, A. M. Casazza, C. Soranzo, and G. Pretesi, *Experientia,* **34**, 1255 (1978).
51. G. Schroeter, *Chem. Ber.,* **54**, 2242 (1921).
52. C. Dufraisse and R. Horclos, *Bull. Soc. Chim. France,* **3**, 1880 (1936).
53. J. P. Marsh, Jr., R. H. Iwamoto, and L. Goodman, *Chem. Comm.,* **589** (1968).
54. C. M. Wong, D. Pipien, R. Schwenk, and T. Raa, *Canad. J. Chem.,* **49**, 2712 (1971).
55. C. M. Wong, R. Schewenk, D. Pipien, and T. L. Ho, *Canad. J. Chem.,* **51**, 466 (1973).
56. A. Suarato, S. Penco, A. Vigevani, and F. Arcamone, *Carbohyd. Res.,* in press.
57. V. Bonfante, G. Bonadonna, F. Villani, G. Di Fronzo, A. Martini, and A. M. Casazza, *Cancer Treat. Rep.,* **63**, 915 (1979).
58. V. Bonfante, G. Bonadanna, F. Villani, and A. Martini, *Recent Results in Cancer Research,* Vol. 74, Springer, Berlin, 1980, pp. 202-209.
59. P. K. Schauer, R. E. Wittes, R. J. Grolla, E. S. Casper, and C. W. Young, *Cancer Clinical Trials,* in press.
60. V. Bonfante, F. Villani, and G. Bonadonna, *Cancer Chemotherapy and Pharmacology,* in press.
61. P. Hurteloup, G. Mathe, and M. Hayat, *Comm. UICC Conference on Clinical Oncology,* Lausanne, Switzerland, Oct. 28-31, (1981).
62. R. De Jager, *Comm. Symp. "Anthracyclines,"* Paris, June 24-25 (1981).
63. A. M. Casazza, *Comm. Symp. "Anthracyclines,"* Paris, June 24-25 (1981).

64. F. C. Giuliani, K. A. Zirvi, N. O. Kaplan, and A. Goldin, *Int. J. Cancer,* in press.
65. A. M. Casazza, C. Bertazzoli, G. Pratesi, O. Bellini, and A. Di Marco, Proceedings of 7th Annual Meeting of AACR, May 16-19, 1979 and of the 15th Annual Meeting of ASCO, May 14-15, New Orleans, U.S., 1979, p. 16, Abstr. 63.
66. M. Verini, S. Kaplan, P. Togni, and F. Cavalli, 3rd NCI-EORTC Sympossium on New Drugs in Cancer Therapy, Brussels, Oct. 15-17, 1981, Abstr. 57.
67. V. Bonfante, F. Villani, and G. Bonadonna, 3rd NCI-EORTC Symposium on New Drugs in Cancer Therapy, Brussels, Oct. 15-17, 1981, Abstr. 61.

# The Nitrosoureas

## 9

John A. Montgomery

The discovery of the antitumor activity of the nitrosoureas was closely associated with the establishment of the Cancer Chemotherapy National Service Center (CCNSC) under the auspices of the National Cancer Institute. Indeed, they were the first class of compounds derived from a lead compound identified by the random screening program of the CCNSC to show useful activity against human cancer.[1] The CCNSC began its activities by establishing a program to screen large numbers of compounds against three murine neoplasms: sarcoma 180, adenocarcinoma 755, and leukemia L-1210. In the first year of operation, 1959, approximately 6500 synthetic chemicals were screened. In 1958 $N$-methyl-$N'$-nitro-$N$-nitrosoguanidine (MNNG, NSC 9369), a chemical precursor of diazomethane supplied to the CCNSC by Dr. Evan C. Horning, then at the National Heart Institute, was one of 7700 synthetics evaluated in the three-tumor screen. Initial testing carried out at the Wisconsin Alumni Research Foundation showed MNNG to be very weakly active against S-180 and Ca-755 but to have significant activity against leukemia L-1210 in BDF1 mice, increasing life span 138% at the optimal dose (7 mg/kg) (Table 1). Unfortunately these favorable results were not confirmed by the Hazelton Laboratories nor by the Southern Research Institute (data not in table). These two laboratories found at best about a 35% increase in life span, indicating that MNNG is barely active in this system. An early clinical trial of the agent was quickly aborted because of toxicity and lack of activity. The original WARF data, however, transmitted by Howard Bond, then head of drug development at the CCNSC, to me, to the late B. R. Baker, and to several other interested parties, caused me to enter into the CCNSC screen another diazomethane precursor, $N$-methyl-$N$-nitrosourea (MNU, NSC 23909),[2] always on hand at that time in the refrigerator of our organic chemistry department for the

## Table 1
### Anticancer Activity of $N$-Methyl-$N'$-Nitro-$N$-Nitroso-Guanidine (NSC-9369)[a]

| Lab | Tumor | Control | Strain | Dose[b] | Animal wt. change | Response (treated/control) Tumor wt. or surv. time[c] | T/C |
|---|---|---|---|---|---|---|---|
| WARF | S-180 | 144(017) | Swiss | 65 | — | — | — |
| | | — | — | 16 | — | — | 0.53 |
| | | 403(097) | — | 16 | −1.0/+0.9 | 487/612 | 0.63 |
| | | 619(048) | — | 14 | +2.7/+4.4 | 655/861 | 0.76 |
| | | 619(048) | — | 9 | +4.1/+4.4 | 590/861 | 0.69 |
| | | 619(048) | — | 6 | +2.8/+4.4 | 527/861 | 0.61 |
| | CA-755 | 109(107) | BDF1 | 14 | −2.4/+1.5 | 371/630 | 0.59 |
| | | 190(048) | — | 14 | −0.1/+0.9 | 235/672 | 0.35 |
| | | 190(048) | — | 9 | +1.4/+0.9 | 483/672 | 0.72 |
| | | 190(048) | — | 6 | +1.6/+0.9 | 351/672 | 0.52 |

| | | | | | |
|---|---|---|---|---|---|
| L-1210 | 96(077) | — | 16 | +0.2/+2.4 | 14.2/8.5 | 1.67 |
| | 112(097) | — | 16 | −1.0/+2.4 | 13.2/7.5 | 1.76 |
| | 123(107) | — | 16 | −0.4/+3.1 | 12.8/7.9 | 1.62 |
| | 173(028) | — | 26 | −1.7/+3.0 | 8.5/7.9 | 1.08 |
| | 173(028) | — | 16 | −1.2/+3.0 | 9.7/7.9 | 1.23 |
| | 173(028) | — | 10.6 | −1.2/+3.0 | 16.6/7.9 | 2.10 |
| | 173(028) | — | 7 | −0.8/+3.0 | 18.8/7.9 | 2.38 |
| Hazelton  L-1210 | 102(038) | — | 26 | −2.5/+0.6 | 7.8/7.4 | 1.05 |
| | 102(038) | — | 16 | −2.6/+0.6 | 10.0/7.4 | 1.26 |
| | 102(038) | — | 10.6 | −2.1/+0.6 | 9.3/7.4 | 1.26 |
| | 102(038) | — | 7 | −1.1/+0.6 | 9.3/7.4 | 1.26 |

[a]From J. Leiter and M. A. Schneiderman, *Cancer Res.*, **19** (3), 2 (1959).

[b]Mg/kg/dose, i.p.: S-180, qd 2-8; CA-755, qd 2-13; L-1210, qd 2-16 or until death.

[c]Tumor weight in mg and survival time in days.

## Table 2
### Anticancer Activity of *N*-Methyl-*N*-Nitrosourea

| Date | Tumor | Dose[a] | Schedule | Animal wt. change[b] | Tumor wt. (mg) or survival time (days)[b] | T/C[b] |
|---|---|---|---|---|---|---|
| 5/7/58 | S-180 | 100 | 2xD | — | Toxic | — |
| | | 25 | 2xD | −5/−1 | 228/595 | 0.38 |
| | | 12.5 | 2xD | −6/−3 | 345/740 | 0.47 |
| 6/30/58 | CA-755 | 22.5 | 1xD | — | Toxic | |
| | | 11 | 1xD | −3/+4 | 308/1397 | 0.22 (Toxic) |
| | | 5 | 1xD | −2/+3 | 1149/1650 | 0.70 |
| 7/14/58 | L-1210 | 25 | 1xD | — | 8.2/14.4 | 0.56 (Toxic) |
| 5/11/59 | | 20 | 1xD | −2.5/+0.1 | 11.3/12.2 | 1.02 |
| | | 15 | 1xD | −0.4/−0.1 | 13.5/12.2 | 1.08 |
| | | 5 | 1xD | −1.2/−0.1 | 13.2/12.2 | 1.11 |
| | | 2.5 | 1xD | −1.1/−0.1 | 12.5/12.2 | 1.02 |

| Date | mg/kg i.p.[a] | | | | Treated/control[b] |
|---|---|---|---|---|---|
| 5/15/59 | 12.5 | 1xD | −2.8/+0.9 | 17/11 | 1.55 |
| 8/10/59 | 14 | 1xD | −1.5/−0.1 | 20.5/11.3 | 1.81 |
|  | 13 | 1xD | −1.7/−0.1 | 17.4/11.3 | 1.54 |
|  | 12 | 1xD | −0.8/−0.1 | 18.7/11.3 | 1.65 |
|  | 11 | 1xD | −1.4/−0.1 | 21.3/11.3 | 1.88 |
| 10/19/59 | 20 | 1xD | −1.9/+0.6 | 13.5/9.7 | 1.39 |
|  | 15 | 1xD | −1.1/+0.6 | 16.2/9.7 | 1.67 |
|  | 10 | 1xD | −1.0/+0.6 | 18.2/9.7 | 1.88 |
|  | 5 | 1xD | −1.0/+0.6 | 12.4/9.7 | 1.28 |
| 10/19/59 | 12 | 1xD | −1.8/+0.1 | 20.2/9.6 | 2.10 |
| 10/26/59 | 12 | 1xD | −1.2/+1.1 | 20.0/9.3 | 2.15 |
| 10/19/59 | 12 | 1xD | −0.7/+2.0 | 16.7/8.0 | 2.09 |
| 11/2/59 | 12 | 1xD | −1.7/+0.6 | 18.0/8.6 | 2.09 |

[a] mg/kg i.p.
[b] Treated/control.

preparation of methyl esters and the like. Initial results (Table 2) were far from encouraging: At nontoxic doses little activity was observed in the three-tumor panel. Since the only dose used in the L-1210 test was toxic, I requested that the MNU be retested at lower doses; they were clearly nontoxic but also inactive. Fortunately, what appeared to be a glimmer of activity to a chemist desperately looking for a lead to a new structural type of anticancer agent caused me to request a retest at a dose intermediate between 5 and 15 mg/kg, namely 12.5 mg/kg. At this level, true but not spectacular activity, a 55% increase in life span, was observed, and the search was on. A number of tests at doses from 10 to 20 mg/kg repeatedly showed significant activity ranging from a high of 88% to a low of 39% increase in life span. The criticism that a test injecting drug i.p. into a mouse with leukemic cells implanted i.p. is "an *in vivo* cell culture system" caused us to test MNU orally, and the activity held up.

It was at this time that the following statement was made: Meningeal leukemia has become increasingly important as a complication in acute leukemia. While chemotherapy has resulted in prolongation of life, the effective antimetabolites do not reach therapeutic levels in the cerebrospinal fluid. As a result meningeal leukemia has become the major therapeutic problem in patients with acute leukemia who are in remission, as well as a serious complication in patients with marrow relapse.[3] This situation caused Skipper et al. to initiate a study to (1) develop a quantitative or semiquantitative bioassay for L-1210 cells, (2) employ such a bioassay in a study of the anatomical distribution of leukemic cells at various periods after inoculation, and (3) determine the relative effectiveness of antileukemic drugs against the disease induced by inoculation of known numbers of L-1210 cells at different sites. If the L-1210 cells were inoculated intracerebrally, none of the standard agents—including methotrexate, 6-mercaptopurine, actinobolen, azaserine, cyclophosphamide, 8-azaguanine, 5-fluorouracil, or mitomycin C—had any effect on the course of the disease. It should be easy to imagine the excitement generated by the results obtained with MNU, which was as active against the i.c. as the i.p. form of the disease.[4] We had discovered that MNU, an old, old compound,[5] possessed unique activity in our animal test system. Although MNU possessed real and reproducible activity, we hesitated to believe that its degree of activity at the optimal dose was great enough to warrant a clinical trial, even though the NCI selected it for development.[1] Later it did receive such a trial in Russia.[6] Preclinical development of MNU proceeded from 1960 to 1962. More important, this discovery provided the impetus for our drug development program on the nitrosoureas, which is still active today.

We mentally divided MNU into three parts that appeared to be amenable to chemical modification. It seemed clear from the beginning that the biologic activity of the compound resulted from its chemical reactivity. At high pH

$$CH_3-N\!-\!\overset{\overset{\textstyle O}{\textstyle \|}}{C}\!-\!NH_2$$
$$\underset{ON}{\phantom{x}}$$

$$\begin{array}{ccc} A & B & C \end{array}$$

(about 12 or more) MNU decomposes to give diazomethane,[7] and the azaserine story[8] probably led some investigators to propose that *in vivo*-generated diazomethane was responsible for its anticancer activity. It seemed unlikely to us that this was the case and our studies on the chemistry of the nitrosoureas[9] showed rather clearly that under physiologic conditions, pH 7.4, methyl-nitrosoureas break down to methanediazohydroxide and isocyanates. It has also been shown that MNU methylates the bases of DNA,[10] and the evidence is accumulating that biological activity is associated with this alkylation.

$$\text{At pH 7.4:}\quad CH_3N\!-\!\overset{\overset{\textstyle O}{\textstyle \|}}{C}\!-\!NH_2 \longrightarrow CH_3N\!=\!N\!-\!OH \;+\; O\!=\!C\!=\!NH \longrightarrow CH_3\!-\!DNA \;+\; N_2 \;+\; H_2O$$
$$\underset{NO}{\phantom{x}}$$

If this postulation were true, then it was logical to first study the effect of alterations in the A moiety, which would give rise to a variety of alkane diazohydroxides, on the activity in the L-1210 system. Most of the alterations in the A moiety were clearly detrimental to L-1210 activity (Tables 3 and 4), decreasing both efficacy and degree of activity. The single exception was the 2-chloroethyl group, which appeared to give a compound somewhat more active than MNU. The importance of the presence of the nitroso group on the 2-chloroethyl side of the molecule was emphasized by the low level of activity exhibited by *N*-(2-chloroethyl)-*N* '-methyl-*N* '-nitrosourea. The next compound prepared, *N,N* '-bis(2-chloroethyl)-*N*-nitrosourea (BCNU),[11] was by far the most active compound to be tested in the L-1210 system[12] and the first one to provide cures of this experimental leukemia, both the i.p. and the i.c. disease.[13] Two lines of investigation were then undertaken: the other halogens, fluorine, bromine, and iodine, were substituted for the chlorines of BCNU, and later CCNU (Table 5) and skeletal variations of the 2-chloroethyl were prepared (Table 6). Again, although most of these variants were inferior to BCNU itself, BFNU[*N,N* '-bis(2-fluoroethyl)-*N* '-nitrosourea, NSC 91728] proved to be just as active and initially appeared to have a greater therapeutic index. Difficulties in obtaining a reproducible $LD_{10}$ can probably be attributed to the complications of fluoroacetate toxicity, since a major decomposition product of BFNU is 2-fluoroethanol,[9,14] which is readily oxidized *in vivo* to fluoroacetaldehyde and hence to fluoroacetate.[15]

## Table 3
### N-Alkyl-N-Nitrosoureas vs. Leukemia L-1210

| | RN(NO)CONH$_2$ | L-1210 (i.p., $10^5$ cells); Rx: i.p., chronic | |
|---|---|---|---|
| NSC no. | R | Optimal dose (mg/kg/day) | % ILS[a] |
| 23909 | Me | 12 | 109 |
| 45403 | Et | 50 | 34 |
| 48390 | CH$_2$=CHCH$_2$ | 100 | 32 |
| 46792 | n-Pr | 100 | 30 |
| 45639 | n-Bu | 200 | 29 |
| 67523 | 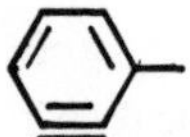 ⬡—CH$_2$ | | Inactive |
| 71911 | 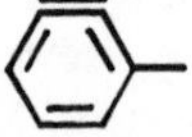 ⬡—(CH$_2$)$_2$ | | Inactive |
| 47547 | Cl(CH$_2$)$_2$ | 0.9 | 157 |

[a]Percent increase in life span.

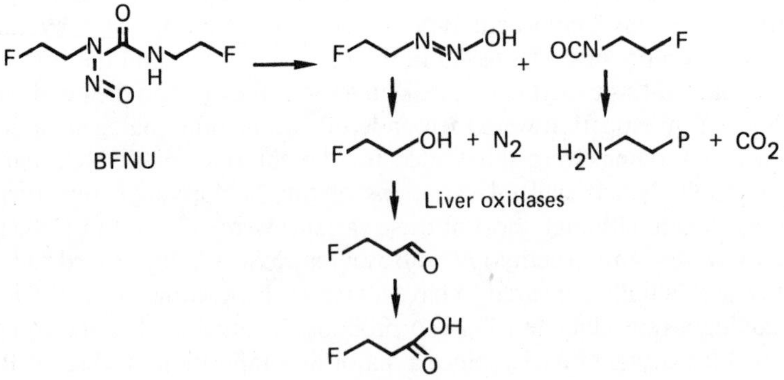

BFNU

Liver oxidases

## Table 4
### Various $N,N'$-Disubstituted Nitrosoureas vs. Leukemia L-1210

| | RN(NO)CONHR' | | L-1210 (i.p., $10^5$ cells) | | |
| | | | Optimal dose | | |
| NSC no. | R | R' | (mg/kg) | % ILS[a] | Rx (i.p.) |
|---|---|---|---|---|---|
| 72721 | NC(CH₂)₂ | (CH₂)₂CN | 150 | 55 | Single dose |
| 409935 | Me | (CH₂)₂Cl | 150 | 46 | Chronic |
| 89402 | MeO(CH₂)₂ | (CH₂)₂OMe | 375 | 45 | Single dose |
| 82190 | Et | Et | 400 | 44 | Single dose |
| 75941 | Cl—⟨ ⟩—CH₂ | CH₂—⟨ ⟩—Cl | 300 | 27 | Chronic |
| 74255 | EtO₂CCH₂ | (CH₂)₂Cl | >100 | >26 | Chronic |
| 103525 | CH₂=CHCH₂ | CH₂CH=CH₂ | | Inactive | |
| 91742 | CF₃CH₂ | CH₂CF₃ | | Inactive | |
| 74705 | HO₂C(CH₂)₃ | (CH₂)₃CO₂H | | Inactive | |
| 80590 | ⟨ ⟩ | ⟨ ⟩ | | Inactive | |
| 82186 | ⟨ ⟩ | ⟨ ⟩ | | Inactive | |

[a]Percent increase in life span.

The decomposition of BCNU (and of the 2-chloroethylnitrosoureas) in buffered media (pH 7.4) is very complex: 16 compounds have been identified from this reaction, but the major products are 2-chloroethanol, acetaldehyde, 2-chloroethylamine, the chloride ion, nitrogen, and $CO_2$.[16]

### Table 5
### $N'$-Substituted $N$-(2-Haloethyl)-$N$-Nitrosoureas vs. Leukemia L-1210 (i.p. or i.c.)

| | RN(NO)CONHR' | | L-1210 (Rx: i.p., single dose) | | | |
| | | | i.p. ($10^5$ cells) | | i.c. ($10^4$ cells) | |
| NSC no. | R | R' | Log kill[a] | % Cures[b] | Log kill[a] | % Cures[b] |
|---|---|---|---|---|---|---|
| 91728 | F(CH$_2$)$_2$ | (CH$_2$)$_2$F | 6 | (50-60)[c] | 5 | 60 |
| 409962 | Cl(CH$_2$) | (CH$_2$)$_2$Cl | 6 | 0-100 | 5 | 0-100 |
| 93184 | [F(CH$_2$)$_2$ / Cl(CH$_2$)$_2$] | [(CH$_2$)$_2$Cl / (CH$_2$)$_2$Cl][d] | 6 | 90-100 | 5 | 50-90 |
| 82189 | Br(CH$_2$)$_2$ | (CH$_2$)$_2$Br | 5 | 20 | 0 | 0 |
| 82183 | [Br(CH$_2$)$_2$ / Cl(CH$_2$)$_2$] | [(CH$_2$)$_2$Cl / (CH$_2$)$_2$Br][d] | 6 | (100) | 0 | 0 |
| 81166 | I(CH$_2$)$_2$ | (CH$_2$)$_2$I | Inactive | | | |
| 87974 | F(CH$_2$)$_2$ | cyclohexyl | 6 | 70-90 | 5 | 60-100 |
| 79037 | Cl(CH$_2$)$_2$ | cyclohexyl | 6 | 80-100 | 5 | 20-100 |
| 82182 | Br(CH$_2$)$_2$ | cyclohexyl | 5 | (30) | 0 | 0 |

[a]Reduction in cell population expressed as a logarithm (see reference 4).
[b]45-Day survival.
[c]Parentheses denote only determination.
[d]Mixture.

## Table 6
## The Effect of Modification of the 2-Chloroethyl Group on Leukemia L-1210 Activity

| | RN(NO)CONHR' | | L-1210 (i.p., $10^5$ cells); Rx: i.p., single dose | |
| NSC no. | R | R' | Optimal dose (mg/kg) | % ILS[a] |
| --- | --- | --- | --- | --- |
| 95465 | ClCHCH₂ (Me) | CH₂CHCl (Me) | 1000 / 750 | 140[b] / 97 |
| 95460 | ClCHCH₂ (Me) | ⬡ (cyclohexyl) | 750 | 87 |
| 81701 | Cl(CH₂)₃ | ⬡ (cyclohexyl) | | Inactive |
| 95462 | ClCH₂CH— (Et) | —CHCH₂Cl (Et) | | Inactive |
| 87426 | ⬡–Cl (chlorocyclohexyl) | ⬡–Cl (chlorocyclohexyl) | | Inactive |
| 102864 | ⬡–NHCONCH₂CHCH₂NCONH–⬡ (NO, Cl, NO) | | | Inactive |

[a]Percent increase in life span.

[b]One of six animals cured.

While we continued to investigate structural alterations that might improve the L-1210 activity of the first curative compound, BCNU, clinical studies of this drug were undertaken under the auspices of the National Cancer Institute.[17,18] In initial trials BCNU showed significant activity against advanced Hodgkin's disease and some activity in other lymphomas. Results in gastrointestinal cancer were similar to those obtained with 5-fluorouracil, the agent of choice at that time. Meningeal leukemia was controlled by BCNU in five of nine patients with advanced acute lymphocytic leukemia, but the most exciting activity was observed in preliminary studies with brain tumors. Responses were also noted in three of eight children with other types of solid tumors. All in all these results, although falling short of expectations based on

## Table 7
### The Effect of Modifying the Carbamoyl Function of Nitrosoureas on Activity Against Leukemia L-1210

| NSC no. | Structure | L-1210 (i.p., $10^5$ cells) % ILS[a] at Optimal dose | Rx (i.p.) |
|---|---|---|---|
| 106633 | $Cl(CH_2)_2\underset{\underset{NO}{\mid}}{N}CONHSO_2$—⟨ ⟩—Me | 207[b] | Single dose |
| 78794 | $Me\underset{\underset{NO}{\mid}}{N}CONHCONH_2$ | 88 | Chronic |
| 83273 | $Cl(CH_2)_2\underset{\underset{NO}{\mid}}{N}CO(CH_2)_4CO\underset{\underset{NO}{\mid}}{N}(CH_2)_2Cl$ | | |
| 77666 | $Me\underset{\underset{NO}{\mid}}{N}CONHCO\underset{\underset{NO}{\mid}}{N}Me$ | 62 | Chronic |
| 409425 | $Me\underset{\underset{NO}{\mid}}{N}CONHNHCO\underset{\underset{NO}{\mid}}{N}Me$ | 52 | Chronic |
| 85387 | $Cl(CH_2)_2\underset{\underset{NO}{\mid}}{N}CONHCONH(CH_2)_2Cl$ | 47 | Single dose |
| 88722 | $Cl(CH_2)_2\underset{\underset{NO}{\mid}}{N}OC$ ⬡ $CO\underset{\underset{NO}{\mid}}{N}(CH_2)_2Cl$ | 46 | Single dose |
| 88719 | $Cl(CH_2)_2\underset{\underset{NO}{\mid}}{N}CO$ ⬡ | Inactive | Chronic |
| 45628[c] | Me—⟨ ⟩—$SO_2\underset{\underset{NO}{\mid}}{N}(CH_2)_2Cl$ | Inactive | Chronic |
| 44575 | $Me\underset{\underset{NO}{\mid}}{N}CSNHMe$ | Inactive | Chronic |

[a]Percent increase in life span.
[b]Four of six animals cured.
[c]See reference 7.

animal data, were certainly encouraging and provided additional impetus to seek via the synthesis program new congeners with improved activity against human cancer.

Results obtained in the L-1210 system to this time led to the synthesis of a variety of 2-chloroethyl and 2-fluoroethyl N-nitroso compounds varying both the B and C moieties (Table 6). Although certain other 2-chloroethyl N-nitroso compounds such as N-nitrosoamides and guanidines had some activity (Table 7), all were clearly inferior to the N-nitrosoureas, causing our synthesis program to focus on variations in the C moiety. The L-1210 leukemia system, both the i.p. and i.c. disease, continued to be the primary means of evaluation of these compounds, and improvement in activity against the i.c. disease was the basic goal. This phase of the work led to N-(2-chloroethyl)-N '-cyclohexyl-N-nitrosourea (CCNU, NSC 79037)[13] and to N-(2-chloroethyl)-N '-2,6-dioxo-3-piperidyl)-N-nitrosourea (PCNU, NSC 95466),[13] both clearly superior to BCNU against i.c. leukemia L-1210, the latter compound still being the most active congener for this disease.

CCNU                    PCNU

At this point two factors influenced the direction of our synthetic efforts. First, we had accumulated 50 or so congeners whose activities were almost indistinguishable in the L-1210 system. Large numbers of cures were obtained at the single dose $LD_{10}$, providing no basis for a selection of the best compounds for clinical trials. Second, emphasis at the National Cancer Institute shifted from the leukemias, for which very effective treatment regimens were being developed, to the solid tumors of humans still largely unresponsive to chemotherapy.

At Southern Research Institute, Frank Schabel and his colleagues selected the Lewis lung carcinoma as a secondary system for the evaluation of the nitrosoureas and other promising agents.[19] The Lewis lung carcinoma is implanted subcutaneously as a fragment weighing approximately 40 mg and then treated the next day (early disease) or allowed to grow to approximately 400 mg (day 6-7 postimplant), at which time metastasis to the lung has occurred (established disease) before treatment. In general, even though there are notable exceptions, compounds most active against the early tumor are most

## Table 8
### Activity[a] of Various Agents vs. Solid Tumors

| Compound | Advanced Lewis Lung | Colon | | | | | | Mammary 16/C | Melanoma B16 | Ovarian M5076 |
|---|---|---|---|---|---|---|---|---|---|---|
| | | 06/A | 07/A | 08/A | 26 | 38 | 51 | | | |
| Methotrexate | – | ND[b] | – | ND | – | – | – | – | – | – |
| 6-Thioguanine | – | – | – | ++ | +++ | +++ | – | – | – | – |
| 5-Fluorouracil | – | ± | ++ | + | + | ++ | ± | +++ | – | – |
| 9-β-D-Arabino-furanosylcytosine | – | +++ | +++ | ++++ | – | + | – | ++ | – | + |
| Hydroxyurea | – | ++ | +++ | + | ND | + | ND | ND | – | ND |
| Vincristine | – | – | – | – | – | – | – | +++ | – | ND |
| Prednisone | – | ND | ND | ND | ND | – | ND | ++ | – | ND |
| Adriamycin | – | + | + | +++ | – | ++ | – | ++++ | – | ± |
| Actinomycin D | – | +++ | – | – | + | ++ | – | ND | – | ND |
| Bleomycin | – | ND | +++ | ND | – – | ± | ++ | – | + | ND |
| Nitrogen mustard | ND | ND | ND | ND | ND | ND | ND | ND | – | ND |
| Melphalan (L-PAM) | ND | +++ | + | +++ | +++ | – | + | +++ | – | ++ |
| Cyclophosphamide | +++ | +++ | + | +++ | ++ | ++ | ++ | +++ | ++ | +++ |
| BCNU | – | + | ND | + | ND | ND | + | – | – | ND |
| CCNU | ++ | – | ++ | + | ND | – | ND | ND | ++ | ND |
| MeCCNU | ++++ | ++ | ++ | – | ++++ | – | ++ | ND | +++ | +++ |
| PCNU | + | ++ | ++ | ND | ND | ND | ++ | – | + | ND |
| Chlorozotocin | – | ND | ND | – | – | ND | + | – | – | ++ |

[a] Activity rating (approximate log₁₀ cell kill): + + + + >2.6, + + + 1.6-2.6, + + 0.9-1.5, + 0.5-0.8, – <0.5.
[b] ND = No data available.

active against the established disease.[20] The advanced disease, capable of more clearly differentiating between the activity of different structural types, responds best to N-(2-chloroethyl)-N'-cyclohexyl-N-nitrosoureas containing a substituent at the 4-position of the cyclohexane ring *trans* to the nitrosourea function, an observation not easily explained but which led to the establishment of N-(2-chloroethyl)-N'-(*trans*-4-methylcyclohexyl)-N-nitrosourea (MeCCNU)[21,22] as one of the most potent compounds for the treatment of a variety of solid tumors in rodents (Table 8) and to its use in the treatment of solid tumors in humans.

MeCCNU (R = Me)

Streptozotocin, a natural glucose-substituted N-methyl-N-nitrosourea,[23] is a broad-spectrum antibiotic[24] and an experimental anticancer agent[25] that has shown diabetogenic activity in animals[26] and clinical activity in the treatment of malignant insulinomas in humans.[27] Based on our structure-activity studies, the synthesis of the 2-chloroethyl analogue of streptozotocin was undertaken via the tetraacetate.[21] Although deacetylation by a variety of methods failed, the tetraacetate itself proved highly active in the L-1210 system[21] and, like streptozotocin, showed reduced bone-marrow toxicity.[28] Since the limiting toxicity of the nitrosoureas in humans is to the marrow, this finding caused renewed interest in the preparation of the deacetylated compound, which was accomplished by the nitrosation of 2-[3-(2-chloroethyl)ureido]-2-deoxy-D-glucopyranose by means of $N_2O_3$ in concentrated hydrochloric acid.[29] The high level of activity of the new compound, named chlorozotocin,[29] coupled with its reduced marrow toxicity[30] and good water solubility led to clinical trials of this agent also.[31]

Streptozotocin (R = Me)
Chlorozotocin (R = $CH_2CH_2Cl$)

BCNU, CCNU, MeCCNU, PCNU, and chlorozotocin have all shown significant activity in clinical trials, with BCNU being the most studied drug of this class.[17,18] Activity has been observed in the treatment of Hodgkin's and non-Hodgkin's lymphomas, lung cancers, brain tumors, tumors of the gastrointestinal tract, malignant melanomas, multiple myeloma, and metastatic sarcomas.[31] BCNU and CCNU are now widely used in drug combinations for the treatment of Hodgkin's disease. BCNU has become the drug of choice to be used concomitantly with and after postoperative radiation therapy of the malignant gliomas. The nitrosoureas, especially CCNU, are included in most of the highly effective combinations used for the treatment of oat-cell lung cancers. Thus, it would appear that the nitrosoureas have earned their place in the armamentarium of clinically useful anticancer agents. Their biggest liability is delayed and cumulative myelosuppression,[31] which clearly limits their use and makes the development of a less toxic analogue a worthy, albeit difficult, goal.

## REFERENCES

1. S. A. Shepartz, *Cancer Treat. Rep.*, **60**, 647 (1976).
2. *Organic Syn.*, Coll. Vol. 2, A. H. Blatt, Ed., John Wiley & Sons, Inc., New York, 1943, p. 461.
3. R. E. Rieselbach, E. E. Morse, D. P. Rall, E. Frei III, and E. J. Freireich, *Cancer Chemother. Rep.*, **16**, 191 (1962).
4. H. E. Skipper, F. M. Schabel, Jr., M. W. Trader, and J. R. Thomson, *Cancer Res.*, **21**, 1154 (1961).
5. G. Von Bruning, *Ber.*, **21**, 1809 (1888).
6. N. M. Emanuel, E. M. Vermel, L. A. Ostrovskaya, and N. P. Korman, *Cancer Chemother. Rep.*, **58**, 135 (1974).
7. *Organic Syn.*, Coll. Vol. 2, A. H. Blatt, Ed., John Wiley & Sons, Inc., New York, 1943, p. 165.
8. I. B. Dawid, T. C. French, and J. M. Buchanan, *J. Biol. Chem.*, **238**, 2178 (1963).
9. J. A. Montgomery, R. James, G. S. McCaleb, and T. P. Johnston, *J. Med. Chem.*, **10**, 668 (1967).
10. A. Loveless and C. L. Hampton, *Mutation Res.*, **7**, 1 (1969).
11. T. P. Johnston, G. S. McCaleb, and J. A. Montgomery, *J. Med. Chem.*, **6**, 669 (1963).
12. F. M. Schabel, Jr., T. P. Johnston, G. S. McCaleb, J. A. Montgomery, W. R. Laster, and H. E. Skipper, *Cancer Res.*, **23**, 725 (1963).
13. T. P. Johnston, G. S. McCaleb, P. S. Opliger, and J. A. Montgomery, *J. Med. Chem.*, **9**, 892 (1966).
14. J. A. Montgomery, R. James, G. S. McCaleb, M. C. Kirk, and T. P. Johnston, *J. Med. Chem.*, **18**, 568 (1975).
15. M. B. Chenoweth, *Pharmacol. Rev.*, **1**, 383 (1949).
16. J. A. Montgomery, in B. Serrou, P. S. Schein, and J.-L. Imbach, Eds., *Nitrosoureas in Cancer Treatment*, Inserm Symposium No. 19, Elsevier/North-Holland Biomedical Press, Amsterdam, 1981, p. 13.
17. R. B. Livingston and S. K. Carter, *Single Agents in Cancer Chemotherapy*, IFI/Plenum, New York, 1970, p. 360.
18. S. K. Carter, F. M. Schabel, Jr., L. E. Broder, and T. P. Johnston, *Advan. Cancer Res.*, **16**, 273 (1972).

19.  J. G. Mayo, W. R. Laster, Jr., C. M. Andrews, and F. M. Schabel, Jr., *Cancer Chemother. Rep.,* Part 1, **56,** 183 (1972).
20.  J. A. Montgomery, G. S. McCaleb, T. P. Johnston, J. G. Mayo, and W. R. Laster, Jr., *J. Med. Chem.,* **20,** 291 (1977).
21.  T. P. Johnston, G. S, McCaleb, P. S. Opliger, W. R. Laster, Jr., and J. A. Montgomery, *J. Med. Chem.,* **14,** 600 (1971).
22.  T. P. Johnston, G. S. McCaleb, S. D. Clayton, J. L. Frye, C. A. Krauth, and J. A. Montgomery, *J. Med. Chem.,* **20,** 279 (1977).
23.  R. R. Herr, H. K. Jahnke, and A. D. Argoudelis, *J. Am. Chem. Soc.,* **89,** 4808 (1967).
24.  J. J. Vavra, C. DeBoer, A. Dietz, L. J. Hanka, and W. T. Sokolski, *Antibiot. Ann.,* 1959-1960, 230 (1960).
25.  B. K. Bhuyan, T. J. Fraser, H. H. Buskirk, and G. L. Neil, *Cancer Chemother. Rep.,* (Part 1), **56,** 709 (1972).
26.  N. Rakieten, M. L. Rakieten, and M. V. Nadkarni, *Cancer Chemother. Rep.,* **29,** 91 (1963).
27.  I. M. Murray-Lyon, A. L. W. E. Eddelston, R. Williams, M. Brown, B. M. Hogbin, A. Bennett, J. C. Edwards, and K. W. Taylor, *Lancet,* **2** (7574), 895 (1968).
28.  P. S. Schein and S. Loftus, *Cancer Res.,* **28,** 1501 (1968).
29.  T. P. Johnston, G. S. McCaleb, and J. A. Montgomery, *J. Med. Chem.,* **18,** 104 (1975).
30.  T. Anderson, M. G. McMenamin, and P. S. Schein, *Cancer Res.,* **35,** 761 (1975).
31.  "Clinical Studies," in A. W. Prestayko, S. T. Crooke, L. H. Baker, S. K. Carter, and P. S. Schein, Eds., *Nitrosoureas: Current Status and New Developments,* Academic Press, New York, 1981, p. 143.

# 10

Amikacin

Hiroshi Kawaguchi
and Takayuki Naito

...orkers in 1957[1] and its introduction ...anamycin has been a valuable ...t of penicillin-resistant staphylococcal ...ulosis, and serious gram-negative infections. The spectrum of kanamycin is somewhat limited, however, in that it is virtually inactive against *Pseudomonas* species, and clinical isolates resistant to other aminoglycoside antibiotics are generally resistant to kanamycin. In contrast, gentamicin C, another important aminoglycoside antibiotic, discovered in 1963,[3] inhibits a broader spectrum of microbes including *Pseudomonas*. Unfortunately, the incidence of gentamicin-resistant strains encountered in the clinic has been rapidly increasing with the increased use of the antibiotic.[4,5]

R-Factor-mediated aminoglycoside resistance was first described by Okamoto and Suzuki in 1965,[6] and the biochemical basis for the mechanisms of resistance to kanamycin was elucidated by Umezawa et al. in 1967,[7,8] Ten years after the discovery of kanamycin. This work has been confirmed and extended in other academic institutions, and it is now well established that the major mechanisms of resistance possessed by aminoglycoside-resistant organisms are inactivation of the antibiotics through *N*-acetylation,[9-13] *O*-phosphorylation,[14-19] and *O*-adenylation.[20-23]

These findings opened a new era in aminoglycoside antibiotic research. Knowledge of the mechanism of resistance to aminoglycosides offered the possibility of synthesizing derivatives that would be effective against resistant organisms, and chemists were encouraged to investigate specific structural modifications of aminoglycoside antibiotics.

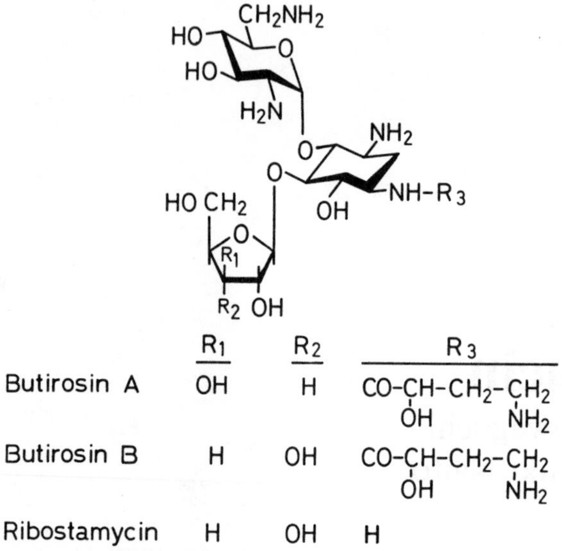

| | $R_1$ | $R_2$ | $R_3$ |
|---|---|---|---|
| Butirosin A | OH | H | $CO-CH-CH_2-CH_2$ with $OH$ and $NH_2$ |
| Butirosin B | H | OH | $CO-CH-CH_2-CH_2$ with $OH$ and $NH_2$ |
| Ribostamycin | H | OH | H |

**Figure 1.**   Structure of butirosins and ribostamycin.

## Table 1
### Comparison of the Antibacterial Spectra
### of Butirosin and Ribostamycin

| | MIC ($\mu g/ml$) | |
|---|---|---|
| Test organism | Butirosin | Ribostamycin |
| *Staphylococcus aureus* Smith | 0.8 | 1.6 |
| *Escherichia coli* Juhl | 0.8 | 1.6 |
| *Escherichia coli* K12 | 0.4 | 0.8 |
| *Escherichia coli* ML-1630[a] | 6.3 | 100 |
| *Escherichia coli* JR35/C600[a] | 1.6 | >100 |
| *Pseudomonas aeruginosa* D15 | 6.3 | >100 |
| *Pseudomonas aeruginosa* H9 | >100 | >100 |

[a]Reported to produce neomycin-kanamycin phosphorylating enzymes.[14,16]

One direction taken for the chemical modification of aminoglycosides was the removal of the functional group that is susceptible to attack by an inactivating enzyme. The 3'-hydroxyl group of aminoglycoside antibiotics has been shown to be the target site of phosphorylating enzymes. Thus, 3'-deoxykanamycin A and 3', 4'-dideoxykanamycin B (dibekacin) were synthesized by Umezawa and coworkers[24-26] and have, in fact, proved to be active against kanamycin-resistant *Escherichia coli* and *Pseudomonas* species.

Another direction for the chemical modification of aminoglycoside antibiotics was the attempt to prevent the inactivating enzymes from binding at the active sites on the aminoglycoside molecule. Amikacin, a semisynthetic derivative of kanamycin, was developed on the basis of this concept.

The chain of events that led to the synthesis of amikacin originated with the discovery of butirosin. In the course of a new antibiotic screening program at Bristol-Banyu Research Institute (BBRI) in Tokyo, it was observed that a bacterial strain isolated from a soil sample collected in Taiwan produced an aminoglycosidic antibiotic complex, designated Bu-1709, that contained 2-deoxystreptamine in its structure. This finding was the first example of aminoglycoside biosynthesis by a member of the order Eubacteriales, since all aminoglycoside antibiotics known at that time were produced by members of the order Actinomycetales, such as *Streptomyces* or *Micromonospora*. More important, the new antibiotic had an interesting antibacterial spectrum and inhibited certain organisms that were known to phosphorylate neomycin and kanamycin. Studies of the molecular structure of Bu-1709 revealed two major components: xylosyl- or ribosyl-neamine and an unusual amino acid, $L$(-)-$\gamma$-amino-$\alpha$-hydroxybutyric acid ($L$-AHBA). Workers at Parke, Davis and Company isolated the identical antibiotic complex from the fermentation broth of *Bacillus circulans* and named it butirosin A and B (originally called ambutyrosin A and B). At the same time that their report appeared in a patent publication,[27] antibiotic chemists at BBRI (Tsukiura, Konishi, and coworkers) had nearly completed the work to elucidate the structure of Bu-1709. Although having lost the chance to patent the antibiotic, they made efforts to utilize and further develop the specific knowledge that they had obtained with this interesting antibiotic.

As shown in Figure 1, butirosin B is closely related structurally to ribostamycin,[28] an aminoglycoside antibiotic produced by a strain of *Streptomyces*,[29] differing from it only in that the specific amino acid $L$-AHBA is attached at the C-1 amino group. Comparison of the antibacterial spectra of butirosin and ribostamycin (Table 1) suggested to us that selective acylation of a particular amino group of an aminoglycoside antibiotic with a specific amino acid might be effective in protecting the antibiotic from the action of inactivating enzymes.

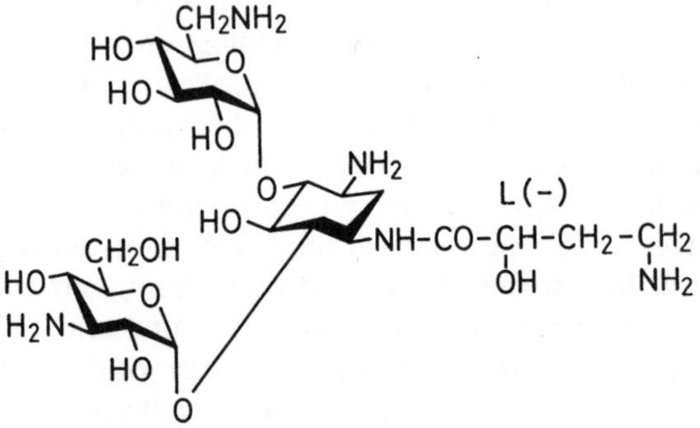

**Figure 2.**   Structure of amikacin (BB-K8).

Taking into consideration the postulated structural requirements for activity against resistant organisms, we planned to investigate new types of chemical modifications of several aminoglycoside antibiotics, particularly kanamycin A. Although the antibacterial spectrum of ribostamycin, a 5,6-disubstituted-2-deoxystreptamine-containing aminoglycoside, was shown to be markedly improved by acylation at the C-1 amino group, it remained to be determined which amino group would be most appropriate for such acylation in kanamycin, a 4,6-disubstituted-2-deoxystreptamine-containing antibiotic. Here the problem posed a challenge to organic chemists, since selective acylation of a specific amino group in an aminoglycoside antibiotic had never been attempted. The solution of this problem resulted in a series of new aminoglycoside derivatives, from which amikacin (Figure 2) was selected because of its desirable biological properties: activity, spectrum, and toxicity.[30],[31],[32]

## 1.   SYNTHESIS OF AMIKACIN AND ITS POSITIONAL ISOMERS

There are four acylable amino groups in the kanamycin molecule (Figure 3), two in the 2-deoxystreptamine (DOS) part and one each in the 6-amino-6-deoxy-D-glucose (6-AG) and 3-amino-3-deoxy-D-glucose (3-AG) moieties. We assumed that the four amino groups of kanamycin are not totally equivalent in their steric environment and hence their reactivity to acylating agents. The 6'-amino group in the 6-AG moiety, located on a methylene carbon, was predicted to be the most reactive amino function, but since the remaining three amino groups were each attached to a methine carbon they were presumed to have a similar level of reactivity. Therefore, specific and well-controlled reac-

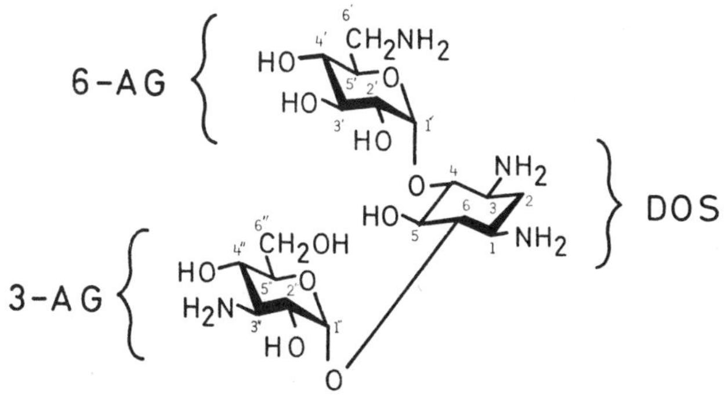

**Figure 3.**   Structure of kanamycin A.

tion conditions seemed necessary for the selective acylation. For this purpose, we first examined the use of $N$-hydroxysuccinimide ester of $L$-AHBA for the acylation of kanamycin.

The acylating agent was prepared by protecting the $\gamma$-amino group of $L$-AHBA with a benzyloxycarbonyl(Cbz) group, followed by reaction with $N$-hydroxysuccinimide(OSu) and dicyclohexylcarbodiimide to form the active ester of $N$-Cbz-protected $L$-AHBA ($N$-Cbz-AHB-OSu).

Figures 4 and 5 illustrate synthetic routes for the selective introduction of $L$-AHBA to kanamycin A to afford amikacin and its positional isomers, respectively. The four amino groups of kanamycin A are designated, for convenience, as $N^1$, $N^2$, $N^3$, and $N^4$ in the order of hypothetical reactivity to acylating agents. Reaction of kanamycin A with an equimolar amount of $N$-Cbz-AHB-OSu followed by removal of the blocking group by hydrogenation resulted in $N$-acylation at the most reactive amino group to give $N^1$-AHB-kanamycin A as a major product, designated BB-K6.[33] The $N^1$-acylated product thus obtained retained only a very weak antibacterial activity compared with kanamycin. However, there was an indication, revealed by thin-layer chromatography (TLC), that the reaction mixture still contained a low level of a new active component that was supposed to be a derivative acylated at one of the three amino groups other than $N^1$. Selective acylation at the second most reactive amino group, $N^2$, required a prior blocking of the $N^1$ amino function. The $N^1$ amino group of kanamycin was protected with the Cbz group by an equimolar reaction with $N$-(benzyloxycarbonyloxy)succinimide (Cbz-OSu). The $N^1$-Cbz-blocked kanamycin thus obtained was then reacted with an equimolar amount of $N$-Cbz-AHB-OSu. Subsequent hydrogenolysis to remove

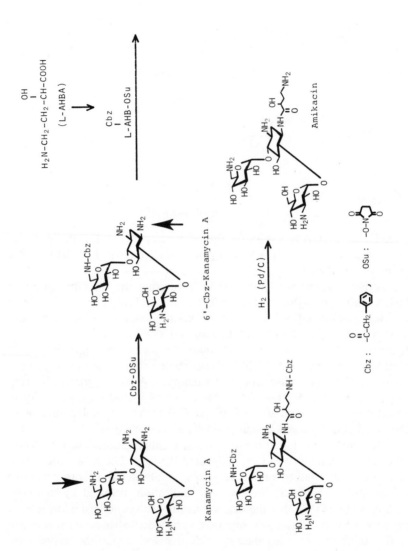

**Figure 4.** Preparation of amikacin.

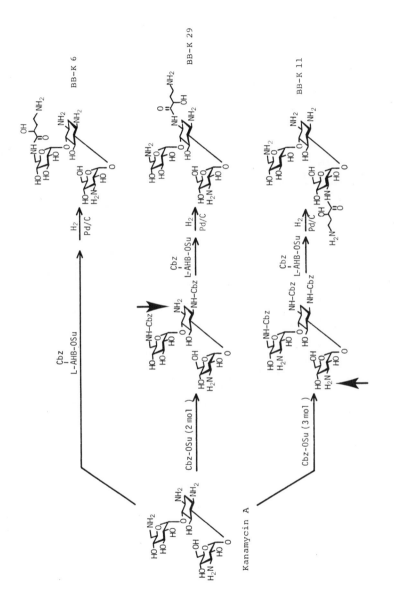

**Figure 5.** Preparation of positional isomers of amikacin.

213

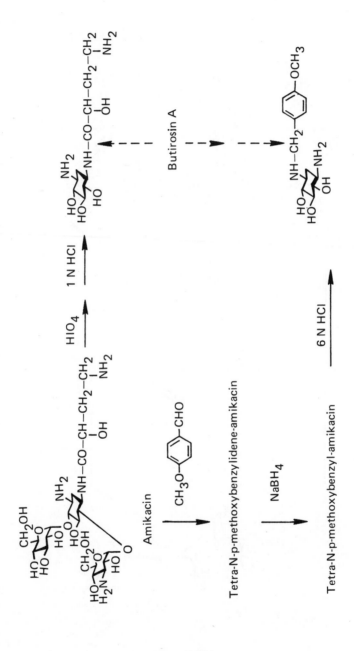

**Figure 6.** Structure determination of amikacin.

214

the two protecting groups on the $N$ and $\gamma$-amino groups, followed by chromatographic purification, yielded $N^2$-AHB-kanamycin A, which was designated BB-K 8 and later named amikacin (Figure 4).

Kanamycin A was reacted with two molar equivalents of Cbz-OSu to give the compound shown in the middle scheme of Figure 5, which had two protective groups at the most reactive and second most reactive amino groups. Acylation of the $N^1$,$N^2$-di-Cbz-kanamycin A with $N$-Cbz-AHB-OSu followed by reductive deblocking afforded $N^3$-AHB-kanamycin A, designated BB-K 29.[33] Similarly, $N^4$-AHB-kanamycin A, designated BB-K 11, was obtained from $N^1$,$N^2$,$N^3$-tri-Cbz-kanamycin A, as shown in Figure 5.

The site of acylation with L-AHBA in the amikacin molecule was determined by the method illustrated in Figure 6.[30] Periodate oxidation of amikacin followed by mild acid hydrolysis afforded an $L$-AHBA-acylated DOS. Upon similar treatment, butirosin yielded the same degradation product,[34] which was identified by TLC and optical rotatory dispersion (ORD). Alternatively, the Schiff's base of amikacin with $p$-methoxybenzaldehyde was reduced with NaBH₄ and then hydrolyzed to give 3-$N$-$p$-methoxybenzyl-DOS, which was identical, by ORD and circular dichroism (CD), with the corresponding product obtained from butirosin A. The 3-$N$-substituted DOS derivative showed a double-positive Cotton effect with peaks at 280 and 332 nm in the ORD, and with positive peaks at 273 and 223 nm in the CD. Thus, the structure of amikacin was unequivocally established to be 1-$N$-[$L$(-)-$\gamma$-amino-$\alpha$-hydroxybutyryl]kanamycin A, and accordingly the C-1 amino group of DOS moiety was proved to be the second most reactive amino function, $N^2$, in kanamycin A.

Determination of the sites of acylation for three amikacin isomers[33] is briefly described below: BB-K 29, the $N^3$-acylated isomer, was subjected to reductive $N$-alkylation with $p$-methoxybenzaldehyde and subsequent hydrolysis by the procedure similar to that used for amikacin. The resulting product was identified by ORD and CD as 1-$N$-$p$-methoxybenzyl-DOS, the enantiomer of that obtained from amikacin. Thus, BB-K 29 is 3-$N$-AHB-kanamycin A. BB-K 6, the $N^1$-acyl isomer, was deaminated by Van Slyke method to give a ninhydrin-negative product. The product was hydrolyzed in 4$N$ HCl affording only 6-AG, with neither 3-AG nor DOS being obtained. Thus, BB-K 6 is 6'-$N$-AHB-kanamycin A. The site of acylation in BB-K 11, the $N^4$-acyl isomer, was determined to be the C-3" amino group in the 3-AG moiety by a method similar to that used for BB-K 6. From the hydrolysate of the deamination product of BB-K 11, 3-AG was isolated and identified but neither 6-AG nor DOS was detected. Thus the structures shown in Figure 5 were assigned to three amikacin isomers, BB-K 6, BB-K 11, and BB-K 29. The physicochemical prop-

**Table 3**

**Resistance of Various Bacterial Species to Aminoglycoside Antibiotics**[a]

| Organism | No. of strains | No. of sources | Resistance to (%) | | | |
|---|---|---|---|---|---|---|
| | | | Kanamycin | Gentamicin | Tobramycin | Amikacin |
| *Escherichia coli* | 34 | 20 | 97.1 | 44.1 | 44.1 | 8.8 |
| *Enterobacter* species | 30 | 13 | 100 | 46.7 | 33.3 | 10 |
| *Klebsiella pneumoniae* | 39 | 13 | 94.9 | 82.1 | 53.8 | 0 |
| *Proteus mirabilis* | 2 | 2 | 100 | 0 | 50 | 0 |
| *Proteus rettgeri* | 29 | 15 | 75.9 | 93.1 | 82.8 | 13.8 |
| *Proteus vulgaris* | 1 | 1 | 100 | 100 | 0 | 0 |
| *Providencia stuartii* | 35 | 9 | 54.3 | 74.3 | 62.9 | 0 |
| *Serratia marcescens* | 38 | 18 | 92.1 | 65.8 | 78.9 | 5.3 |
| *Salmonella* species | 7 | 3 | 100 | 42.9 | 14.3 | 0 |
| *Pseudomonas aeruginosa* | 65 | 25 | 100 | 98.5 | 56.9 | 32.3 |
| *Pseudomonas maltophilia* | 5 | 3 | 100 | 100 | 100 | 100 |
| *Pseudomonas* species | 6 | 3 | 100 | 100 | 100 | 33.3 |
| *Alcaligenes* species | 9 | 7 | 100 | 100 | 100 | 100 |
| *Acinetobacter* species | 5 | 3 | 40 | 80 | 80 | 40 |
| *Flavobacterium* species | 2 | 2 | 100 | 50 | 50 | 50 |
| *Staphylococcus aureus* | 9 | 3 | 100 | 0 | 0 | 0 |
| *Staphylococcus epidermidis* | 3 | 2 | 100 | 0 | 33.3 | 0 |
| Total | 319 | | 90% | 72.7% | 58.6% | 16.3% |

[a]From K. E. Price et al.[36]

## Table 2
## Physicochemical Properties of Amikacin
## and Its Position Isomers

| Compound | Site of acylation | mp (°C, dec) | $[\alpha]_D$ (H$_2$O) | TLC$^a$ (Rf) |
|---|---|---|---|---|
| Amikacin | C-1 | 203-204 | + 99° | 0.17 |
| BB-K6 | C-6′ | 184-187 | + 109° | 0.29 |
| BB-K11 | C-3″ | 202 | + 92° | 0.15 |
| BB-K29 | C-3 | 181-183 | + 83.5° | 0.24 |

$^a$Silica gel plate: CHCl$_3$-CH$_3$OH-NH$_4$OH (28%)-H$_2$O (1:4:2:1).

erties of amkacin and its positional isomers are shown in Table 2. Assignments of the $^{13}$C-NMR spectra of amikacin, its isomers, and related compounds have been described by Toda et al. of BBRI.[35]

## 2.   ANTIMICROBIAL ACTIVITY OF AMIKACIN

Amikacin exhibits a broad-spectrum antimicrobial activity against kanamycin-sensitive and resistant organisms including *Pseudomonas* species. The intrinsic activity of amikacin against kanamycin-sensitive strains is equal to or higher than that of kanamycin. Amikacin is active against various types of aminoglycoside-resistant organisms because of its high degree of resistance to the action of inactivating enzymes produced by the resistant organisms.[30,31]

Price et al.[36] carried out an extensive study comparing the inhibitory action of amikacin with currently used aminoglycoside antibiotics, utilizing a total of 319 clinical isolate known to be resistant to one or more aminoglycosides. The results of the study are summarized in Table 3. The percentages of isolates found by an agar dilution method to be susceptible were: amikacin, 83,7%; tobramycin, 41.4%; gentamicin C, 27.3%; kanamycin A, 10.0%. This extension in the spectrum of amikacin, which results in the inhibition of various strains of gentamicin-resistant and tobramycin-resistant organisms, has also been described by many clinical investigators.[37-42]

It has been shown that resistance to aminoglycoside antibiotics is largely due to the presence of plasmids that code for aminoglycoside-modifying enzymes.[43] A number of different aminoglycoside-modifying enzymes have been identified, 12 of which are known to be capable of inactivating kanamycin A (Figure 7) and six of which can inactivate gentamicin C$_1$ (Figure 8). The antimicrobial

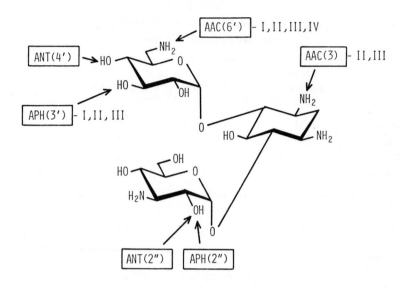

**Figure 7.**   Enzymatic inactivation of kanamycin A.

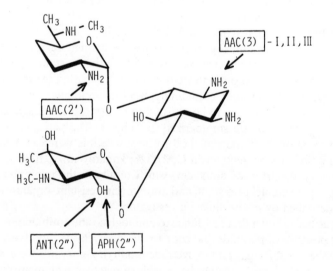

**Figure 8.**   Enzymatic inactivation of gentamicin $C_1$.

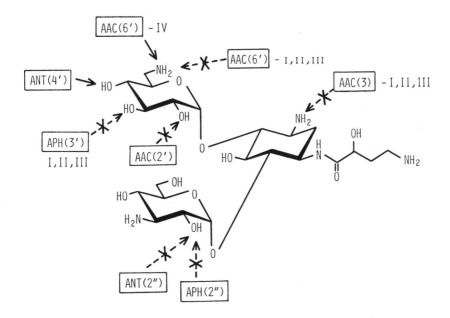

**Figure 9.** Resistance of amikacin to aminoglycoside-modifying enzymes.

activity of amikacin has been found to be affected by two enzymes, AAC(6′)-IV and ANT(4′).* However, as shown in Figure 9, amikacin is not inactivated by 12 aminoglycoside-modifying enzymes that affect the activity of kanamycin, tobramycin and/or gentamicin, indicating that *L*-AHBA-acylation at the C-1 amino group of kanamycin produced an inhibitory effect on the action of this group of enzymes.

The importance of the site of acylation in the kanamycin molecule for expressing desirable biological properties is recognized by comparing the activity and spectrum of amikacin with those of three of its positional isomers. The antibacterial activity of amikacin and its isomers, BB-K 6, BB-K 11, and BB-K 29, was determined with the use of 20 strains of kanamycin-sensitive organisms comprising seven bacterial genera. The results are summarized in Table 4 in terms of the geometric mean of MICs for each of the genera tested. The relative activity of each compound compared with kanamycin A is also shown in the table. Amikacin is generally more active than kanamycin A against kanamycin-

---

*See footnote of Table 5 for abbreviations of aminoglycoside-modifying enzymes.

## Table 4

### In vitro Activity of Amikacin and Its Isomers Against Kanamycin-Sensitive Organisms

| Organism | No. of strains tested | Geometric mean MIC (mcg/ml) | | | | | Relative activity (kanamycin = 100) | | | | |
|---|---|---|---|---|---|---|---|---|---|---|---|
| | | Kana- mycin | Amikacin (1-N) | BB-K6 (6'-N) | BB-K11 (3"-N) | BB-K29 (3-N) | Kana- mycin | Amikacin | BB-K6 | BB-K11 | BB-K29 |
| Escherichia coli | 5 | 2.07 | 1.03 | 174 | 66 | 50 | 100 | 200 | 1 | 3 | 4 |
| Klebsiella pneumoniae | 3 | 2.48 | 1.57 | 159 | 79 | 79 | 100 | 160 | 2 | 3 | 3 |
| Proteus mirabilis | 2 | 1.10 | 0.55 | 71 | 35 | 35 | 100 | 200 | 2 | 3 | 3 |
| Shigella species | 2 | 2.21 | 1.57 | 142 | 71 | 50 | 100 | 140 | 2 | 3 | 4 |
| Enterobacter species | 2 | 4.43 | 3.13 | 401 | 100 | 100 | 100 | 140 | 1 | 4 | 4 |
| Staphylococcus aureus | 4 | 0.93 | 0.78 | 84 | 35 | 42 | 100 | 120 | 1 | 3 | 2 |
| Bacillus species | 2 | 0.78 | 0.28 | 50 | 25 | 25 | 100 | 280 | 2 | 3 | 3 |
| Total | 20 | 1.68 | 1.00 | 128 | 54 | 50 | 100 | 170 | 1 | 3 | 3 |

## Table 5

## *In vitro* Activity of Amikacin and Its Isomers Against Aminoglycoside-resistant Organisms

| Aminoglycoside-modifying enzyme produced[a] | No. of strains tested | Geometric mean MIC (mcg/ml) | | | | | Relative activity (kanamycin = 100) | | | | |
|---|---|---|---|---|---|---|---|---|---|---|---|
| | | Kana-mycin | Amikacin (1-N) | BB-K6 (6'-N) | BB-K11 (3"-N) | BB-K29 (3-N) | Kana-mycin | Amikacin | BB-K6 | BB-K11 | BB-K29 |
| APH(3')-I | 6 | 250 | 0.45 | 1,000 | 200 | 71 | 100 | 55,000 | 25 | 125 | 350 |
| APH(3')-II | 4 | 200 | 1.1 | 670 | 480 | 84 | 100 | 18,000 | 30 | 40 | 240 |
| ANT(2") | 2 | 71 | 0.1 | 200 | 140 | 35 | 100 | 71,000 | 35 | 50 | 200 |
| ANT(4') | 3 | 630 | 10 | 800 | 2,500 | 630 | 100 | 6,300 | 80 | 25 | 100 |
| AAC(6') | 3 | 100 | 10 | 250 | 800 | 400 | 100 | 1,000 | 40 | 13 | 25 |
| AAC(3)-II | 2 | 400 | 8.9 | 1,600 | 1,600 | 400 | 100 | 4,500 | 25 | 25 | 100 |

[a]Abbreviations for aminoglycoside-modifying enzymes[44]: APH = aminoglycoside phosphotransferase; ANT = aminoglycoside nucleotidyl-transferase; AAC = aminoglycoside acetyltransferase; number in parentheses indicates the site of modification; roman numeral distinguishes different types of enzyme.

**Table 6**

**Aminoglycoside Modification by 1-$N$ Acylation
with $L$-AHBA or Its Congeners**

| Parent antibiotic | Year | Reference |
|---|---|---|
| Kanamycin A | 1972 | 30 |
| Ribostamycin | 1972 | 45 |
| Kanamycin B | 1973 | 46, 47 |
| Dibekacin | 1973 | 48 |
| Lividomycin A | 1973 | 49, 50 |
| Gentamicin $C_1$ | 1973 | 51, 52 |
| Tobramycin | 1974 | 53 |
| Gentamicin $C_{1a}$ | 1974 | 54 |
| Gentamicin $C_2$ | 1974 | 55 |
| Neomycin B, C | 1974 | 56 |
| Paromomycin | 1974 | 57 |
| Lividomycin B | 1975 | 58 |
| Sagamicin | 1975 | 59 |
| Sisomicin | 1976 | 60 |
| Verdamicin | 1976 | 60 |
| Gentamicin B | 1977 | 61 |

sensitive organisms and shows, on an average, 170% of the intrinsic anti-bacterial activity of kanamycin A, whereas the three positional isomers of amikacin are only 1-3% as active as kanamycin A. The activity against 20 strains of aminoglycoside-resistant organisms is shown in Table 5. The resistant organisms are classified into six groups according to the type of aminoglycoside-modifying enzymes produced. Amikacin is highly active against the aminoglycoside-resistant organisms that produce APH(3′) or ANT(2′). Some strains that produce ANT(4′) or AAC(6′) are still fairly susceptible to amikacin. The three amikacin isomers, especially BB-K 29, are relatively more resistant than kanamycin to the enzymatic action of resistant organisms when their weak intrinsic activities against kanamycin-sensitive bacteria are taken into account.

## 3. AMIKACIN ANALOGUE AND DERIVATIVES

In recognition of the striking effect of acylation with *L*-AHBA at the C-1 amino group of kanamycin, a number of DOS-containing aminoglycoside antibiotics have been modified in similar fashion. Table 6 lists the aminoglycoside derivatives reported to date that are acylated at the C-1 amino group with *L*-AHBA or its congeners. These derivatives were shown, in fact, to be active against aminoglycoside-resistant organisms that were not inhibited by the parent antibiotics. The last compound in the table, which is designated Sch 21420 and has a structure of 1-*N*-(S)-3-amino-2-hydroxypropionyl]-gentamicin B,[61] appears to be an interesting compound in view of its improved spectrum[62] and favorable toxicity profile.[63]

The configurational isomers of amikacin, which are acylated at the C-1 amino group of kanamycin A with *DL*- or *D*(+)-AHBA, instead of *L*-(-)-AHBA in amikacin, were prepared by essentially the same method as that used for amikacin.[33] These configurational isomers have an antibacterial spectrum similar to that of amikacin. However, the intrinsic activity of the *DL*-isomer (BB-K 19) is approximately one-half that of amikacin, while the *D*-isomer (BB-K 31) is only one-fourth as active as amikacin (Table 7).

A series of amikacin analogues were prepared by the procedure similar to that used for amikacin synthesis.[64] The major modifications made on the amikacin side chain involved the $\alpha$-hydroxyl and $\gamma$-amino groups and the length of the alkyl chain. Structures and activities of representative analogues are shown in Table 7. Any modification of the $\alpha$-hydroxyl group, such as elimination (BB-K 9), replacement with an amino group (BB-K 13), or shift to the $\beta$-position (BB-K 14), reduced the activity to less than 5% that of amikacin. Removal of the terminal basic function (BB-K 20) resulted in nearly complete loss of activity. However, the derivatives having both the $\alpha$-hydroxyl and terminal amino groups retained a substantial proportion of the activity of amikacin, with amikacin still the best followed by its next higher and next lower homologues (BB-K 23) and (BB-K 101).

Further studies of the modification of aminoglycoside antibiotics at the C-1 amino group have been extended to *N*-alkylation. Scientists at Schering synthesized 1-*N*-ethylsisomicin, netilmicin, which is highly active against sisomicin-resistant organisms and has a reduced potential for toxicity in animal models.[65] The effect of 1-*N*-alkylation in kanamycin antibiotics was studied by Nakagawa et al. of BBRI.[66] Richardson et al. at Pfizer Central Research in England prepared 1-*N*-[(S)-4-amino-2-hydroxybutyl]kanamycin A by diborane reduction of amikacin.[67] This compound, designated UK-18892 and now called butikacin, is reported to have an antibacterial spectrum similar to that of amikacin[68] and a relatively low level of cochlear toxicity.[69]

**Table 7**

**Physicochemical Properties and Relative Activity
of Amikacin Analogs**

| Code no. | 1-$N$ Acyl residue | | mp (°C) | TLC (Rf)[a] | Relative activity[b] |
|----------|---------|-----------------|---------|-------------|---------------------|
| | Structure | α-Configuration | | | |
| Amikacin | | $L$ | 203-204 | 0.16 | 100 |
| BB-K31 | | $D$ | 179-180 | 0.16 | 26 |
| BB-K19 | | $DL$ | 180-181 | 0.17 | 47 |
| BB-K9 | | — | 175-180 | 0.22 | 4.0 |
| BB-K13 | | $L$ | 185 | 0.18 | 3.5 |
| BB-K14 | | $\beta$-$DL$ | 174-180 | 0.31 | 4.5 |
| BB-K20 | | $DL$ | 190-193 | 0.54 | 0.8 |
| BB-K101 | | $L$ | 200-205 | 0.33 | 57 |
| BB-K23 | | $L$ | 214-215 | 0.18 | 84 |
| BB-K30 | | $L$ | 220-203 | 0.23 | 9 |

[a]Silica gel plate; $CHCl_3$-$CH_3OH$-28% $NH_4OH$-$H_2O$ (1:4:2:1).

[b]Relative to amikacin: assigned on the basis of geometric mean of MICs for 32 test organisms, including 23 aminoglycoside-sensitive and 10 resistant strains.

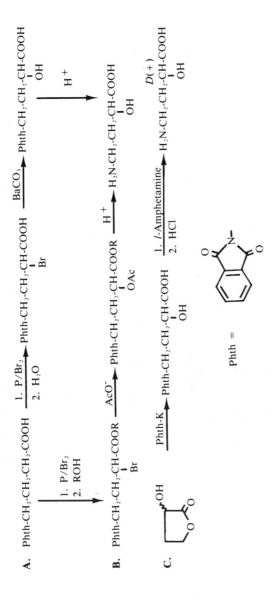

**Figure 10.** Historical preparation of γ-amino-α-hydroxybutyric acid (~ 1970).

225

**I.** Butirosin $\xrightarrow{\text{0.5 } N \text{ NaOH}}$ L-AHBA

**II.** 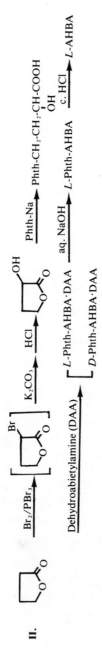 $\xrightarrow{\text{Br}_2/\text{PBr}_3}$ $\xrightarrow{\text{K}_2\text{CO}_3, \text{ HCl}}$ $\xrightarrow{\text{Phth-Na}}$ Phth-CH$_2$-CH$_2$-CH-COOH (OH) $\xrightarrow{\text{aq. NaOH}}$ L-Phth-AHBA $\xrightarrow{\text{Dehydroabietylamine (DAA)}}$ $\Big[$ L-Phth-AHBA·DAA / D-Phth-AHBA·DAA $\Big]$  L-Phth-AHBA $\xrightarrow{\text{c. HCl}}$ L-AHBA

**III.** DL-AHBA $\xrightarrow{Acetobacter \ sp. \ (\text{ATCC 21780})}$ L-AHBA

**IV.** HOOC-CH$_2$-CH$_2$-CH-COOH (NH$_2$) L(+) $\xrightarrow[\text{(Schmidt R.)}]{\text{HN}_3}$ H$_2$N-CH$_2$-CH$_2$-CH-COOH (NH$_2$) L(+) $\xrightarrow{\text{HNO}_2}$ L-AHBA

**V.** HOOC-CH$_2$-CH$_2$-CH-COOH (NH$_2$) L(+) $\xrightarrow{\text{HNO}_2}$ 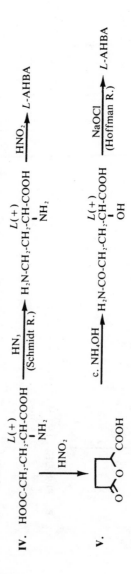 $\xrightarrow{\text{c. NH}_4\text{OH}}$ H$_2$N-CO-CH$_2$-CH$_2$-CH-COOH (OH) L(+) $\xrightarrow[\text{(Hoffman R.)}]{\text{NaOCl}}$ L-AHBA

**Figure 11.** Development of L-AHBA preparation at BBRI (1970-1974).

## 4. CHEMICAL DEVELOPMENT IN AMIKACIN SYNTHESIS

From the time of the first synthesis of amikacin in a test tube in December, 1970, a number of developments in chemical technology have made it feasible to produce it at a commercially useful level. The following description is a brief review of the developments achieved in preparing the optically active side chain acid of amikacin, L-AHBA, and the progress reported relating to the selective acylation in amikacin synthesis.

### 4.1 Developments in the Preparation of L(-)-γ-Amino-α-hydroxybutyric Acid (L-AHBA)

The initial sample of amikacin was prepared by utilizing the side chain acid of butirosin (Bu-1709), obtained by mild alkaline hydrolysis of Bu-1790. It soon became essential to make L-AHBA in larger quantities at a more reasonable cost. The synthesis of DL-AHBA was first described by Fischer and Goddertz in 1910,[70] starting from γ-phthalimidobutyric acid followed by α-bromination, hydroxylation, and hydrolysis, as shown in Figure 10 (route A). Tanable and colleagues improved the α-hydroxylation step (route B) to obtain DL-AHBA with an overall yield of 55%.[71] The preparation of D(+)-AHBA was described by Saito et al.,[72] starting from 2-hydroxybutyrolactone, with optical resolution accomplished by using l-amphetamine (route C). At the time of amikacin discovery, the desired L(-)-isomer of AHBA had never been synthesized.

The developmental work carried out at BBRI for the preparation of L-AHBA is summarized in Figure 11. The first synthesis of L-AHBA (route II) was undertaken starting from commercially available γ-butyrolactone to obtain 2-hydroxybutyrolactone.[33] Then, the above-described route C was followed to give a racemic α-hydroxy-γ-phthalimidobutyric acid (DL-Phth-AHBA), which was readily separated into diastereomers with the use of dehydroabietylamine (DAA). The overall yield of L-AHBA from γ-butyrolactone was 22% by route II.

The microbiological resolution of DL-AHBA was studied by Miyaki and Matsumoto of BBRI.[73] A number of microorganisms were examined for their ability to metabolize D-AHBA without consuming the L-isomer. The one found to be suitable for the purpose was a bacterial strain called No. C286-B3, which had been isolated from a soil sample collected at Hachijo-jima Island, Japan, and was subsequently identified as a species of Acetobacter. The culture (deposited as ATCC 21780) was incubated in a defined inorganic medium supplemented with DL-AHBA as a sole carbon source. After 3 days of incubation at 28 °C most of the D-isomer was consumed and L-AHBA was isolated in 40.7% yield by weight, or 81.4% theoretically (route III).

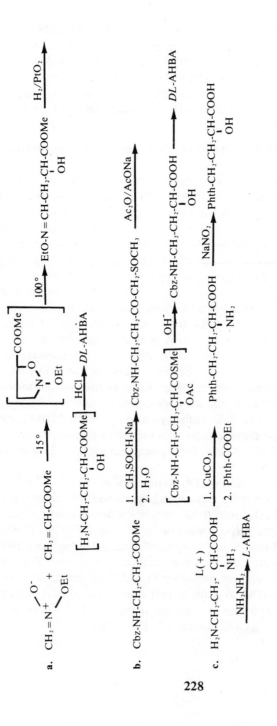

**Figure 12.** Recent syntheses of AHBA (1975-1978).

228

The preparation of L-AHBA via the racemic mixture appeared to be unsatisfactory for large-scale processing because of the lengthy resolution procedure involved, and an alternative stereospecific synthetic route was sought. As shown in route **IV** of Figure 11, commercially available $L(+)$-glutamic acid was converted by the Schmidt reaction to $L$-$\alpha,\gamma$-diaminobutyric acid, the $\alpha$-amino group of which was displaced to give L-AHBA (overall yield) 32% with the retention of the $\alpha$-configuration.[74] Although route **IV** was more economical than the former process, the use of a hazardous reagent (hydrazoic acid) in the Schmidt reaction seemed disadvantageous for industrial scale-up. An alternative new process (route **V**) was then developed.[75] Deamination of L-glutamic acid with nitrous acid afforded $L$-$\gamma$-carboxy-$\gamma$-butyrolactone with full retention of the configuration.[76] Subsequent ammonolysis of the lactone proceeded well with concentrated ammonia at room temperature, giving $L$-$\alpha$-hydroxyglutaric acid $\gamma$-amide. The Hoffmann rearrangement was successfully applied for the conversion of the $\gamma$-amide group to an amine, giving L-AHBA (overall yield 40%). The new three-step synthesis, route **V**, provided a practical route to L-AHBA and was found suitable for large-scale production.

Four additional synthetic methods for DL- or L-AHBA have been reported since 1974 (Figure 12). DL-AHBA was prepared by the 1,3-dipolar addition of a nitronic ester to methyl acrylate followed by catalytic hydrogenation (route **a**),[77] or by the Pummerer reaction of $\beta$-ketosulfoxide with acetic anhydride (route **b**).[78] Route **c**[79] is a modification of route **IV** in which the $\gamma$-amino group of diaminobutyric acid is protected with a phthalimido group. L-Asparagine was used as a starting material in route **d**.[80] Displacement of the $\alpha$-amino group of L-asparagine, acetylation, and subsequent catalytic hydrogenation afforded L-AHBA in an overall yield of 30%.

## 4.2 Progress in the Technology of Selective Acylation

The active ester method, using N-hydroxysuccinimide (OSu), was successfully applied to the early synthesis of amikacin for selective protection of the C-6′ amino function of kanamycin with a Cbz group and also for the selective acylation of the C-1 amino group with L-AHBA. It was found subsequently that the esters of N-hydroxy-5-norbornene-2,3-dicarboximide (ONB) were more suitable than the OSu esters for both the protection and acylation steps in amikacin synthesis.[81] The significantly improved yield obtained in the 6′-N protection step with a Cbz-ONB reagent (56% yield, vs. 45% by the Cbz-OSu process) is probably due to the bulkiness of the acylating agent, which may enhance the differentiation of the steric environment between the 6′-amino group located on a methylene carbon and other amino groups on methine carbons. The beneficial effect of ONB ester was less pronounced for the subsequent 1-N-acylation process compared with the OSu ester method.

Miyano and coworkers of Banyu[82] reported that the 6'-$N$ blocking step was improved by using a Cbz active ester with $p$-hydroxybenzoic acid. This reagent was reported to be more selective than Cbz-ONB and afforded 6'-$N$-Cbz-kanamycin in 70.5% yield (52.5% by the Cbz-ONB process). Another advantage of this reagent was that its property of water solubility enabled the benzyloxycarbonylation process to be conducted in an aqueous solution.

Schreiber and Keil of Bristol-Myers[83] attempted to increase selectivity in the 1-$N$-acylation process by prior formation of Schiff bases of 6'-$N$-Cbz kanamycin at the C-1, C-3, and C-3" amino groups. An improved yield of amikacin was reported with simultaneous decrease in the production of the undesirable isomers, BB-K 11, BB-K 29, and diacyl derivatives.

Since the deblocking of CBz groups involved in the above synthetic routes required catalytic hydrogenation, a photosensitive $o$-nitrobenzyloxycarbonyl (NBOC) group was investigated on a laboratory scale at BBRI as an alternative $N$-blocking group.[84] 6'$N$-NBOC-kanamycin A, prepared from kanamycin A and the OSu or ONB active ester of NBOC, was acylated with the active ester of $\gamma$-$N$-NBOC-protected $L$-AHBA. The two $N$-blocking groups at C-6' and $\omega$-amino groups were finally removed by irradiation with a high-pressure mercury lamp to give amikacin in an optimal yield of 29%.

Millon et al. of Pfizer[85] described the preparation of 6',3"-di-$N$-trifluoroacetylkanamycin A as a useful precursor for amikacin synthesis. Horii et al. at Takeda[86] reported that the 1-$N$-formyl group of per-$N$-formylated kanamycin was preferentially removed by mild alkaline hydrolysis to give 3,6',3"-tri-$N$-formylkanamycin A, which was acylated with $N$-Phth-$L$-AHB-OSu to afford amikacin in a good yield (66% for 1-$N$-acylation step).

Cron et al. of Bristol-Myers[87] reported a unique process for amikacin synthesis. Kanamycin A was refluxed in acetonitrile with hexamethyl disilazane to give a polytrimethylsilylated derivative, which was dissolved in acetone and treated with 10 molar equivalents of water under nitrogen atomosphere. The resulting partially trimethylsilylated kanamycin was acylated with $N$-Cbz-AHB-OSu to afford amikacin in 50% yield. A notable advantage of this process was the lack of formation of the 3"-$N$-acyl isomer BB-K 11, the separation of which requires additional steps in amikacin production.

Nagabhushan et al. of Schering[88] reported that certain pairs of amino and hydroxyl groups in aminoglycoside antibiotics could form complexes with divalent transition metal cations such as $Cu^{2+}$, $Ni^{2+}$ and $Co^{2+}$. As illustrated in Figure 13, kanamycin A formed a complex with $Ni^{2+}$, which chelated with 1-amino/2"-hydroxy and 3"-amino/4"-hydroxy pairs. Benzyloxycarbonylation of the complex afforded 3,6'-di-$N$-Cbz-kanamycin in high yield, which is a useful intermediate for amikacin synthesis. Hanessian and Patil of Montreal

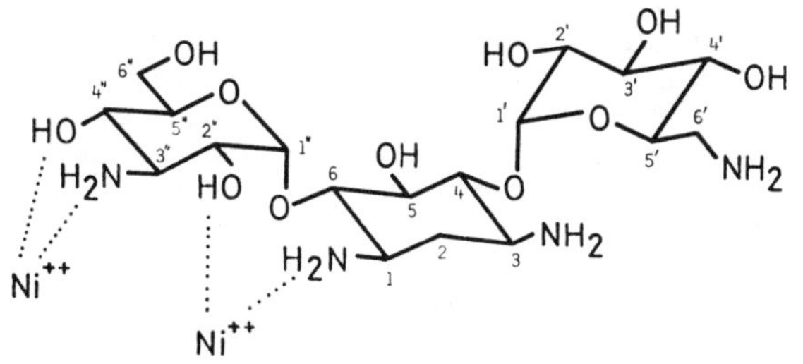

**Figure 13.** Complex formation of kanamycin A with Ni$^{++}$. From Nagabhushan et al.[88]

University[89] described the preparation of 6'-N-Cbz-kanamycin A via the temporary protection of vicinal amino alcohol functions at C-3" and C-4 as the Cu$^{2+}$ chelate. Tsuchiya et al. of Institute of Bioorganic Chemistry[90] reported a similar chelation of kanamycin A with Zn(OAc)$_2$ followed by treatment with Cbz-OSu to give 3,6'-di-N-Cbz-kanamycin A. Subsequent treatment with ethyl trifluoroacetate protected the 3"-amino group regiospecifically to afford 3,6'-diN-Cbz-3"-trifluoroacetyl-kanamycin A, a key intermediate in amikacin preparation.

## REFERENCES

1. H. Umezawa, M. Ueda, K. Maeda, K. Yagishita, S. Kondo, Y. Okami, R. Utahara, Y. Osato, K. Nitta, and T. Takeuchi, *J. Antibiot.,* **10**, 181 (1957).
2. T. Ichikawa, *J. Japan. Med. Assoc.,* **39**, 730 (1958).
3. M. J. Weinstein, G. M. Luedemann, E. M. Oden, G. H. Wagman, J. P. Rosselet, J. A. Marquez, C. T. Coniglio, W. Charney, H. L. Herzog, and J. Black, *J. Med. Chem.,* **6**, 463 (1963).
4. Ç. M. Martin, N. S. Ikari, J. Zimmerman, and J. A. Waitz, *J. Infect. Dis.,* **124**(suppl.), S24 (1971).
5. C. F. T. Snelling, A. R. Ronald, C. Y. Cates, and W. C. Forsythe, *J. Infect. Dis.,* **124**(Suppl.), S264 (1971).
6. S. Okamoto and Y. Suzuki, *Nature,* **108**, 1301 (1965).
7. H. Umezawa, M. Okanishi, S. Kondo, K. Hamana, R. Utahara, K. Maeda, and S. Mitsuhashi, *Science,* **157**, 1559 (1967).
8. H. Umezawa, M. Okanishi, R. Utahara, K. Maeda, and S. Kondo, *J. Antibiot.,* **20**, 136 (1967).
9. M. Brzezinska, R. Benveniste, J. Davies, P. J. L. Daniels, and J. Weinstein, *Biochemistry,* **11**, 761 (1972).
10. H. Umezawa, M. Yagisawa, Y. Matsuhashi, H. Naganawa, H. Yamamoto, S. Kondo, and T. Takeuchi, *J. Antibiot.,* **26**, 612 (1973).

11.  M. Chevereau, P. J. L. Daniels, J. Davies, and F. LeGoffic, *Biochemistry,* **13,** 598 (1974).
12.  H. Kawabe, S. Kondo, H. Umazawa, and S. Mitsuhashi, *Antimicrob. Agents Chemother.,* **7,** 494 (1975).
13.  J. Davies and S. O'Connor, *Antimicrob. Agents Chemother.,* **14,** 69 (1978).
14.  M. Okanishi, S. Kondo, R. Utahara, and H. Umezawa, *J. Antibiot.,* **21,** 13 (1968).
15.  H. Umezawa, O. Doi, M. Ogura, S. Kondo, and N. Tanaka, *J. Antibiot.,* **21,** 154 (1968).
16.  B. Ozanne, R. Benveniste, D. Tipper, and J. Davies, *J. Bacteriol.,* **100,** 1144 (1969).
17.  J. Davies, M. Brzezinska, and R. Benveniste, *Ann. N. Y. Acad. Sci.,* **182,** 226 (1971).
18.  M. Yagisawa, H. Yamamoto, H. Naganawa, S. Kondo, R. Takeuchi, and H. Umezawa, *J. Antibiot.,* **25,** 748 (1972).
19.  M. Brzezinska and J. Davies, *Antimicrob. Agents Chemother.,* **3,** 266 (1973).
20.  H. Umezawa, S. Takasawa, M. Okanishi, and R. Utahara, *J. Antibiot.,* **21,** 81 (1968).
21.  R. Benveniste and J. Davies, *F.E.B.S. Lett.,* **14,** 293 (1971).
22.  M. Yagisawa, H. Naganawa, S. Kondo, M. Hamada, T. Takeuchi, and H. Umezawa, *J. Antibiot.,* **24,** 911 (1971).
23.  P. Santanam and F. H. Kayser, *J. Infect. Dis.,* **134**(Suppl.), S333 (1976).
24.  S. Umezawa, T. Tsuchiya, R. Muto, Y. Nishiyama, and H. Umezawa, *J. Antibiot.,* **24,** 274 (1971).
25.  H. Umezawa, S. Umezawa, T. Tsuchiya, and Y. Okazaki, *J. Antibiot.,* **24,** 485 (1971).
26.  S. Umezawa, H. Umezawa, Y. Okazaki, and T. Tsuchiya, *Bull. Chem. Soc. Jpn.* **45,** 3624 (1972).
27.  P. W. K. Woo, H. W. Dion, G. L. Coffey, S. A. Fusari, and G. Senos, Ger. Offen. 1,914,529 (October 9, 1969); *Chem. Abstr.* **72,** 41742 (1970).
28.  E. Akita, T. Tsuruoka, N. Ezaki, and T. Niida, *J. Antibiot.,* **23,** 173 (1970).
29.  T. Shomura, N. Ezaki, T. Tsuruoka, T. Niwa, E. Akita, and T. Niida, *J. Antibiot.,* **23,** 155 (1970).
30.  H. Kawaguchi, T. Naito, S. Nakagawa, and K. Fujisawa, *J. Antibiot.,* **25,** 695, 709 (1972).
31.  K. E. Price, D. R. Chisholm, M. Misiek, F. Leitner, and Y. H. Tsai, *J. Antibiot.,* **25,** 709 (1972).
32.  J. C. Reiffenstein, S. W. Holmes, G. H. Hottendorf, and M. E. Bierwagen, *J. Antibiot.,* **26,** 94 (1973).
33.  T. Naito, S. Nakagawa, Y. Abe, S. Toda, K. Fujisawa, T. Miyaki, H. Koshiyama, H. Ohkuma, and H. Kawaguchi, *J. Antibiot.,* **26,** 297 (1973).
34.  P. W. K. Woo, H. W. Dion, and Q. R. Bartz, *Tetrahedron Lett.,* 2625 (1971).
35.  S. Toda, S. Nakagawa, T. Naito, and H. Kawaguchi, *Tetrahedron Lett.,* 3913 (1978).
36.  K. E. Price, M. D. DeFuria, and T. A. Pursiano, *J. Infect. Dis.,* **134**(Suppl.), S249 (1976).
37.  G. P. Bodey and D. Stewart, *Antimicrob. Agents Chemother.,* **4,** 186 (1973).
38.  L. S. Young and W. L. Hewitt, *Antimicrob. Agents Chemother.,* **4,** 617 (1973).
39.  S. Mitsuhashi, H. Kawabe, S. Iyobe, T. Tanaka, and M. Inoue, *Jpn. J. Antibiot.,* **27,** 189 (1974).
40.  R. M. Kluge, H. C. Standiford, B. Tatem, V. M. Young, W. H. Greene, S. C. Schimpff, F. M. Calia, and R. B. Hornick, *Antimicrob. Agents Chemother.,* **6,** 442 (1974).
41.  H. Knothe, *J. Infect. Dis.,* **134**(Suppl.), S271 (1976).
42.  J. F. Acar, J. L. Witchitz, F. Goldstein, J. N. Talbot, and F. le Goffic, *J. Infect. Dis.,* **134**(Suppl.), S280 (1976).
43.  R. Benveniste and J. Davies, *Ann. Rev. Biochem.,* **42,** 471 (1973).
44.  S. Mitsuhashi, S. Yamahishi, T. Sawai, and H. Kawabe, in S. Mitsuhashi, Ed., *R Factor: Drug Resistance Plasmid,* Japan Scientific Societies Press, Tokyo, 1977, pp. 195-251.

45.  D. Ikeda, T. Tsuchiya, S. Umezawa, and H. Umezawa, *J. Antibiot.,* **25**, 741 (1972).
46.  H. Kawaguchi, T. Naito, and S. Nakagawa, U.S. Patent 3,781,268 (Dec. 25, 1973).
47.  S. Kondo, K. Iinuma, M. Hamada, K. Maeda, and H. Umezawa, *J. Antibiot.,* **27**, 90 (1974).
48.  S. Kondo, K. Iinuma, H. Yamamoto, K. Maeda, and H. Umezawa, *J. Antibiot.,* **26**, 412 (1973).
49.  I. Watanabe, T. Tsuchiya, S. Umezawa, and H. Umezawa, *J. Antibiot.,* **26**, 310 (1973).
50.  T. Naito, S. Nakagawa, and S. Toda, U.S. Patent 3,808,198 (Apr. 30, 1974).
51.  M. Konishi and H. Tsukiura, U.S. Patent 3,780,018 (Dec. 18, 1973).
52.  P. J. L. Daniels, J. Weinstein, and T. L. Nagabhushan, *J. Antibiot.,* **27**, 889 (1974).
53.  T. Naito and S. Nakagawa, U.S. Patent 3,872,079 (Mar. 18, 1975).
54.  T. Naito, S. Nakagawa, and Y. Abe, U.S. Patent 3,796,699 (Mar. 12, 1974).
55.  T. Naito, S. Nakagawa, and Y. Abe, U.S. Patent 3,796,698 (Mar. 12, 1974).
56.  T. Naito, S. Nakagawa, and M. Oka, U.S. Patent 3,860,574 (Jan. 14, 1975).
57.  T. Naito and S. Nakagawa, U.S. Patent 3,897,412 (July 29, 1975).
58.  T. Naito, S. Nakagawa, and S. Toda, U.S. Patent 3,896,106 (July 22, 1975).
59.  K. Shirahata, S. Tomioka, T. Nara, H. Matsushima, and I. Matsubara, *Jpn. Kokai,* 50-88,050 (July 15, 1975).
60.  J. J. Wright, A. B. Cooper, P. J. L. Daniels, T. L. Nagabhushan, D. Rane, W. N. Turner, and J. Weinstein, *J. Antibiot.,* **29**, 714 (1976).
61.  T. L. Nagabhushan, A. B. Copper, H. Tsai, and P. J. L. Daniels, 17th Intersci. Conf. Antimicr. Agents & Chemother., New York, Oct. 12-14, 1977, Abstr. No. 249.
62.  P. K. W. Yu and J. A. Washington II, *Antimicrob. Agents Chemother.,* **13**, 891 (1978).
63.  L. I. Rankin, F. C. Luft, M. N. Yum, R. S. Sloan, C. B. Dinwiddie, Jr., and L. L. Isaacs, *Antimicrob. Agents Chemother.,* **16**, 491 (1979).
64.  T. Naito, S. Nakagawa, Y. Narita, S. Toda, Y. Abe, M. Oka, H. Yamashita, T. Yamasaki, K. Fujisawa, and H. Kawaguchi, *J. Antibiot.,* **27**, 851 (1974).
65.  J. J. Wright, *J. Chem. Soc., Chem. Comm.,* 206 (1976).
66.  S. Nakagawa, S. Toda, Y. Abe, H. Yamashita, K. Fujisawa, T. Naito, and H. Kawaguchi, *J. Antibiot.,* **31**, 675 (1978).
67.  K. Richardson, S. Jevons, J. W. Moore, B. C. Ross, and J. R. Wright, *J. Antibiot.,* **30**, 843 (1977).
68.  R. J. Andrews, K. W. Brammer, H. E. Cheeseman, and S. Jevons, *Antimicrob. Agents Chemother.,* **14**, 846 (1978).
69.  A. J. Carter, *Antimicrob. Agents Chemother.,* **16**, 362 (1979).
70.  E. Fischer and A. Goddertz, Ber., **43**, 3272 (1910).
71.  K. Tanabe, R. Takasaki, and T. Hashimoto, Jpn. Patent 37-17,962 (1962).
72.  Y. Saito, M. Hashimoto, H. Seki, and T. Kamiya, *Tetrahedron Lett.,* **1970**, 4863 (1970).
73.  T. Miyaki and K. Matsumoto, U.S. Patent 3,923,069 (July 9, 1974).
74.  T. Naito and S. Nakagawa, *Jpan. Kokai* 49-24,914 (Mar. 5, 1974).
75.  T. Naito and S. Nakagawa, U.S. Patent 3,923,187 (July 9, 1974).
76.  K. Koga, M. Taniguchi, and S. Yamada, *Tetrahedron Lett., 263 (1971).*
77.  *H. Sato, T. Kusumi, K. Imaye, and H. Kakisawa, Chem. Lett.,* **1975** 965; *Bull. Chem. Soc. Jpn.,* **49**, 2815 (1976).
78.  S. Iriuchijima, K. Maniwa, and G. Tsuchihashi, *J. Am. Chem. Soc.,* **97**, 596 (1975).
79.  Y. Horiuchi, E. Akita, and T. Ito, *Agr. Biol. Chem.,* **40**, 1649 (1976).
80.  T. Yoneta, S. Shibahara, S. Fukatsu, and S. Seki, *Bull. Chem. Soc. Jpn.,* **51**, 3296 (1978).
81.  T. Naito, S. Nakagawa, and M. Oka, *Jpn. Kokai* 50-77,345 (June 24, 1975).
82.  T. Miyano, S. Tomisaka, F. Sasaki, and I. Matsumoto, *Jpn. Kokai* 51-54,536 (May 13, 1976).

83.  R. H. Schreiber and J. G. Keil, *Jpn. Kokai* 49-102,644 (Sept. 27, 1974).
84.  T. Naito, S. Nakagawa, and M. Oka, unpublished data (1973).
85.  W. A. Millon, R. M. Plews and K. Richardson, U.S. Patent 4,160,082 (July 3, 1979).
86.  S. Horii, H. Fukase, Y. Kameda and N. Mizokami, *Carbohyd. Res.,* **60**, 275 (1978).
87.  M. J. Cron, J. G. Keil, J-S. Lin, M. V. Ruggeri, and D. Walker, *J. Chem. Soc., Chem. Comm.,* **266** (1979).
88.  T. L. Nagabhushan, A. B. Cooper, W. N. Turner, H. Tsai, S. McCombie, A. K. Mallams, D. Rane, J. J. Wright, P. Reichert, D. L. Boxler, and J. Weinstein, *J. Am. Chem. Soc.,* **100**, 5253 (1978).
89.  S. Hanessian and G. Patil, *Tetrahedron Lett.,* 1035 (1978).
90.  T. Tsuchiya, Y. Takagi, and S. Umezawa, *Tetrahedron Lett.,* 4951 (1979).

# The Azole Story

# 11

## K. H. Büchel and M. Plempel

### 1. INTRODUCTION

Clotrimazole was the first step in the development of a large class of anti-mycotic and fungicidal agents generally known as the azoles. The discovery of this drug can be attributed to the combined efforts of a chemist who was following a structure-activity concept over the course of several years and a newly formed mycological testing laboratory whose optimal capability was just being realized. Certain lucky events that could be called fortune played a decisive part.

We reconstruct here the clotrimazole story as it developed, from the viewpoints of both the chemist and the microbiologist in charge of testing. The microbiological aspect predominates, but it should be borne in mind that each microbiological test result, particularly if it was problematic, was discussed with the chemist and reconsidered in the light of his structure-activity concept. This then led to a reappraisal of the test data and to new test designs.

### 2. THE CHEMICAL CONCEPT

Our work on azole antimycotics and fungicides originated from the hypothesis that compounds which are capable of forming reactive carbenium ions *in vivo* possess biological activity.[1] It is assumed that such active intermediates will intervene in nucleic acid synthesis or in the regulating actions of messenger RNA; the carbenium ion, for example, could suffer nucleophilic attack.

This hypothesis is supported by literature reports of the various biological effects of certain compounds. Examples are triphenylmethane derivatives of primary[2] and secondary[3] amines of the Frescon type (see formulas **1** and **2**, Figure 1), which are active against various species of aquatic snails (such as

---

*This chapter is dedicated to Prof. Dr. Herbert Grunewald on the occasion of his 60th birthday.

235

Structures:

$(C_6H_5)_3C-N-CH_2-CH(CH_3)_2$ with H on nitrogen and $CH_3$ groups

**1** I.C.I. experimental molluscicide

$(C_6H_5)_3C-N$ (morpholine ring with O)

**2** Frescon (Shell)

**3** (cycloheptatriene)—OR

**4** (cycloheptatriene)—$N\langle{R \atop R}$

**5** X = $BrI_2^-$, $BrCl_2^-$ $ICl_4^-$, $I_7^-$ (tropylium cation) $X^-$

*Australorbis glabratus*) but which lack fungicidal and antimycotic properties. A series of triphenylmethane dyes has been reported to possess parasitological activity.[4]

Our own initial experiments with cycloheptatriene and tropylium derivatives (**3-5**) were based on the same concept.[1,5] These compounds are indeed somewhat active as fungicides, plant-growth inhibitors, and molluscicides. The naturally occurring tropolone derivatives $\alpha,\beta,\gamma$-thujaplicin, from the heartwood of *Thuja plicata*,[6] and the alkaloid colchicine are physiologically active compounds that also belong in this category. In view of the biological activity of potential carbenium ions, we surmised that trityl-imidazoles might have interesting properties.

According to H. A. Staab, the activity of the acyl carbon atom in acyl derivatives of imidazoles (**6**) is enhanced by involvement of the amide nitrogen electron pair in the $\pi$-system of the imidazole ring.[7] We expected much the same to be true of 1-trityl-imidazoles (**7**). Therefore, bearing in mind the biological activity of potential carbenium ions, we synthesized a series of substituted 1-trityl-imidazoles, triazoles and other $\pi$-excessive azoles. The very first examples showed strong activity *in vitro* and *in vivo* against pathogenic fungi and yeasts.[8-11]

The trityl-imidazoles, and even more so the 1,2,4-triazoles, were also found to be highly effective against phytopathogenic fungi, notably the powdery mildews (*Erysiphe*).[12-14] Following this lead, we undertook a series of systematic structure/activity-oriented syntheses in close and fruitful cooperation with medical and biological testing specialists. In the course of this work and in the light of the test results obtained, it was soon discovered that the biological activity of the trityl-imidazoles is not linked to the formation of a free tritylium ion inasmuch as substitutions in the imidazole ring, for example

O=C–CH₃

H₅C₆–C–C₆H₅
C₆H₅

6             7

with a single methyl group, rendered the compounds completely inactive but did not greatly affect carbenium ion formation.[15] Among other azoles, 1,2,4-triazoles were effective whereas pyrazoles and benzimidazoles were not. It thus became necessary to revise the working hypothesis by postulating a decisive role for the potential carbenium moiety with the imidazole as the leaving group. It is now believed that the trityl-azole molecule as a whole needs to be bound to the site of action and that a reaction then occurs in this close proximity, which may in fact involve carbenium ion formation.

### 3. THE BASIS OF MYCOLOGICAL TESTING

In 1963 a special mycological medical laboratory was set up at Bayer's pharmaceutical research center. This step was taken in view of the situation then existing with regard to the therapy of human mycotic infections: Parenteral mycoses could be treated only with the relatively toxic compound amphotericin B. Two chemically related antibiotics, nystatin and pimaricin, could be used with limited success for the topical treatment of yeast infections of mucous membranes. Griseofulvin, the orally effective but not completely satisfactory agent for the treatment of dermatophytosis and onchomycoses, and tolnaftate, the topically applied agent effective only against dermatophytosis, constituted the only other drugs in this field.[16] In addition, there were a number of topical antimycotics that were essentially disinfectants, and they were unsatisfactory in terms of therapeutic reliability and efficacy.[17]

Antimycotic research was given three assignments:

1. To find a topical antimycotic possessing broad activity against pathogenic fungi. A broad antimycotic spectrum is important because diagnostic problems hindered the timely and appropriate use of narrow-spectrum drugs.

2. To search for an oral or parenteral antimycotic agent whose spectrum would encompass the opportunistic mycoses of internal organs of worldwide occurrence, such as candiosis and aspergillosis, as well as the endemic primary mycoses such as histoplasmosis, coccidioidomycosis, and paracoccidioidomycosis.

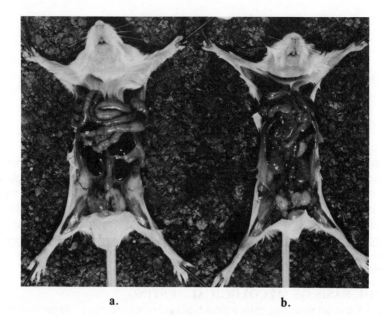

a.                    b.

**Figure 1.**   Renal candidosis in mice after i.v. infection with *Candida albicanas:* **(a)** uninfected control animal, **(b)** infected animal.

3.   To search for a "better griseofulvin", that is, for an oral dermatological agent that would be effective against dermatophyte and *Candida* infections of the skin and mucous membranes.

Until mid-1966, our mycological laboratory was engaged in the development and standardization of screening techniques and tests, the few known active antimycotics serving as positive controls.

*In vitro,* the following test models were available to us:[18]

1. Serial dilution and agar diffusion tests.
2. Respiration tests according to Warburg.
3. Intermittent and continuous nephelometry.
4. Tests of fungicidal action.

*In vivo,* the following test models were available to us:

1. Mouse candidosis after i.v. infection. The disease picture developing in these mice after i.v. infection with *Candida albicans* consists of a brief period of sepsis followed by renal candidosis with multiple candidal abscesses, mostly in the renal cortex (Figure 1). In this model infection, 90-95% of the animals die between the 3rd and 6th days post infection (p.i.).

For a more precise evaluation of the chemotherapeutic activity of test compounds, this experiment was supplemented by cell counts performed on the renal homogenates of infected animals at different infection times. The number of *Candida* organisms found, after plating-out and incubation, in aliquots of the renal homogenates from the treated as compared with the untreated animals served as a measure of the tissue diffusion and therapeutic efficacy of the test compounds.[19-22]

2. Guinea pig trichophytosis. Guinea pigs are highly susceptible to dermatophyte infections. We infect the animals by lightly rubbing a fully germinated microconidium suspension of the dermatophytes onto the shaved dorsal skin. The developing dermatophytosis reaches a maximum 14-16 days after infection and then heals spontaneously at a slow rate. Depending on whether *Trichophyton mentagrophytes* or *T. quinckeanum* is the infecting organism, varying disease pictures are seen (Figures 2 and 3).

The test model of guinea pig dermatophytosis is nearly 100% reproducible and is characterized by a high interindividual consistency in the course of infection.[11,23] We evaluate and rate the course of infection by assigning grades 0 to 5: grade 0 stands for no signs of infection, grades 1 to 4 identify intermediate stages, and grade 5 designates the extreme phase of the infection. The model is adapted to the testing of topical as well as oral antimycotics.

Possible relapses after initially successful treatment are easily detectable if the animals are followed for a period of 4 weeks after the conclusion of the treatment. The frequency of such relapses is taken as a measure of the fungistatic or fungicidal efficacy of an active ingredient.

3. Mouse cryptococcosis. This is one of our most interesting test models. Depending on the capsule size of the *Cryptococcus neoformans* strain employed, i.v. infection of the mice leads to:
   (a)   Septic cryptococcosis, which proves fatal within 4-6 days p.i.
   (b)   Pulmonary cryptococcosis, with protracted mortality between the 4th and 12th days p.i.
   (c)   Hepatic cryptococcosis, of which only about 50% of the animals die within 14 days p.i.
   (d)   Fulminating meningoencephalic cryptococcosis, with 100% mortality within 3-4 days p.i.

When properly used, this model of infection with its variable infection sites provides important information about tissue distribution and cerebrospinal fluid (CSF) passage of an orally or parenterally administered active ingredient.[20]

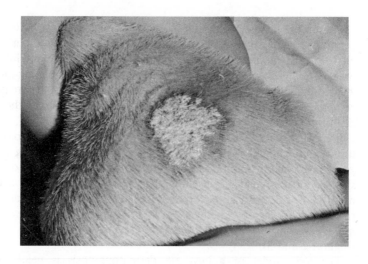

**Figure 2.** Guinea pig, infected with *Trichophyton mentagrophytes.*

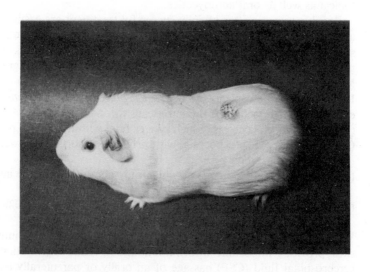

**Figure 3.** Guinea pig, infected with *Trichophyton quinckeanum.*

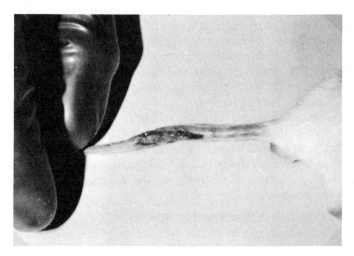

**Figure 4.** Experimental mouse-tail sporotrichosis, 16th day postinfection.

**4.**   Mouse aspergillosis. This test model using the organism *Aspergillus fumigatus* is poorly reproducible. An i.v. infection with the conidia (asexually reproducing spores) of the fungus results, after a brief phase of fungemia, in a necrotizing pyelonephritis which, with the use of more than $5 \times 10^5$ spores, leads to the death of 75-85% of the animals 8 to 15 days p.i. The infective pattern of mouse aspergillosis is so far removed from that of human aspergillosis, which is nearly always pulmonary, that it can serve only as a rough model for the general *in vivo* efficacy of a potential antimycotic against *Aspergillus fumigatus*.[24,25]

Intratracheal mouse infections with *Aspergillus fumigatus*, after producing a very short initial effect, run an aberrant course, healing spontaneously within 2 days postinfection.[24]

The above-described mouse test models refer to infections with opportunistic fungi. To round out our test program, we needed a model involving a primarily biphasic pathogenic fungus.

*Histoplasma capsulatum* and *Coccidioides immitis* as well as *Paracoccidioides brasiliensis* are so highly pathogenic that routine laboratory handling of these organisms is very hazardous to laboratory personnel unless costly special equipment is at hand. We therefore decided to use sporotrichosis as a model. Mouse-tail sporotrichosis is readily reproducible and its course and response to therapy can be evaluated very easily.

An infectious wheal is produced by means of a careful intracutaneous injection of a suspension of the mycelial form of *Sporothrix schenkii* into the upper third of the mouse tail. Within 6 to 8 days the wheal develops into an ulceration with deep necroses, which finally leads to mutilation of the tail by loss of its proximal part. The infection progresses distally. It can be observed for about 3 weeks (Figure 4), after which the animals are so gravely ill that it would be inhumane to prolong the test further.

This was our test program up to the middle of 1966. Today, in contrast to that time, most of these tests and model infections belong to the tools that any good mycological medical laboratory has at its disposal.

We no longer have any doubt that the uncommon breadth of our test repertory, for 1966, contributed decisively to the discovery of the first active imidazole compounds.

## 4.   TEST RESULTS AND CONSEQUENCES

In our random screening procedures, we first tested compounds *in vitro* for effectiveness against dermatophytes, *Candida* species, and *Aspergillus* and *Penicillium* species, and we usually employed serial dilution and agar diffusion techniques. Substances that proved effective *in vitro* at dilutions that seemed therapeutically attainable (e.g., <10 μg/ml substrate) were tested further on animal models appropriate to their *in vitro* activity. We were convinced that this sequence:

$$\textit{in vitro} \text{ test} \longrightarrow \text{activity} \longrightarrow \textit{in vivo} \text{ test}$$

was the correct one.

In that year, 1966, we received a sample of 5-fluorocytosine, a substance then being tested as an antimycotic at Hoffman-La Roche in Basel for internal testing. In the initial *in vitro* tests on our customary complex culture media, the compound showed no effect whatever at concentrations up to 200 μg/ml. Nevertheless, contrary to our usual procedure we ran the mouse aspergillosis and mouse candidosis tests with the product, using oral doses of 12.5, 25, and 50 mg/kg body weight, without placing great hopes on the outcome. The result was that at the oral dose of 12.5 mg/kg (and, as we saw later, at doses down to 1 mg/kg), 5-fluorocytosine had a curative effect in mouse candidosis, and doses between 25 and 50 mg/kg effected a cure in mouse aspergillosis. This striking discrepancy between an absence of activity *in vitro* and curative efficacy *in vivo* at very low doses prompted us to conduct blood level studies in mice after oral doses of 5-fluorocytosine. The blood concentrations determined by chemical methods were far below 200 μg/ml, the active threshold in our *in vitro* tests, and so could not explain the good effects obtained *in vivo*.

This was a severe blow for our assumption of a correlation between *in vitro* and therapeutic effects and, consequently, for our testing policy. We revised our procedure so as to test compounds concurrently *in vitro* and *in vivo*. Not until several months after this change in procedure, which required a great deal more work but which was also more satisfying and reassuring, did we learn that 5-fluorocytosine only has competitive, antagonist-dependent activity *in vitro*. We learned that the drug can be effective against *Candida* and *Aspergillus* on culture media free of antagonists, even in our *in vitro* tests, at concentrations of less than 1 $\mu$g/ml.

We nonetheless continued our concurrent *in vitro* and *in vivo* testing and added to our *in vitro* test program a partly synthetic culture medium besides the complex Sabouraud medium. We also tried to develop routinely usable microbiological methods for determining serum and urine levels of systemically administered investigational compounds.

## 5.   SYNTHESIS AND TESTING OF TRITYL-IMIDAZOLES AND THE DISCOVERY OF CLOTRIMAZOLE

### 5.1   The Timetable of the First Year

Unsubstituted triphenylmethyl-imidazole, synthesized by Büchel in December 1966, was sent to the mycological laboratory. Test results became available at the beginning of February 1967: Triphenylmethyl-imidazole was active. The compound exhibited moderate to weak activity *in vitro* against dermatophytes, yeasts, and *Aspergillus,* showing minimum inhibitory concentration (MIC) values between 8 and 32 $\mu$g/ml. *In vivo,* however, the compound was effective when 1% suspensions were applied topically in guinea pig trichophytosis due to *Trichophyton mentagrophytes*. It was particularly exciting to find that after repeated oral administration of 100 mg/kg the substance had a partially curative effect in the mouse candidosis model. We repeated the tests and confirmed the results and determined the serum level 2,4, and 8 hours after single oral doses of 100 mg/kg. It showed a peak value of 6 $\mu$g/ml and thus fell slightly short of the compound's *in vitro* MIC for *Candida albicans,* though within a range allowing a causal explanation. Chemists and microbiologists met to discuss these data.

The following laboratory log entries illustrate the enthusiasm, cooperation, and productiveness of these discussions:

| | |
|---|---|
| August 1966 | Synthesis of first triphenylmethyl-imidazole. |
| February 1967 | Test results available. |
| February 1967 to August 1967 | Synthesis and testing of additional imidazoles. |
| September 1967 | Application for Patent: German Patent 1,617,481 (15 Sept. 1967). |

The patent application already identified clotrimazole by name and described its effects.

## 5.2   Comments on the Synthesis of Trityl-Azoles and of Clotrimazole

In principle, the trityl-imidazole system can be varied in many ways. However, after modifications to the amine or azole component, we found that on the whole only trityl derivatives of the unsubstituted imidazole, of 1,2,4-triazole, and to a limited extent of 1,2,3-triazole have high efficacy against fungi pathogenic to humans, animals, or plants. Less effective are trityl derivatives of substituted imidazoles, benzimidazoles, other heterocyclic compounds, homologous open chain amidines, hydrazones, and anilines.[26,27] Substitution on the triphenylmethyl group can, however, be varied with retention of activity. New types of syntheses, particularly for derivatives of 1-trityl-imidazole, had to be developed, since known synthetic methods tended to give only moderate yields.

**5.2.1   The Preparation of Precursors.**   Conventional Grignard synthesis can be used for the preparation of triphenylmethylchlorides as starting materials. In these, phenylmagnesiumbromide is reacted with benzophenone and the carbinol formed after hydrolysis is chlorinated with $SOCl_2$ or HCl. The starting components can carry one or more substituents in any position. For the

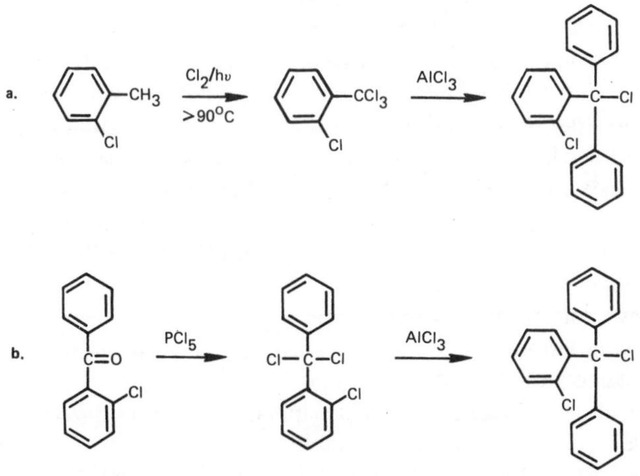

**Figure 5.**   Reaction sequences for the preparation of o-chlorotriphenylmethyl-chloride, the precursor of clotrimazole.

tritylchlorides monosubstituted by halogen in one phenyl ring, we found a very elegant route in the Friedel-Crafts reaction of the benzotrichlorides with 2 mol of benzene. Figure 5 shows the reaction sequence for the preparation of o-chlorotriphenylmethylchloride, the precursor of clotrimazole.

**5.2.2 The Tritylation of Imidazole.** We developed a number of pathways for the synthesis of the trityl-azolides, the particular value of which depends on the substitution pattern of the reaction components. Tritylchlorides react with imidazole in polar organic solvents in the presence of equimolar amounts of a tertiary amine or of an excess imidazole to give the azolides.[28]

In the case of R = ortho-Cl, clotrimazole is obtained. Products are generally very pure. The yields are highly dependent on the type of solvent used. For example, only small yields of the azolide are formed in benzene, whereas particularly good yields are obtained in solvents with high dielectric constants.

There are several other attractive routes to convert the tritylcarbinols into the azolides, as summarized in Figure 6.[8,29-31]

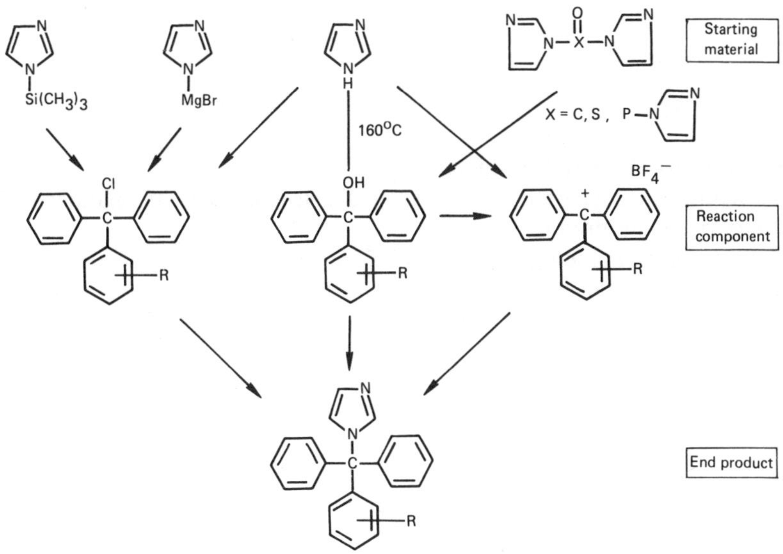

**Figure 6.** Conversion of tritylcarbinols into the azolides.

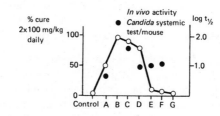

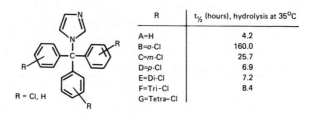

| R | $t_{1/2}$ (hours), hydrolysis at 35°C |
|---|---|
| A=H | 4.2 |
| B=o-Cl | 160.0 |
| C=m-Cl | 25.7 |
| D=p-Cl | 6.9 |
| E=Di-Cl | 7.2 |
| F=Tri–Cl | 8.4 |
| G=Tetra–Cl | |

**Figure 7.** Biological data taken from a *Candida* systemic test with mice.

### 5.3 Structure-Activity Considerations

Several attempts have been made to elucidate structure-activity relations in the series of azole antimycotics and fungicides.

A study with a homologous series of chlorine-substituted trityl-imidazoles arrived at some conclusions that suggested further synthesis.[32]

Biological data were taken from the *Candida* systemic test with mice, and the data were expressed as percentage cured. The lipophilicity increases with the chlorine content of trityl-azoles and the activity reaches a maximum at ortho-monochlorination, so that, with respect to activity, there is an optimum for lipophilicity (see Figure 7). The rate constants and half-lives of the proton-catalyzed hydrolysis have their highest values in the case of o-chloro substitution (clotrimazole), coinciding with the highest activities.

The following parameters contribute *inter alia* to the structure-activity relation:
1.  The hydrolysis rate of the C-N bond, corresponding to the extent of formation of the carbenium ion.

2. The lipophilicity of the molecule, corresponding to transport.
3. The steric structure of the whole molecule, resulting from certain sub-stituents responsible for the fit on the site of action.

Except within narrow ranges of molecular variation, none of the individual parameters can be correlated directly with the biological effects.

In another study, 34 compounds were selected from the viewpoint of maximum possible variation in chemical structure, including 80% of the trityl-imidazoles with high *in vivo* activity.[33] For the compounds selected, the following physicochemical parameters were determined:

1. The rate constants of acid hydrolysis at 35° and 50 °C.
2. The $R_f$ values in a reversed-phase thin-layer chromatography system.

The result of this comparison can be described as follows:

1. No clear-cut effect of the hydrolysis rate on the activity can be seen; at most, there is a small excess number of compounds with local activity against *Trichophyton* among the rapidly hydrolyzed compounds. The hypothesis that the activity depends on the formation of carbenium ions is not supported because the proportion of active compounds among the compounds that are particularly stable towards hydrolysis ($K_{35} = 0.0018$-$0.026$, or half-lives between 27 and 390 hours) corresponds to the average.
2. There is also no marked effect of the lipophilicity on the activity. However, the compounds with systemic or oral activity, such as clotrimazole, are found primarily in the groups with slight to moderate lipophilic properties.
3. A marked excess number of compounds active in all three tests is found in the group of ortho-substituted compounds, which also includes clotrimazole. Despite the small numbers involved, this finding is probably not of random origin.

The special role of the ortho substituents was also seen in the discussion of hydrolysis rate and lipophilicity parameters. Although there is no direct connection between these effects and the significance of ortho substitution for activity, the common cause for these should probably be sought in the fact that an ortho substituent affects the conformation of the total molecule to a considerable extent through its spatial arrangement. The propeller-form arrangement of the rings in triphenylmethyl compounds, which is normally present, is exaggerated in *o*-substituted 1-trityl-imidazoles. The resulting conformation possibly favors the binding of the molecule at the site of action.

The results of these studies should not mean that quantitative structure-activity correlation methods are of little value. Both the Hansch and the Free-Wilson method require biological data of some precision. Our biological data

| Rank Sum | $R_{1,2,3}$ |
|----------|-------------|
| 29 | 2–Cl |
| 54 | 2–CH$_3$ |
| 56 | 3–Cl |
| 59 | 2–F |
| 59 | 3–F |
| 65 | 2,5–(CH$_3$)$_2$ |
| 67 | 2–C$_2$H$_5$ |
| ⋮ | ⋮ |
| 94 | H |
| ⋮ | ⋮ |
| 188 | 4–N(CH$_3$)$_2$ |

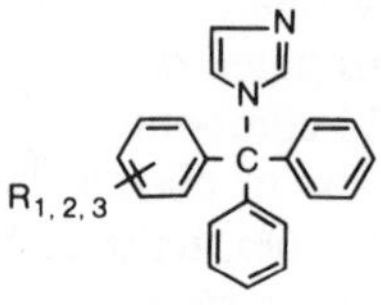

Conclusions:

1. Ortho-substitution favours activity.
2. Clotrimazole ($R_1$ = 2–Cl) has the best rank sum.

**Figure 8.**  Rank sums obtained by summation of the rank numbers from four biological tests and hydrolysis rates. Conclusions: (1) Ortho-substitution favors activity. (2) Clotrimazole ($R_1$ = 2—Cl) has the best rank sum.

| Rank Sum | $R_1$ |
|----------|-------|
| 35 | 4–Cl |
| 35.5 | 2–C$_6$H$_5$ |
| 40 | H |
| 47 | 4–Br |
| 48 | 4–F |
| ⋮ | |
| 124 | 4–SO$_2$C$_6$H$_5$ |
| 127 | 4–CH$_2$C$_6$H$_5$ |
| 128.5 | 4–NH$_2$ |
| 139 | 4–COC$_6$H$_5$ |

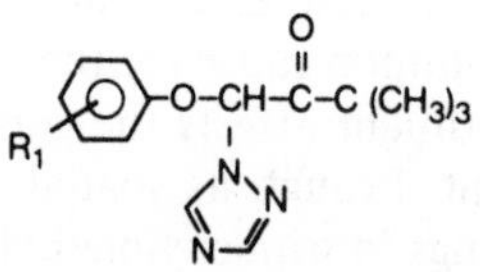

**Figure 9.**  Phenoxy-triazolyl-methanes, rank sums.

lack some properties that are required for fruitful application of regression analysis; many *in vitro* data were not available as minimum inhibitory concentrations (MIC's) but rather as upper limits of the true MIC. In a strict sense the application of a statistical method such as regression analysis is only permissible when the distribution over the whole data range resembles a Gaussian curve. This does not apply to our data. For such data, nonparametric methods like discriminant analysis or rank correlation have been suggested.[34] In a set of 34 selected trityl-imidazoles we calculated Spearman's rank correlation coefficients, $r_s$, for all our ranked variables.[27]

Figure 8 shows some of the results obtained by summing the rank numbers of each compound and then ranking the compounds again, according to their rank sums. The rank table reveals an interesting result. Among the most active compounds at the top of the table, those with an ortho-substituent accumulate. Furthermore, clotrimazole is the compound with the highest rank (= lowest rank sum). Retrospectively, this confirms the choice to develop this compound.

As already mentioned, we found high activities against powdery mildew in the series of trityl-azoles, particularly among triazole derivatives. An example is the mildew fungicide Persulon. Variations of the substituents in the trityl moiety, for example, replacement of the phenyl residues by alkyl and keto groups, led to the very interesting systemic agricultural fungicides such as Bayleton, Baytan, and Baycor, the so-called triazolyl-*O,N*-acetals.

Structure-activity correlations were also studied in this group.[35] Again, at first a rank correlation was checked with 26 compounds, and as biological data, values for 50% inhibition against *Erysiphe cichoracearum* in a greenhouse test were incorporated.

Activity as a function of substitution may also be deduced from Spearman's rank numbers. Addition of the rank numbers from all fungi tested shows the excellent activity of triadimefon (Bayleton) from its rank sum. The breadth of activity against these fungi decreases in the series from 4-chloro over 2-phenyl, hydrogen, 4-bromo, 4-fluoro, down to 4-amino and 4-carbonyl-phenyl (see Figure 9).

In search of a quantitative correlation, $R_f$ values obtained on Merck paraffin-coated silica gel plates $Pf_{254}$ with the solvent dioxan/acetone/water 1:1:2 were included in the QSAR as an experimental physicochemical parameter. The parameters $\pi$, $\pi$-, and $F$, $R$, and $MR$ were taken from Norrington's review.[36] The steric parameters $L$, $B_1$, $B_2$, $B_3$, $B_4$ were obtained from publications of Verloop and coworkers.[37] The steric Taft parameter $E_S$ from Craig's paper[38] was taken. Whereas no correlation was obtainable between Taft's steric parameter $E_S$ and the Hammet $\delta$ constant or the electronic parameters $F$ and $R$ from Swain and Lupton,[39] a good correlation of biological

(1) $\log pI_{50} = 5.38 + 0.55\ \pi\ -0.35\ B_4$
$\qquad\qquad\quad (0.09)\quad\ (0.05)$

$n = 24 \quad r = 0.868 \quad s = 0.373 \quad F = 31.9$

(2) $\log pI_{50} = 5.46 + 1.80\ R_M - 0.35\ B_4$
$\qquad\qquad\qquad (0.32)\qquad (0.05)$

$n = 26 \quad r = 0.847 \quad s = 0.389 \quad F = 28.0$

**Figure 10.**  Inhibition of *Erysiphe cichoracearum* by phenoxy-triazolyl-methanes; quantitative structure-activity relationships.

activity was found with the lipophilicity data $\pi$, $R_M$, and Verloop's steric parameter $B_4$ (Figure 10. From this correlation it may be deduced that a highest possible lipophilicity of the substituents in the phenyl ring coupled with a lowest possible steric factor for these substituents is decisive for activity in the triazolyl-*O,N*-acetals series.

## 6.  THE DEVELOPMENT OF THE AZOLE ACTIVITY PRINCIPLE

One result from correlation studies is that the variation of the stability of the C-N bond is an important consideration with regard to the synthesis of further compounds. In the trityl system a phenyl ring may be replaced by any 5- or 6-membered heterocycle or by two open-chain aliphatic groups.[40,41] The resulting group of N-substituted imidazoles include many highly effective antimycotics and plant fungicides (Figure 11). The mixed alkane-alkyne JAE 0472 has optimal activity in the plant protection sector against *Helminthosporium* diseases of barley. BAY d 9603 is of interest as a technical microbicide in view of its optimal activity against *Trichophyton* and mold species. An important variation consists of the replacement of phenyl by a ketone, carboxylic ester, nitrile, or carboxylic amide.[42]

In the course of further studies, we found that the ether-ketones[43] represented an especially active and versatile azolide system. Here the trityl phenyl groups are completely replaced by other substituents. Several synthesis routes are possible. In the example shown in the formula-scheme for Bayleton (Figure 12), the ether-ketone can be rehalogenated and reacted with triazole to give the systemic fungicides of the triadimefon type. This series represents the first highly systemic fungicides to be found in the azole group[44] (see also Section 11.2).

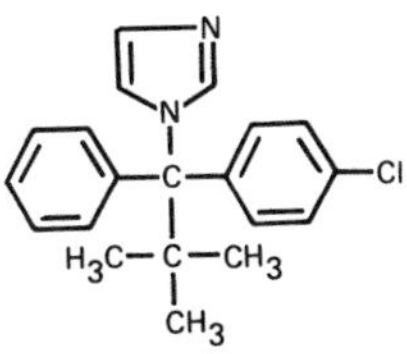

BAY c 7720

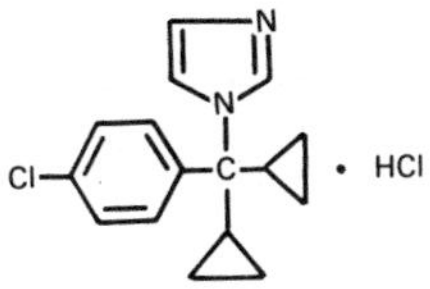

BAY d 6995

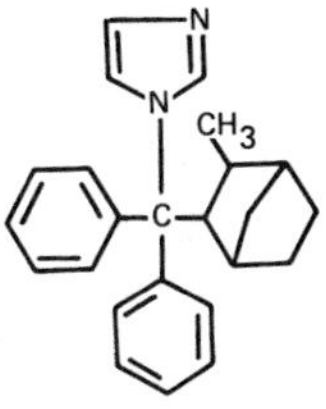

BAY d 6890

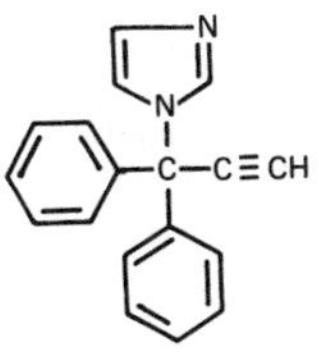

BAY d 9603

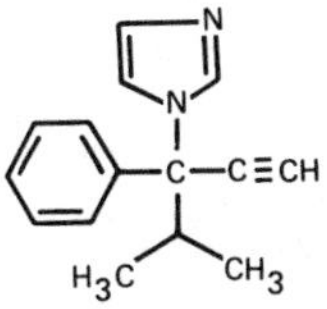

JAE 0472

Figure 11. N-substituted imidazoles.

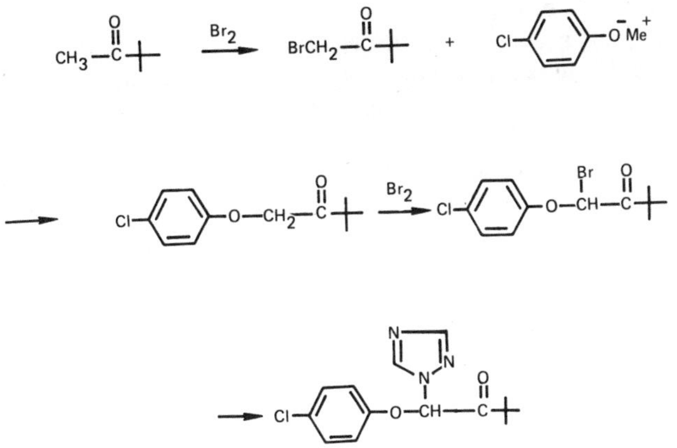

MEB 6447
Triadimefon
Bayleton

Figure 12. Synthesis of Bayleton.

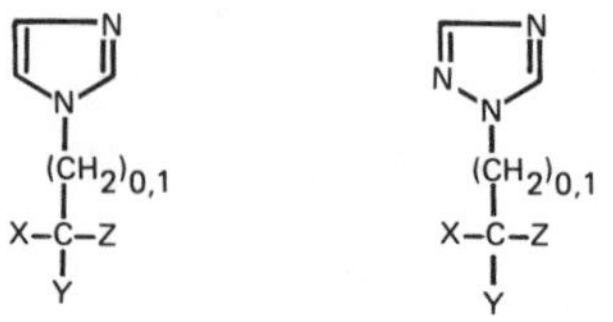

$(CH_2)_{0,1}$

$X–C–Z$

$Y$

$(CH_2)_{0,1}$

$X–C–Z$

$Y$

$$N = 4\ \frac{n}{3} + \frac{n^2}{2} + \frac{n^3}{6}$$

$N$ = Number of possible active compounds in the azole group [for imidazoles and 1,2,4-triazoles and $(CH_2)_{0,1}$].
$n$ = Number of different substituents $X$, $Y$, and $Z$.
Examples:

| $n$ | 10 | 50 | 100 | 200 |
|---|---|---|---|---|
| $N$ | 880 | 88,400 | 688,800 | 5,413,600 |

**Figure 13.**   Variability of the azole system.

The example of the ether-ketones demonstrates the extreme variability of the azole system to give biologically active compounds (Figure 13). The number of possible variations according to the calculation in Figure 13 is extremely large. Where $n = 200$, for example, which is not exaggerated given the variability of $X$, $Y$, $Z$, and $CH_2 = 0$ or 1, the $N$ represents more than 5.4 million possible active structures in which imidazole or triazole form the amine part. We call this generalized structure the Azole Activity Principle. It is thus no wonder that there is still worldwide synthetic activity in the azole class of fungicides.

## 7. PROBLEMS OF MYCOLOGICAL TESTING AND THEIR SOLUTIONS

During the period of the chemical optimization efforts, approximately until early 1969, an average of 10-15 newly synthesized products per month were tested at any one time in the mycological laboratory. Most of these products were quite effective *in vivo* when administered topically and orally in mouse candidosis and guinea pig trichophytosis. The tests revealed certain common properties of the imidazole derivatives:

1. Very broad antimycotic spectrum encompassing four large groups: dermatophytes, yeasts (Candida species, *Torulopsis* and *Cryptococcus*

species), molds (*Aspergillus, Cladosporium, Geotrichum, Saprolegnia,* and *Penicillium* species but no *Mucor* species), and biphasic fungi (*Histoplasma, Coccidioides, Paracoccidioides, Blastomyces, Sporothrix*).

2. *In vivo* efficacy against mycoses due to these organisms after oral, parenteral, or topical administration.
3. Primarily fungistatic activity *in vitro*.[21-23]

When compared with other compounds that had shown efficacy, clotrimazole showed the best spectrum of activities in the various tests; some surprising paradoxes showed up, however, during the testing program.[45-48]

### 7.1 Effect of Inoculum Size

We noted in many comparative studies that *in vitro* MIC values, particularly in the case of yeasts and biphasic fungi in the yeast phase, varied widely from one test to another, with values ranging from 0.062 $\mu$g/ml to 32 $\mu$g/ml on identical fungus strains. As one important cause we traced a pronounced effect of the inoculum size.

When inoculum effects are of the observed magnitude, the microbiologist, in the light of his experience with bacteria and antibacterial agents, immediately suspects that the organisms develop resistance or that primarily resistant variants are being selected from among a susceptible population of organisms. We were able to clear the product of the suspicion of resistant selection, which would have been fatal for the compound, by demonstrating in turbidimetry and respiration tests that subcultures from such test populations that appeared insensitive in the presence of large inocula showed the normal, high sensitivity to clotrimazole when again subjected to MIC determination with small inocula amounting to $10^4$ organisms/ml.

To date, as a matter of fact, no clotrimazole-resistant yeasts have been observed anywhere in the world. The reasons for the effect of inoculum size on imidazoles remains obscure.

### 7.2 Effect of Incubation[45-47]

It was noted in agar dilution tests (for example by the Multipointer technique) that were carried out with clotrimazole and yeasts of the species *Candida albicans* and *Torulopsis glabrata* that after a prolonged incubation period initially inhibited colonies would grow again. After 140-150 hours of incubation, the extent and density of this regrowth approached that of the untreated control colonies, which were fully grown after 48 hours. Isolates obtained from such regrown colonies interestingly showed normal MIC values of clotrimazole when retested, that is, nonresistance.

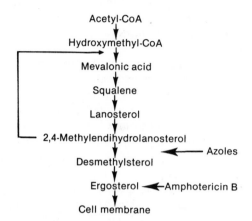

**Figure 14.** Suggested mode of action of clotrimazole in yeasts.

Even at that time, early in 1968, we interpreted this effect of the incubation time by assuming that, as in the case of the action of sulfonamides on bacteria, growth of the organisms after the lag phase is considerably slowed but not completely inhibited by the action of clotrimazole within the range of the minimum inhibitory concentration.

If we view the phenomena of lag phase and effect of incubation time from the vantage point of our present knowledge about the probable mode of the antifungal action of clotrimazole (Figure 14), the two effects can easily be explained: before clotrimazole — and other imidazoles — can become effective against fungi, the sterol pool in the cytoplasm of the fungi has to be consumed down to the end product, ergosterol. For this reason, the activity of clotrimazole is restricted to proliferating organisms.[46]

Our working hypothesis explaining the inoculum effect has been published.[19,22,47,49]

## 8. PROBLEMS OF *IN VIVO* TESTING

Orally administered clotrimazole gave evidence of very good, dose-dependent effectiveness in our standard model infections of mouse candidosis and guinea pig trichophytosis. Figure 15 presents the therapeutic efficacy of various oral doses in *Candida albicans* infections.

Fifty mg/kg body weight given once daily may be said to be an effective threshold concentration with animal survival rates in excess of 60% on the 6th postinfection day. At daily doses of 75 and 100 mg/kg, 90-100% of the treated

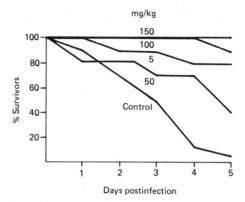

**Figure 15.** Mortality curves of *Candida*-infected mice dependent on various oral doses of clotrimazole.

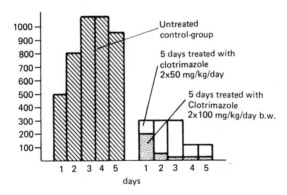

**Figure 16.** *Candida* cell-counts in kidney-homogenates of mice (diluted 1:5000).

256     Chronicles of Drug Discovery

animals survived (Figure 16). These results are quite consistent with those obtained by comparing renal homogenates of infected and treated animals with
those of untreated controls on the 5th day after infection.[46],[47],[49]

Reflecting the effect of the therapy, the count of *Candida* organisms in the
renal tissue of animals treated, i.g. with 100 mg/kg, had dropped to about
1-5% of the organism counts in untreated control animals. Clotrimazole levels
in the blood of mice after oral administration of different clotrimazole doses
showed good correlation with the therapeutic effect and the organism count.
The results of blood levels tested with agar diffusion test after single oral doses
of clotrimazole are given in Figure 17.[21],[46],[49]

Clotrimazole levels determined this way in pooled 6- and 12-hour urine of
mice following oral doses showed that only a small fraction of the orally
administered clotrimazole was excreted renally in microbiologically active
form. Inasmuch as microbiological testing of pooled mouse feces following
oral administration of clotrimazole also detected only very small quantities of
the microbiologically active substance, we had to infer that clotrimazole
undergoes a high degree of metabolism in mammals. These initial data and
pharmacokinetic studies of orally administered clotrimazole proved to be most
helpful later on.

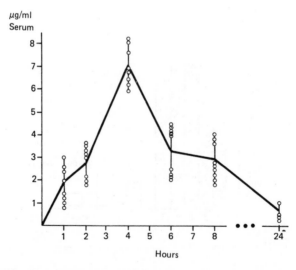

**Figure 17.** Concentrations of clotrimazole in the blood of mice and rats after a
single oral dose of 100 mg/kg.

In guinea pig trichophytosis due to *Trichophyton mentagrophytes,* daily oral doses of 50 mg/kg, given from the day of infection to the 10th postinfection day, produced a rapid remission of the dermatophytosis. The therapeutic effect became clearly discernible beginning with the 5th day of treatment. We were particularly excited to find that from that day on clotrimazole became detectable in the newly grown hair of the animals by means of microbiological test methods.[50]

We drew the conclusion that after oral administration to guinea pigs and dogs, clotrimazole is excreted via sweat and sebum and/or incorporated into the keratin of the hairs that regrow during treatment. Comparable findings had been made with orally administered griseofulvin. This finding was reported in mice after administration of single 100 mg/kg doses for 5 or 6 days. This confirmed that orally administered clotrimazole reaches the site of dermatophyte infections, skin and hair, in microbiologically active form (Figure 18).

Clotrimazole also proved very effective after topical application of 1% formulations, cream and solutions, in the model of guinea pig trichophytosis due to all three *Trichophyton* species and in the *Microsporum canis* model. Figures 19 and 20 show an untreated control animal and an animal with a *Trichophyton mentagrophytes* infection that was treated eight times with clotrimazole cream, once daily from the 3rd to the 10th postinfection day. Even 0.5% formulations proved quite effective, but 0.1% formulations had less marked therapeutic effects.[22]

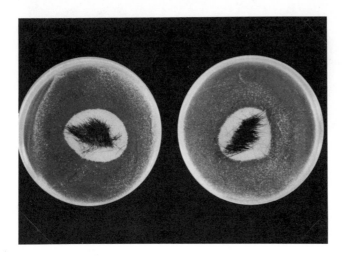

**Figure 18.**   Microbiological detection of clotrimazole in hairs of orally treated dogs.

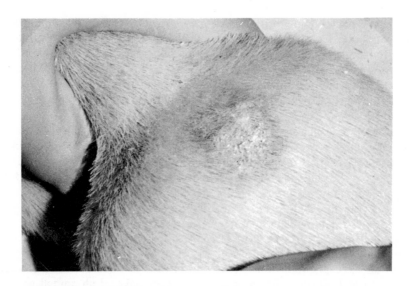

**Figure 19.**   Guinea pig trichophytosis. Untreated control animal 12 days postinfection.

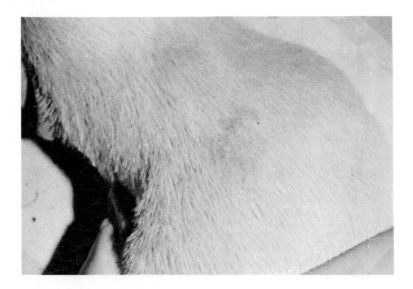

**Figure 20.**   Effect of topical treatment with clotrimazole in guinea pig trichophytosis 12 days postinfection.

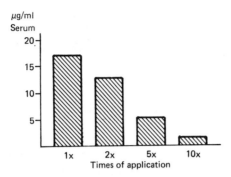

**Figure 21.**  Enzyme induction by clotrimazole. Serum levels of clotrimazole in mice 2 hours after application. Repeated oral doses of 100 mg/kg b.w. Evaluation-method: colorimetric, after extraction of serum.

We worked at the time with Prof. K. Bartmann, an inventive and extremely well-read colleague. He called our attention to several recently published papers by Remmer on the enzyme-inducing capacity of lipophilic drugs. Figure 21 presents the results of our initial experiments on enzyme induction by clotrimazole.

We gave mice daily 100 mg/kg of clotrimazole each, on 10 consecutive days, and determined the serum levels of clotrimazole 2 hours after administration each day. On the 10th day of administration, the serum levels had fallen to 1/15th of the concentration after the first dose, showing that orally administered clotrimazole had an enzyme-inducing effect in mice.[45,46]

The fact that oral clotrimazole is effective in guinea pig trichophytosis, and is apparently not affected by decreased levels caused by enzyme induction, may be due, in our opinion, to the rapid incorporation of clotrimazole, before it is metabolized, into skin and hair keratin; drugs from those stores cannot rediffuse to the liver to be metabolized.

We were able to arrive at an adequate quantification of the enzyme-inducing power of clotrimazole (and other imidazole derivatives) for screening and comparative purposes by two test methods:

1.  The Hexobarbital Test (modified by Remmer), measuring the individual sleeping time after administration of hexobarbital with and without treatment with clotrimazole.

2.  The Pretreatment Test, treating half of the test animals with clotrimazole before infection.

The latter test appeared especially suitable for additional screening and optimization of imidazole derivatives.

Meanwhile, several independent microbiologists had gained some initial experience with clotrimazole in animal studies. Vanbreuseghem (Antwerp) reported on initial therapeutic results in mouse coccidioidomycosis but he was disappointed by the final outcome of his studies, which involved treatment periods of 3 weeks.[51] Drouhet (Paris) found clotrimazole only slightly effective on his model of protracted candidosis.[52] We were able to explain these results on the basis of our new knowledge of enzyme induction by clotrimazole. However, we still remained somewhat concerned.

Waitz and Weinstein (U.S.), on the other hand, obtained good results with clotrimazole,[53] in agreement with our observations, in their septic candidosis model as well as in guinea pig trichophytosis, and Smith-Shadomy[54] (U.S.) and Hoeprich (U.S.) confirmed and extended our *in vitro* findings with clotrimazole. Scholer[55] (Switzerland) and Dittmar[52] (West Germany), too, were able to reproduce our *in vitro* and *in vivo* data with clotrimazole. In addition, we learned of the initial favorable effects of another imidazole, miconazole, newly developed by Janssen (Belgium).

We still had to settle the question whether imidazoles are also effective in animal infections involving biphasic fungi. The *in vitro* data for *Coccidioides immitis, Paracoccidioides brasiliensis, Histoplasma capsulatum,* and *Sporothrix schenckii* showed activity from 0.1 to 1 $\mu$g/ml of substrate and were encouraging.[21]

We therefore used clotrimazole orally in our mouse-tail sporotrichosis model. On the basis of our experience with enzyme induction by clotrimazole, we began with a 5-day treatment two days after the animals' infection; this was followed by a 5-day treatment pause and then another 5-day treatment period. The results obtained at the end of the study were satisfactory.

In contrast with the far-advanced disease in the untreated controls, the inter-mittently treated animals showed a definite therapeutic effect of clotrimazole (Figure 22), even though the sporotrichosis was not cured.[20]

We had now demonstrated that besides their broad antimycotic spectrum *in vitro,* clotrimazole and several of its derivatives had nearly as broad a therapeutic spectrum *in vivo*. It was found *very* effective in mouse candidosis, guinea pig trichophytosis, and septic and pulmonary cryptococcosis of the mouse; effective in mouse sporotrichosis as a model infection of mycoses due to biphasic fungi; and slightly effective or ineffective (for pharmacokinetic rather than microbiological reasons) in mouse aspergillosis and hepatic and meningoencephalic cryptococcosis.

## 9.   AZOLES: A NEW GROUP OF BIOACTIVE COMPOUNDS IN MEDICINE AND PLANT PROTECTION

The part of the azole story we have described covers the period from December 1966 until 1972.

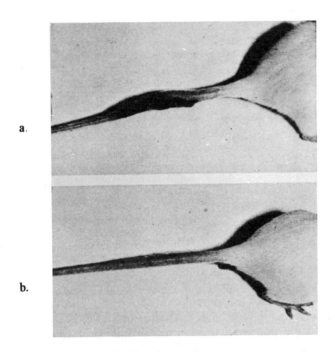

**Figure 22.** (a) Experimental mouse-tail sporotrichosis on the 14th postinfection day. (b) Mouse-tail sporotrichosis following clotrimazole treatment on the 10th postinfection day.

Besides clotrimazole, the chemists had prepared more than 2000 new azole derivatives and turned them over for testing to the plant protection division as well as the pharmaceutical division. In our tests more than half of these derivatives showed antimycotic activity. We were right to assume that we had found a new class of chemotherapeutic agents. As a group, the imidazole antimycotics exhibited the characteristics seen in Figure 23.

We had meanwhile selected clotrimazole for use as a human antimycotic on the basis of numerous comparative studies of antimycotic imidazole derivatives, examples of which we have described here.

Although clotrimazole was not the best product in all the tests, it gave evidence of impressive balanced efficacy in nearly all parameters without showing an extreme in individual properties, such as blood levels, absorption rate, penetrating ability, tissue distribution, and type of action. This was a good

| | |
|---|---|
| 1 | Broad spectrum of activity *in vitro*, including dermatophytes, yeasts, biphasic fungi and moulds |
| 2 | Low MIC-values — depending on culture media |
| 3 | Partial fungicidal type of action |
| 4 | No detectable development of resistance |
| 5 | Enzyme induction with increasing catabolism by repeated doses |
| 6 | Nearly complete metabolism in the liver to microbiological inactive or partially active derivatives |

**Figure 23.**    Group qualities of azole antimycotics.

foundation for pharmacological and toxicological studies to document its safety for therapeutic use. Findings made with several azole derivatives in plant protection research, which led to important commercial products (see Section 11.2), represented additional and interesting evidence in support of the chemists' working hypothesis for the medical-mycological team.

## 10.   EFFICACY AND BEHAVIOR IN HUMANS

Results of toxicologic and pharmacologic studies of clotrimazole in several species (small rodents, dogs, monkeys) had yielded results that permitted the initial use of clotrimazole in humans. Clotrimazole was to be administered orally in mycoses of internal organs as well as topically in cutaneous and mucosal mycoses to be evaluated with regard to its therapeutic efficacy. No problems were encountered in clinical trials of topical dosage forms of clotrimazole. In agreement with the results of our animal studies, the product showed great effectiveness and therapeutic reliability in dermatophytoses, candidal skin infections, mucosal mycoses due to *Candida* and *Torulopsis* species, and ocular mycoses due to yeasts and molds. Clotrimazole for these indications was marketed worldwide under the trade names of Canesten, Lotrimin, Empecid, and Mycelex, beginning in 1973.

Detailed study of the fate of clotrimazole in humans was made possible by a very sensitive specific color spray detection method for use in conjunction with TLC. It was quickly found that the drug undergoes very extensive first-pass hepatic metabolism to inactive species.

Despite this, in trials involving enteric infections, clotrimazole showed efficacy comparable with that of Amphotericin B.

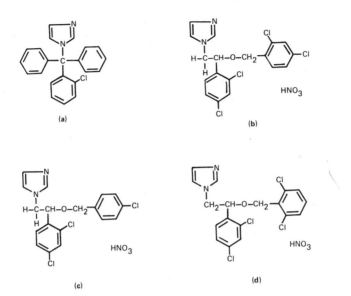

**Figure 24.**   Chemical structures of commercially available imidazole antimycotics (1980). **(a)** Clotrimazole (Bayer) 1967: Canesten, Empecid, Mycelex, Lotrimin. **(b)** Miconazole (Janssen) 1968: Epi/Gyno-Monistat. **(c)** Econazole (Cilag/Janssen) 1968: Pevaryl. **(d)** Isoconazole (Schering, Berlin) 1979: Fazol, Travogen.

By 1972, about 450 patients had been treated with clotrimazole, apart from further studies in volunteers. Two problems arose in the course of these clinical studies:

1.   Considerable uncertainty in the diagnosis of organ mycoses.
2.   A serious pharmacokinetic insufficiency of orally administered clotrimazole (extensive first-pass hepatic metabolism to inactive species).

For these two reasons and because we believed, and are today convinced, that we can find better oral drugs among the imidazoles, we decided not to continue the development of oral clotrimazole.[46,49,56-62]

## 11.   THE AZOLE ANTIMYCOTICS AND FUNGICIDES TODAY

Even while we were developing clotrimazole, the first papers were published on miconazole, an imidazole derivative discovered and developed by Janssen in Belgium. Its properties conform precisely to our description of the characteristics of the imidazole group of antimycotics. Besides clotrimazole, miconazole, econazole, and isoconazole are the three other imidazole derivatives at present being marketed as antimycotics (see Figure 24).

Tioconazole (Pfizer) and butoconazole (Syntex) and, as an antimycotic for organ mycoses, ketoconazole (Nizoral, Janssen) were undergoing clinical trial. The international patent literature on new imidazole derivatives with antimycotic activity is growing steadily.

For these compounds, too, problems of testing and evaluation, such as *in vitro* and *in vivo* determination of MIC values and their correlation with therapeutic activity, enzyme induction and metabolism, and toxicological evaluation have not yet been solved. This task has, however, been greatly facilitated by our early experience with clotrimazole. The imidazole derivatives have gained worldwide acceptance as a new class of chemotherapeutic and plant-protection agents.

## 11.1 Antimycotics

Medical mycology is making impressive advances, partly owing to the new therapeutic approaches made possible by the imidazoles. The new therapeutic modalities have called for improved methods of diagnosis and monitoring of therapy as well as for additional studies on the pathogenesis and epidemiology of mycotic infections. Our current research interest is focused increasingly on fast-acting compounds for topical use and azoles suitable for oral and parenteral use in mycoses of the skin, mucous membranes, and internal organs. Figure 25 gives the structures of three interesting antimycotics that are in the clinical development stage. They demonstrate the variability of the antimycotic and pharmacokinetic characteristics of the azole drugs.[63]

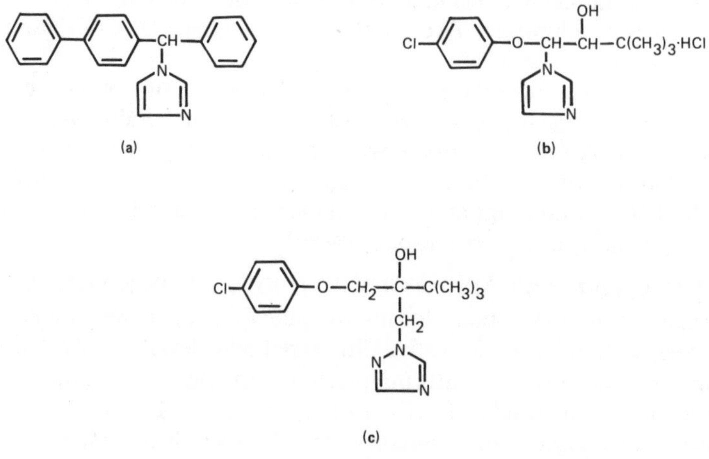

Figure 25.   (a) Bifonazole (Mycospor); (b) Bay 1 9139; (c) Bay n 7133.

Bifonazole is a topical antimycotic with a very good *in vivo* efficacy, due among other things to its long life-time in the skin of animals and humans after application. Bay l 9139 is an oral dermal agent for mycotic infections of the skin, nails, and mucous membranes caused by dermatophytes and candida species. Bay n 7133 is a broad spectrum, systemic antimycotic for oral and parenteral use with an extended efficacy spectrum against aspergillosis.

Individual azole derivatives are distinguished by peak effects against specific organisms. Thus, Baypival, Bay e 6975 (Figure 26), has an MIC of 0.5-1 $\mu g/ml$ for *Pityrosporum ovale* and other *Pityrosporum* species (clotrimazole 20 $\mu g/ml$).[64] *Pityrosporum* species are found very frequently in individuals suffering from unsightly dandruff. This correlates with the assumption voiced in the older dermatological literature that there are etiologic interrelations between the presence of *Pityrosporum* on and in the cells of the scalp and dandruff formation.

Baypival has been used, in a 1% concentration, in lotions and shampoos for the control of dandruff. It has proved as effective in these dosage forms and concentrations as 2% zinc pyrithione, the most effective dandruff control agent thus far. Baypival has been on the market for this indication in Germany and Italy as Ceox shampoo since 1979.

An azole synthesized in 1977, Bay h 6020, at a lower *in vitro* activity against *Candida* species shows maximal activity against *Corynebacterium* acnes and *Corynebacterium granulosum* and is roughly equivalent in its effectiveness against these organisms to erythromycin and tetracycline hydrochloride (MIC 1 $\mu g/ml$). In addition, it is active against streptococci (excepting enterococci) and *Staphylococcus albus* and *Pityrosporum* species. It seemed plausible, considering the classic etiologic concepts regarding acne vulgaris and juvenilis, to use this product as a prophylactic and cosmetic agent for incipient acnelike skin alterations in combination with conventional skin-care products. Bay h 6020 (lombazole) is now commercially available in Germany as a component of the cosmetic product Twent.

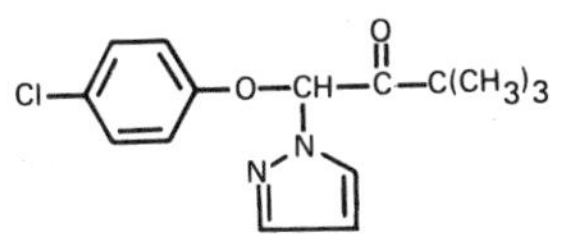

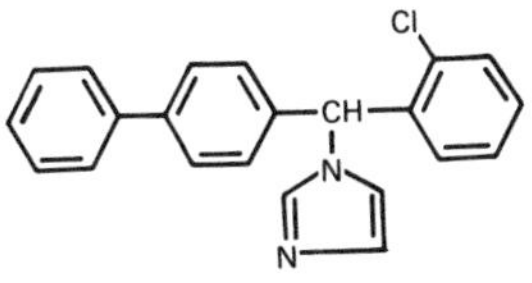

**Figure 26.** (a) Baypival, climbazole, Bay e 6975, active compound in Ceox shampoo. (b) Bay h 6020, lombazole, active compound in Twent, a cosmetic product.

## 11.2   Fungicides in Plant Protection

The class of *N*-alkyl-azole derivatives has opened up new horizons in the control of phytopathogenic fungi. During the testing of compounds out of the triarylmethyl-azole type, we were already struck by the high fungicidal activity of these compounds, particularly against fungicidal organisms of the genus *Erisiphe*. Unlike the antimycotic imidazole derivatives of the clotrimazole type, the optimal activity here for control of plant diseases was found among the triazole derivatives. Optimizing of fungicidal activity and nonphytotoxicity through variation of substituents within the trityl-triazoles led to the development of fluotrimazole (Persulon).[65,66]

This highly active nonsystemic fungicide is active mainly against powdery mildew and is especially suitable for practical use in the cultivation of cereals, vegetables, and beets.

Triadimefon (Bayleton),[65,67,68] triadimenol, (Baytan)[68,69], and bitertanol (Baycor)[68,70] are representative of another group of highly active alkyltriazole fungicides, fully developed for practical use.

Triadimefon, systemic fungicide, is especially suitable for the control of powdery mildew and rust fungi. In dosages of 125-250 g/ha it may be used for the control of disease caused by these phytopathogens in cereals, vegetables, coffee, soft and pome fruit, grapes, sugarcane, and various other crops as well as ornamentals.

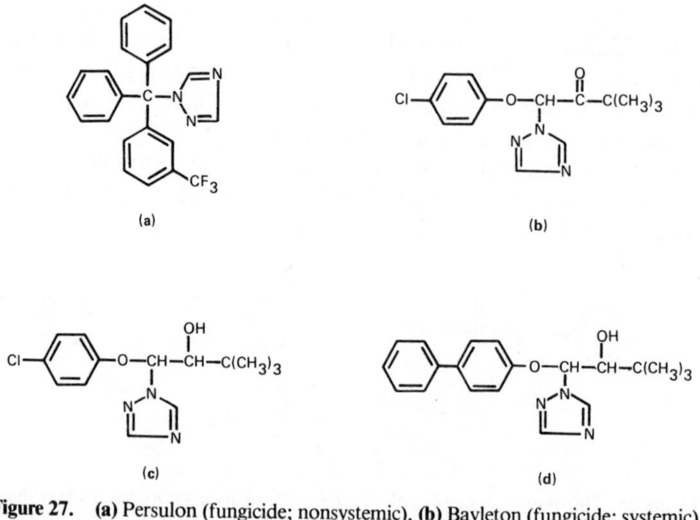

**Figure 27.**   **(a)** Persulon (fungicide; nonsystemic), **(b)** Bayleton (fungicide; systemic), **(c)** Baytan (seed dressing), **(d)** Baycor (leaf fungicide; curative).

Owing to its good systemic properties and broad spectrum of activity, including smuts, mildews, rusts, *Septoria* and *Rhynchosporium,* triadimenol is suitable as a seed dressing for cereals. In dosages of 30-50 g active ingredient/100 kg seed, young plants are protected from seed-borne and soil-borne diseases; a significant increase in crop yields is thus obtained.

Bitertanol is a highly active foliar fungicide with good penetration. Its additional curative and eradicative properties make it much more effective than a protective fungicide when application rates are taken into consideration. Its maximum activity is in the control of powdery mildew, rust, scab, and other pathogenic fungi that cause leaf- and fruit-spot diseases.

In this chapter, we have described the discovery, elaboration, and utilization of a new class of active compounds in human medicine, plant protection, and cosmetics from the standpoint of the laboratory workers directly involved. The story of the azoles has taught us once again to appreciate the role of feelings, apart from the detached scientific attitude, as a driving force in scientific endeavors. Judging from the synthesis and testing programs carried out to date, extrapolation to the number of new azole derivatives that can yet be synthesized allows us to hope that remaining therapeutic problems in mycoses of the skin and its appendages, the mucous membranes, and internal organs, and perhaps some other related problems, will be solved in the foreseeable future.

## REFERENCES

1.  K. H. Büchel and A. Conte, *Z. Naturforsch. B,* **21,** 1110-1111 (1966); *Chem. Abstr.,* **66,** 65,261t (1967).
2.  U.S. Patent 2,938,830 (May 31, 1960), Imperial Chemical Industries Ltd, Inv.: D. G. Davey, N. Greenhalgh, and R. F. Homer; *Chem. Abstr.,* **54,** 17,783d (1960).
3.  Belg. Patent 625,441 (May 28, 1963), "Shell" Research Ltd, *Chem. Abstr.,* **61,** 3120h (1964).
4.  E. F. Elslager, F. W. Short, D. F. Worth, J. E. Meisenhelder, H. Najarian, and P. E. Thompson, *Nature (London),* **190,** 628 (1961).
5.  K. H. Büchel, W. Draber, E. Regel, and M. Plempel, *Arzneim.-Forsch.,* **22,** 1260-1272 (1972).
6.  E. Rennerfelt, *Proc. Int. Bot. Congr.* (7th Congr. Stockholm, 1950), **7,** 316-317 (1953); *Chem. Abstr.,* **48,** 12,251d (1954).
7.  H. A. Staab, *Angew. Chem.,* **74,** 407 (1962).
8.  Belg. Patent 720,801 (Sept. 13, 1968), Ger. Appl. Sept. 15, 1967, Farbenfabriken Bayer A.-G., Inv.: K. H. Büchel, E. Regel, and M. Plempel.
9.  M. Plempel, K. Bartmann, K. H. Büchel, and E. Regel, *Dtsch. Med. Wochenschr.,* **94,** 1356 (1969).
10.  K. H. Büchel, W. Draber, E. Regel, and M. Plempel, *Drugs Made Ger.,* **15,** 79-94 (1972).
11.  K. H. Büchel, M. Plempel, and K. Bartmann, *Ther. Ber.,* **39,** 39-48 (1973).
12.  Neth. Appl. 6,901,307 (Jan. 27, 1969), Ger. Appl. Jan. 29, 1968, Farbenfabriken Bayer A.-G., Inv.: K. H. Büchel, E. Regel, F. Grewe, H. Scheinpflug, and H. Kaspers.
13.  Neth. Appl. 6,901,308 (Jan. 27, 1969), Ger. Appl. Jan. 29, 1968, Farbenfabriken Bayer A.-G., Inv.: K. H. Büchel, E. Regel, F. Grewe, H. Scheinpflug, and H. Kaspers.

14. Belg. Patent 738,095, Aug. 26, 1969, Ger. Appl. Aug. 27, 1968, Farbenfabriken Bayer A.-G., Inv.: K. H. Büchel, F. Grewe, and H. Kaspers.
15. K. H. Büchel and W. Draber, *Med. Chem.*, **5**, 441-450 (1977).
16. H. Otten and M. Plempel in H. Otten, M. Plempel, W. Siegenthaler, Eds. *Antibiotika-Fibel*, 4th ed., Thieme, (Stuttgart), 1975, p. 666.
17. M. Plempel, *Dtsch. Med. J.,* 18, 19, 565 (1967).
18. K. Bartmann and M. Plempel, *Muench. Med. Wochenschr.,* **118** (Suppl. 1), 6 (1976).
19. M. Plempel, K. Bartmann, K. H. Büchel, and E. Regel, *Postgrad. Med. J.,* July Suppl., 11-12 (1974).
20. M. Plempel and K. Bartmann, *Proceedings of the 2nd International Special Symposium on Yeasts,* Univ. Tokyo Press, 1972, p. 305.
21. M. Plempel, K. Bartmann, K. H. Büchel, and E. Regel, *Antimicrob. Agents Chemother.,* 271 (1970).
22. M. Plempel, K. Bartmann, K. H. Büchel, and E. Regel, *Ger. Med.,* **14**, 11, 532 (1969).
23. M. Plempel and K. Bartmann, *Drugs Made Ger.,* **15**, 103 (1972).
24. I. Haller, *Dermatologia 1959,* Suppl. 1, 187-190 (1979).
25. H. J. Scholer, *Proceedings of the 5th Congress for Mycology,* Paris, 1971.
26. K. H. Büchel, W. Meiser, W. Krämer, and F. Grewe, *8th International Congress of Plant Protection,* Moscow, 1975, Section III, 112; *Chem. Abstr.,* **88**, 190,618v (1978).
27. K. H. Büchel and W. Draber, *Med. Chem.,* **5**, 442 (1977).
28. Neth. Appl. 6,813,715 (Sept. 24, 1968), Ger. Appl. Sept. 26, 1967, Farbenfabriken Bayer A.-G., Inv.: K. H. Büchel.
29. Ger. Offen. 1,940,626 (Feb. 11, 1971, Appl. Aug. 9, 1969), Farbenfabriken Bayer A.-G. Inv.: G. Jäger and K. H. Buchel; *Chem. Abstr.,* **74**, 112,048f (1971).
30. Ger. Offen. 1,940,628 and 1,940,627 (Feb. 11, 1971, Appl. Aug. 9, 1969), Farben-fabriken Bayer A.-G., Inv.: K. H. Büchel and W. Draber; W. Draber, K. H. Büchel, *Chem. Abstr.,* **74**, 125,698t, 125,697s (1971).
31. Ger. Offen. 2,009,020 (Nov. 18, 1971, Appl. Feb. 26, 1970), Farbenfabriken Bayer A.-G., Inv.: W. Draber and E. Regel; *Chem. Abstr.,* **76**, 59,632e (1972).
32. K. H. Büchel, *J. Pestic. Sci.,* **2**, (Japan; Special Issue), 576-582 (Dec. 1977).
33. K. H. Büchel, W. Draber, E. Regel, and M. Plempel, *Drugs Made Ger.,* **15**, 79-94 (1972).
34. J. Gibbons, *Nonparametric Statistical Inference,* McGraw-Hill (New York), 1971.
35. W. Krämer, K. H. Büchel, W. Meiser, W. Brandes, H. Kaspers, and H. Scheinpflug, Plenary Lect. Symp. Pap., 4th International Congress of Pesticide Chemistry, *Adv. Pestic. Sci.,* pp. 274-279 (1978).
36. F. E. Norrington, R. M. Hyde, S. G. Williams and R. Wootton, *J. Med. Chem.,* **18**, 604-607 (1975).
37. A. Verloop, W. Hoogenstraaten, and J. Tipker, in E. J. Ariens, Ed., *Drug Design,* Vol. 7, Academic Press, New York, 1976, pp. 165-207.
38. P. N. Craig, *J. Med. Chem.,* **14**, 680-684 (1971).
39. C. Gardner Swain, E. C. Lupton, Jr., *J. Am. Chem. Soc.,* **90**, 4328 (1968).
40. U.S. Patent 3,737,531 (Jan. 5, 1973), Ger. Appl. July 20, 1968, Farbenfabriken Bayer A.-G., Inv.: W. Draber, K. H. Büchel, and M. Plempel, *Chem. Abstr.,* **73**, 35,370e (1970).
41. U.S. Patents 3,709,901 and 3,764,690 (Jan. 9, 1973, and Oct. 9, 1973), Ger. Appl. Mar. 7, 1969, Farbenfabriken Bayer A.-G., Inv.: W. Draber, E. Regel, K. H. Büchel, and M. Plempel; *Chem. Abstr.,* **73**, 120,623j (1970).

42. Belg. Patents 750,724 and 770,662 (May 21, 1970, and July 29, 1971), Farbenfabriken Bayer A.-G., Inv.: K. H. Büchel, W. Meiser, C. Metzger, and M. Plempel; H. Timmler, W. Draber, K. H. Büchel, and M. Plempel.

43. Belg. Patent 778,973 (Feb. 4, 1972), Ger. Appl. Feb. 5, 1971, Farbenfabriken Bayer A.-G., Inv.: W. Meiser, K. H. Büchel, and M. Plempel.

44. Belg. Patent 804,092 (Aug. 28, 1973), Ger. Appl. Aug. 29, 1972, Bayer A.-G., Inv.: K. H. Büchel, W. Krämer, and W. Meiser; Ger. Offen. 2,201,063 (July 26, 1973, Appl. P 2201063.5, Jan. 11, 1972), Bayer A.-G., Inv.: W. Meiser, K. H. Büchel, W. Krämer, and F. Grewe; *Chem. Abstr.*, **79**, 105,257y (1973).

45. M. Plempel and K. Bartmann, *Proceedings of the 7th International Congress of Chemotherapy*, Prague, 1971, p. 949.

46. M. Plempel, *Postgrad. Med. J.*, **55**, 662 (1979).

47. I. Haller and M. Plempel, *Curr. Med. Res. Opin.*, **5**, 315, (1978).

48. I. Haller, *Postgrad. Med. J.*, **55**, 681 (1979).

49. P. Savoyer, R. N. Brogden, R. M. Pinder, T. M. Speight, and G. S. Avery, *Drugs*, **9**, 424 (1975).

50. M. Plempel and K. H. Büchel, *Recent Advances in Medical and Veterinary Mycology*, Vol. III, Univ. Tokyo Press, 1976.

51. A. Vanbrenseghem, *Verh.-Ber. der deutschsprachigen Mykolog. Ges.*, Frankfurt, 1971.

52. Drouhet, personal communication.

53. J. A. Waitz, E. L. Moss, and M. Weinstein, *Appl. Microbiol.*, **22**, 891-898 (1971).

54. S. Smith-Shadomy, *Infect. and Immunity*, **4**, 143-148 (1971).

55. H. Scholer, *Verhandlungsber. Intern. Kongress f. Mykologie*, Paris (1971).

56. H. Oberste-Lehn, I. Baggesen, and M. Plempel, *Mykosen*, **13**, 1 (1970).

57. H. Oberste-Lehn, I. Baggesen, and M. Plempel, *Dtsch. Med. Wochenschr.*, **94**, 26, 1365 (1969).

58. W. Marget and D. Adam, *Med. Klin.* (Munich), **64**, 27, 1235 (1969).

59. H. Schwacke, *Dtsch. Med. Wochenschr.*, **95**, 48, 2437 (1969).

60. H. Weuta, *Postgrad. Med. J.*, **50** (Suppl. I), 45 (1974).

61. J. Bennett, M. Plempel, D. Stevens, and H. Scholer, *Curr. Chemother.*, **53**, (1978).

62. M. Plempel, *Verh. Dtsch. Ges. Inn. Med.*, **84**, 443 (1978).

63. M. Plempel, K. H. Büchel, and E. Regel, Report on the 8th Congress ISHAM, Feb. 8-12, 1982, Palmerston North, New Zealand.

64. M. Plempel, *Der Hautarzt*, **28** (Suppl. 2), 189 (1977).

65. K. H. Büchel, W. Meiser, W. Krämer, and F. Grewe, *8th International Congress of Plant Protection*, Moscow, 1975, Section III, 111-118, *Chem. Abstr.*, **88**, 190,618v (1978).

66. F. Grewe and K. H. Büchel, *Mittl. Biol. Bundesanst. Land-Forstwirtsch.* (Berlin-Dahlem), **59**, 652-655 (1975).

67. H. Kaspers, F. Grewe, W. Brandes, H. Scheinpflug, and K. H. Büchel, *8th International Congress of Plant Protection*, Moscow, 1975, Section III, 398-401; *Chem. Abstr.*, **88**, 190,618v (1978).

68. K. H. Büchel, W. Krämer, W. Meiser, W. Brandes, P. E. Frohberger, and H. Kaspers, *9th International Congress of Plant Protection*, Washington, D.C., 1979, Abstract of Paper No. 475.

69. P. E. Frohberger, *Pflanzenschutz-Nachr. Bayer* (Ger. Ed.), **31**, 11-24 (1978).

70. W. Brandes, H. Kaspers, and W. Krämer, *Pflanzenschutz-Nachr. Bayer* (Ger. Ed.), **32**, 1-16 (1979).

# INDEX